Mobilizing Mutations

Mobilizing Mutations

Human Genetics in the
Age of Patient Advocacy

DANIEL NAVON

The University of Chicago Press   Chicago and London

The University of Chicago Press, Chicago 60637
The University of Chicago Press, Ltd., London
© 2019 by The University of Chicago
Published 2019
Printed in the United States of America

28 27 26 25 24 23 22 21 20 19   1 2 3 4 5

ISBN-13: 978-0-226-63809-6 (cloth)
ISBN-13: 978-0-226-63812-6 (e-book)
DOI: https://doi.org/10.7208/chicago/9780226638126.001.0001

Library of Congress Cataloging-in-Publication Data

Names: Navon, Daniel, author.
Title: Mobilizing mutations : human genetics in the age of patient
    advocacy / Daniel Navon.
Description: Chicago : The University of Chicago Press, 2019. |
    Includes bibliographical references and index.
Identifiers: LCCN 2019009779 | ISBN 9780226638096 (cloth :
    alk. paper) | ISBN 9780226638126 (e-book)
Subjects: LCSH: Human chromosome abnormalities. | Medical
    genetics. | Human genetics. | Mutation (Biology)
Classification: LCC RB155.5 .N38 2019 | DDC 616/.042—dc23
LC record available at https://lccn.loc.gov/2019009779

♾ This paper meets the requirements of ANSI/NISO Z39.48-1992
(Permanence of Paper).

for Claire Bear

Contents

Acknowledgments

The first note of thanks goes to the many researchers, clinicians, caregivers, and patient advocates who took the time to share their perspectives and their stories with me. Above all, I am enormously grateful for the opportunity to meet so many people and families dealing with the genetic conditions discussed in this book. Although I was not able to formally interview patients themselves, spending time with them and their families enriched my thinking and my understanding immeasurably. I hope that this book helps open the door for research that directly addresses their perspectives and starts to unpack important policy questions about the way our knowledge about genetic mutations is shaping their lives.

I am grateful for research support from the Robert Wood Johnson Foundation, the UC San Diego Hellman Fellows Program, and the Binational Science Foundation. In addition, Columbia's Mellon Foundation Fellows Program and Lindt and Lazarsfeld Fellowships, as well as its Institute for Social and Economic Research and Policy and Department of Sociology, provided crucial support at an earlier stage of this project.

Various parts of this book were presented at dozens of conferences, workshops, and talks over the years—thank you to everyone who posed challenging questions or provided helpful feedback. Parts of chapter 1 were published in much earlier form as follows: Daniel Navon, "Genomic Designation: How Genetics Can Delineate New, Phenotypically Diffuse Medical Categories," *Social Studies of Science* 41, no. 2 (2011): 203–26; and Daniel Navon and Uri

Shwed, "The Chromosome 22q11.2 Deletion: From the Unification of Biomedical Fields to a New Kind of Genetic Condition," *Social Science & Medicine* 75, no. 9 (2012): 1633–41. Most of chapter 4 is composed of revised versions of Daniel Navon and Gil Eyal, "The Trading Zone of Autism Genetics: Examining the Intersection of Genomic and Psychiatric Classification," *BioSocieties* 9, no. 3 (2014): 329–52; and Daniel Navon and Gil Eyal, "Looping Genomes: Diagnostic Change and the Genetic Makeup of the Autism Population," *American Journal of Sociology* 121, no. 5 (2016): 1416–71. My thanks go to the anonymous reviewers and journal editors who helped further my thinking.

My editor, Karen Merikangas Darling, deftly guided this book through to publication, and the anonymous reviewers for the University of Chicago Press provided a series of extremely helpful suggestions that made for a much stronger manuscript. Nicholas Murray's meticulous copyediting, along with the contributions of the rest of the production team, helped to bring the book past the finish line and into print.

A number of scholars at Columbia and elsewhere read my early work on this topic and provided sage advice about the best ways forward. I am especially grateful to Sarah Franklin, Herbert Gans, Dani Lainer-Vos, Uri Shwed, Shamus Khan, Eviatar Zerubavel, Bill McAllister, Martine Lappé, Amy Hinterberger, Brendan Hart, Des Fitzgerald, Nikolas Rose, Charles Tilly, Diane Vaughan, and Nadia Abu El-Haj.

More recently, I was very fortunate to receive incisive feedback from Hannah Landecker, Aaron Panofsky, James Evans, Adrian Johns, Peter Marsden, Jason Beckfield, Kathy Swartz, Ilana Löwy, Mattias Smångs, Eric Engles, Fernando Domínguez Rubio, Kwai Ng, Jeff Haydu, and John Evans. A special note of thanks goes to Stefan Timmermans, Sara Shostak, and Alberto Cambrosio for their incredibly generous feedback and advice over the past few years.

Peter Bearman helped a recovering philosophy student learn how to think like a sociologist, albeit an unusual one. He also made a spirited case for writing this book. For that and much more I am very grateful.

I owe an extraordinary debt of gratitude to my advisor, Gil Eyal. From the very beginning of this project, Gil was unwaveringly generous with his time, his feedback, and his advice on matters big and small. This book would be far poorer were it not for his brilliant input, guidance, and encouragement. Suffice it to say I can only hope to one day be such a mentor.

Endless thanks go to the many friends and colleagues who have provided support and advice over the years. You are too many to name, but you have enriched my work and my life in countless ways. I cannot resist singling out a few especially supportive colleagues and cherished friends: Amy Binder, Kevin Lewis, Juan Pablo Pardo-Guerra, Akos Rona-Tas, John Evans, Abigail Andrews, Saiba Varma, Aftab Jassal, Cathy Gere, Laleh Khalili, John Chalcraft, Roz Redd, Jeffrey Lenowitz, Dan Meller, Matt Spooner, Isabel Harland de Benito, Phil Bachelor, Eilidh McPherson, Tom Scott-Smith, James Golden, Cynthia Littlestone, Zac McGowan, and John Keefe.

To my family—especially Larry, Simone, Joshua, and Jimby Navon; Pam, Bill, and Billie Edington; Lisa Clarke; Zev Weiser; and Henry and Renee Bernstein—thank you for your understanding and encouragement throughout this process. Special thanks go my parents, Larry and Simone, and my grandfather, Howard Weiser, for instilling an enduring curiosity about the world and the drive to pursue it.

Finally, I can barely even begin to express what my partner and wife, Claire Edington, has meant to me throughout this process. Claire read drafts of almost every chapter and helped to make each one more elegant and more cogent. She helped me overcome obstacles and frustrations big and small, and together we have safely navigated the early stages of this strange career. Most of all, from the time we met just over a decade ago, Claire has made me a better and far happier person. I can hardly imagine a life without her and our amazing baby girl, Lyla Navon.

Introduction:
From Mutations to
New Kinds of People

The rapid expansion of DNA testing continues apace. With every passing year, more and more people learn that they, their child, or their fetus carry a genetic mutation. But what does finding a mutation actually mean for the way we understand a person? What does it tell us about her fate? Despite all the ink that has already been spilt answering that question, this book shows how having a genetic mutation can mean even more than we realized.

Take the example of someone who is missing a segment of DNA at site 11.2 (pronounced one-one-point-two) on the long arm of one of their twenty-second chromosomes. The 22q11.2 microdeletion is often detected via a fluorescence in situ hybridization, or FISH, test that binds bright probes to a particular location on a chromosome. The absence of a probe indicates a missing segment of a chromosome that would otherwise be too small to see under a microscope. If one of the 22q11.2 probes is missing, as seen in figure 1, then the person in question probably has a 22q11.2 microdeletion—a mutation that likely affects nearly every cell of her body.

Today, finding this mutation means that a person has 22q11.2 Deletion Syndrome, one of the most common genetic disorders after Down syndrome (Bassett et al. 2011; Grati et al. 2015). It means that she and her family have access to a growing network of care, support, advocacy, and

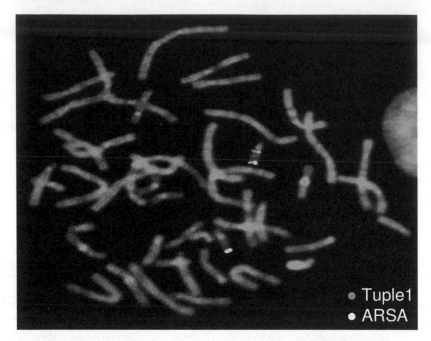

FIGURE 1. A fluorescence in situ hybridization (FISH) test indicating a microdeletion at 22q11.2. The absence of a "Tuple 1" probe on one of the copies of chromosome 22, along with the presence of the ARSA control probe, indicates a missing segment of DNA at site q11.2 (Tonelli et al. 2007). (Image reproduced under the Creative Commons Attribution License; http://creativecommons.org/licenses/by/2.0)

biomedical research headlined by the International 22q11.2 Foundation. Despite its genomic specificity, 22q11.2 Deletion Syndrome (DS) affects people in dramatically different ways. They can have medical issues ranging from schizophrenia and autism to constipation, malar flatness, and hypocalcemia. Congenital heart defects and developmental delays may also result from 22q11.2DS, or it may produce such a mild phenotype that no one will ever even think to refer the patient for genetic testing (McDonald-McGinn et al. 2001). Finally, finding the microdeletion at 22q11.2 is increasingly likely to mean that parents face a dilemma about whether to terminate a pregnancy (Bretelle et al. 2010; chapter 8 below). Numbers are rising fast, mostly in North America and Europe, but also in India, Thailand, Chile, and elsewhere, and 22q11.2DS is the focus of a growing network of specialist clinics, support groups, pharmaceutical trials, and advocacy organizations.

I want to explain how the absence of a bright dot on an image of

stained chromosomes—or any other test indicating a genetic mutation—can distinguish between two clinically indistinguishable patients and provide entrée to a burgeoning network of research, care
and activism. This is not social science fiction, but a way of classifying
people with a sixty-year history. By studying that history, I argue, we
can better grasp how, when and why genetics can radically reshape the
way we understand and act on human difference.

Ever since human geneticists started discovering people with abnormal genomes, they have used two different strategies to make sense of
the relationship between mutations and disease. The first strategy is
easy to grasp. In March 1959, a team of human geneticists in Paris reported that all nine of their patients with Mongolian Idiocy had three
copies of chromosome 21 rather than the normal two (Lejeune, Gautier,
and Turpin 1959). They had discovered a fairly clear-cut chromosomal
explanation of an established medical condition—the first "gene for"
an important category of human difference. The association between
Mongolian Idiocy, now known as Down syndrome, and trisomy 21 was
a true game-changer. It catapulted the field of cytogenetics—the study
of chromosomes—into medical salience and helped lay the foundation
for the rise of medical genetics (Harper 2006; Neri and Opitz 2009).
Decades later, the idea that genetic mutations might explain many important medical conditions helped animate the Human Genome Project, not to mention our broader turn-of-the-century fascination with
the "book of life." These grand hopes for medical genetics were significantly bolstered by a handful of findings in the late 1980s and early
1990s, not least the discoveries of the genes that cause Tay-Sachs disease, cystic fibrosis, and Huntington's disease.

Yet if we have learned anything about human genetics since the op-
timistic 1990s, it is that surprisingly *few* important questions of health
and illness find straightforward answers in our DNA (Check Hayden
2008; Kolata 2012b; Lock 2005; Wade 2009). For the most part, the
relationship between our genomes and the traits or diseases that shape
our lives is just far more complex and uncertain than almost anyone
anticipated. Simply put, there is no "gene for" the vast majority of common medical conditions. The front line of clinical genomics for the
general population is instead about reporting variants in several dozen
genes that mostly confer risk for cancers and heart issues, such as car-
diomyopathies or Long QT syndrome (Trivedi 2017). Nevertheless, the
1959 discovery of trisomy 21 continues to shape our thinking about
what genetics can and should do for our understanding of disease and
difference.

The second strategy for making sense of genetic mutations came into view just months after the first. In September 1959, a team of researchers in Scotland found a "super female" with three X chromosomes instead of the normal female complement of two (Jacobs, Baikie, et al. 1959). Then, in April 1960, the *Lancet* published back-to-back reports of two new chromosomal abnormalities: a team based in Wisconsin reported a patient with trisomy 13, while another group in England reported one with trisomy 18 (Edwards et al. 1960; Patau et al. 1960). It turned out that most of the approximately one in one thousand women who have trisomy X are so mildly affected that they never come to the attention of a medical geneticist. By contrast, trisomy 13 and 18 tend to cause severe malformations that usually lead to prenatal or early childhood death. However, all three chromosome abnormalities had one thing in common: unlike trisomy 21, none of them lined up with an established disorder. The XXX abnormality was clearly not a "gene for" an already-recognized disorder. Triple X syndrome, as it came to be known, was a *new* condition that could never have been discovered or diagnosed until we were able to find and identify people with three X chromosomes. Genetics had shown that it could do more than help us explain, predict, or treat the medical conditions we already know and care about. Almost as soon as we began to find people with abnormal genomes, a wave of new genetic disorders started coming into view.

In this book, I show how knowledge about genetic mutations is being used to carve out new and otherwise unthinkable medical conditions that are shaping people's lives in ever more powerful ways. I call this way of classifying people "genomic designation." The stakes are high. 22q11.2DS and Triple X syndrome are just two among a rapidly growing number of conditions that are delineated strictly according to genetic mutations. Many have become powerful categories of human difference in recent years, even though they lack the distinctive phenotype of a condition like Down syndrome. Although statistics are not available, there is no question that many thousands of people have been diagnosed with genomically designated conditions and that many millions are so diagnosable. This turn to genomic classification has gained considerable steam in just the last few years, and there is good reason to believe that it will come to occupy a far greater role in the way we understand people who are disabled or developmentally different in the coming decades. Most of these mutations are rare, but cumulatively they are not rare at all. With recent advances in genetic testing (both pre- and postnatal), the number of people actually being diagnosed with genomically designated conditions is skyrocketing. Meanwhile, new mutations are joining the fray all the time. We also need to keep in mind how quickly things are moving. It is becoming ever easier to identify mutations and then use databases and communications technologies to create cohorts of patients, even if they are, quite literally, very few and far between.

This new way of classifying human difference has now gained traction far afield from the pages of genetics journals. From 5p– and XYY syndrome to Fragile X and *NGLY1* deficiency, growing networks of research, clinical practice and advocacy are being organized around specific genetic mutations. Throughout this book, I trace the way some of these genomically designated conditions have given rise to innovative patient advocacy movements, new hybrid communities, perplexing biosocial identities, exacting clinical guidelines, and newfangled approaches to human difference. In some cases, knowing that a person has a genetic mutation can destabilize the thresholds of clinical significance—the very boundary between the normal and the pathological—for issues like IQ and childhood growth.

The significance of these mostly rare genetic disorders goes far beyond the people and families directly affected by the discovery of this or that mutation. We will see how a growing number of researchers and pharmaceutical companies are turning their attention to genomically designated conditions in the hope that they can *leverage* them as genetic models and thereby unlock the biological basis of common conditions like autism, schizophrenia, and heart disease, or even our human capacities for things like language or aggression. In this way, research on people with the mutations discussed in this book is often undertaken in pursuit of dual goals: understanding and helping people with a rare genetic disorder while simultaneously trying to get at less biologically tractable but much broader questions about human health, illness, and difference. In a way, my goals are not all that different. I argue that the mutations discussed throughout this book are important not only because they shape so many people's lives, but also because their histories as objects of knowledge and practice help us get at a series of key issues in the social studies of science and medicine.

Genetics, Medical Classification, and Social Mobilization

Throughout this book, I show how genetic mutations can give rise to what philosopher Ian Hacking would call new "kinds of people": the sort of classifications that really change the people they are applied to, even as the categories themselves are constantly changing as well. We will see how some mutations have become powerful objects of bio-scientific research, clinical practice, social mobilization, and identity formation, even though experts could never pick their bearers out of a crowd based on what they are actually like—that is, their phenotype. But more than that, this book explains *how* genetic mutations can come to mean so much. I trace the way a mutation can begin its social career as a thin case report about a child with developmental delay and a handful of congenital abnormalities, but then metamorphose into a bona fide medical condition and eventually a richly detailed kind of person with a whole community built up around it. But how did this come to pass? What lessons does this new way of classifying disease hold for the way we understand the impact of genetics research on medicine and society?

Genomic designation opens the door for the social studies of science and medicine to follow the field of medical genetics away from a century-plus old Mendelian paradigm to a truly genomic one. We have begun to think seriously about genetic complexity in the sense of many genomic variants combining with a host of other factors to produce traits and disease outcomes. But that is just one side of the coin. We have barely scratched the surface of the way researchers are uncovering incredible complexity and far-reaching insights in single pathogenic mutations. Most genetic mutations—whether whole chromosome duplications or tiny DNA variants—do not line up with existing categories of human difference. From a Mendelian or "gene-for" perspective, this represents a gnarl of genetic complexity. From a genomic perspective, by contrast, it is nothing more than variable expressivity. The *real* disease is designated by the mutation—if it turns out to be less clear-cut than we thought, then so be it. This approach comes naturally enough to geneticists, but many physicians and even patient advocates have now embraced genomic designation as well.

Even when a newly discovered mutation seems to straightforwardly explain an older medical condition, further research almost inevitably produces important discrepancies between the people who have the mutation and the condition's clinical diagnostic criteria. This can lead to a different variety of genomic designation where long-standing disorders are recalibrated and reclassified according to genetic mutations. Sometimes, experts and advocates embrace this sort of genomic designation even at the expense of patients who had received an older clinical diagnosis like Williams syndrome or DiGeorge syndrome, but do not have the mutation in question. In this way, genomic designation can turn patients who do not have a particular mutation into nosological orphans.

This turn to the genome as a locus of classification is perhaps best understood according to a series of ideal types. Genetic mutations are variously used to delineate entirely new medical conditions *or* to split, lump, and recalibrate more long-standing clinical categories. Genetic reductionism, or "geneticization"—that old friend of the human sciences—is only very rarely the best way to understand the relationship between mutations and kinds of people, and it is *never* perfectly realized. We need a new toolkit if we want to effectively grapple with twenty-first-century genomic medicine.

At the same time, we will see very clearly that genetics research on its own can only go so far. Just because a researcher talks about a new "syndrome" in the pages of a prestigious biomedical journal does not mean that it will ever inform clinical practice, never mind collective action and identity formation. A newly discovered mutation can indeed be seamlessly cast as a new disorder or syndrome in the esoteric field of human genetics research. And yet it still takes very particular historical conditions and years of painstaking work in order to make a mutation truly matter to a general practitioner, a behavioral psychologist, an educator, a biotech company, a concerned parent, or the people who are diagnosed with a funny-sounding genetic disorder. Whether or not a genetic mutation becomes salient in clinical practice or patient communities is never a given. It takes social mobilization to turn a mutation into a powerful category of identity and community formation— that much is obvious. But it also takes alliances of experts and activists to build up an understanding of the very phenotype of the mutation, develop effective treatment strategies, establish specialist clinics, and garner the resources necessary for a full-fledged research program.

In other words, what it means to have a genetic mutation is as much a sociological phenomenon as it is a biomedical one. What do I mean by that? We sociologists are increasingly refusing to confine ourselves to things we usually think of as "social."[1] My aim here is to examine the admixture of processes and "associations" (Latour 2007:5–9) spanning a dizzying array of fields, objects, and actors that determine what it means to have a mutation. I do not try to explain away changes in what it means to have a mutation by making recourse to hidden social forces exerting an independent power over science and medicine. While I occasionally discuss the role of social processes in a mutation's career, or even the relationship between genetics and society, these sorts of terms should be treated as convenient demarcations within a messier reality. A sociological approach will therefore help us understand what it means to have a mutation today, not because social factors exert some sort of dark power over biology, but because sociology can help us trace a host of key relations that biomedicine itself cannot. The mutations I discuss throughout this book make it abundantly clear that the distinction between biology and society is not a thing out there to be discovered, but a constantly shifting outcome of action and negotiation.

So Much Genomic Data, but What Is to Be Done with It?

We are in the midst of an enormous proliferation of data about our genomes. In 2001, it cost somewhere between $500 million and $1 billion to generate the first "reference" sequence of the roughly three billion bases in a human genome (National Human Genome Research Institute 2016); in late 2007, a somewhat lower-quality sequence of all three billion base pairs was $10 million; today it can be done for less than a thousand dollars, with a *hundred*-dollar genome promised in the very near future (Illumina 2017). That thousand-dollar figure has long been considered the threshold at which whole genome scans for mass consumption would begin to enter the market (Mardis 2006; Service 2006). With clear, quantitative improvements in existing technologies driving further reductions in cost, there is every reason to expect the price to continue its precipitous decline. We may well be on the cusp of the long-anticipated juncture where millions of people own annotations of their three billion DNA base pairs sequence. In any case, clinicians can already order a host of genomic assays capable of detecting thousands of mutations and variants for a fraction of what a test for a limited panel of genes cost just a few years ago. All this takes place against a backdrop where genetics has captured the public imagination and become a powerful component of both disease advocacy and perceptions of health and illness more generally (e.g., Condit 2010; Hacking 2006a; Nelkin and Lindee 2004).

Meanwhile, researchers are finding a far greater range and incidence of potentially pathogenic abnormalities than anticipated, even in seemingly normal people. Our current "mutational repertoire" includes tens of thousands of structural variants like copy number variants, or CNVs (see Lappé and Landecker 2015), and chromosomal abnormalities, as well as millions of smaller mutations. We all harbor numerous variations in our genomes that can shape what we are like.

An average person may bear something like ten thousand DNA variants that affect protein production, several hundred more functionally powerful variants, such as indels and deletions, and fifty to one hundred variants in genes associated with inherited disorders (The 1000 Genomes Project Consortium 2010:1066). The average human genome also contains several rare copy number variants, with 5–10% carrying CNVs where more than five hundred thousand base pairs are either missing or duplicated, and 1–2% carrying CNVs of more than a million base pairs (Harel and Lupski 2018; Sebat et al. 2004). There is clearly no shortage of genetic difference out there.

At the same time, having that complete annotation of your genome is unlikely to tell you anything especially meaningful about your health. Most common medical conditions are genetically complex: researchers may find plenty of genes that are associated with this or that ailment, but each variant will only account for a tiny fraction of a common disease's incidence. Most of them cause the disease in question only some of the time, and most are associated with other diseases and traits as well. To top it all off, even putting all these sorts of genomic variants together tends to leave the large bulk of the common disease's incidence unexplained. Genetics is still a long way from providing convincing answers to questions about most common forms of disease and illness.

Nevertheless, genomic tests are being incorporated into clinical practice, despite the often ambiguous medical implications of the results they produce (Kohane, Masys, and Altman 2006; Manolio et al. 2013). Many mutations, it turns out, have expansive and multivalent spectrums of expression. Some can range from no symptoms at all to benign tumors and certain forms of cancer, heart malformations, autism, and developmental delay (e.g., Varga et al. 2009). Although attempts to standardize the interpretation of these kinds of tests have been published by the relevant professional organizations (ACMG Board of Directors 2012; Green et al. 2013; South et al. 2013), they remain limited to a prescribed list of well-characterized conditions. Beyond that, it takes considerable case-by-case deliberation among expert practitioners to decide which mutations to actually report to physicians, patients, and their families (Timmermans 2014). Even genetic markers that were thought to invariably cause specific disorders like phenylketonuria and cystic fibrosis are often found in people who do not have the expected clinical phenotype once screening is implemented, forcing researchers and clinicians to rethink established disease categories (Timmermans and Buchbinder 2013; Vailly 2008). And yet, genomic diagnoses are increasingly used to guide prognosis and care as part of a broader turn toward "personalized medicine," especially when it comes to children with developmental disabilities and unexplained congenital malformations (Miller et al. 2010).

On the one hand then, we now look back at the euphoria animating late twentieth-century endeavors to pry open the "book of life" as an episode of remarkable hubris. For any given person, DNA is *not* likely to yield clear predictors for her future health (Kolata 2012a; Roberts et al. 2012). Simply put, long-standing questions about disease and difference rarely find clear answers in the Cs, Gs, As, and Ts that make up our genomes. On the other hand, staggering volumes of resources and an abundance of hope continue to be invested in genomics. The Human Genome Project has given way to its natural successor: the turn to using knowledge about people's *particular* genomes, alongside the many factors that shape gene expression, to get at a range of questions about human health, illness, difference, and identity. This broader, "postgenomic" enterprise absorbs billions of dollars in funds across a panoply of fields. Genomics is therefore poised to exert a growing influence on people's lives in the coming years, even though the project of making sense of all this DNA data is still in its infancy. So, with genetic testing becoming ever more rapid, precise, and affordable, what is to be done with all this knowledge about our surprisingly anomaly-ridden genomes?

Going Beyond "Geneticization"

The social sciences are currently at something of a loss when it comes to this important question. This is not because anyone doubts that genomics will continue to have profound social reverberations, nor is there any shortage of work on genetics and society. In fact, a significant interdisciplinary subfield has addressed not only the manifold implications of genetic testing, but also the way that social processes shape the production, diffusion, and use of knowledge about the human genome (for reviews, see Freese and Shostak 2009; Fujimura, Duster, and Rajagopalan 2008).

The problem, rather, is a seductive conceptual error that has guided the field since its earliest stirrings. The social studies of science and medicine have assumed that genetics must work in and through existing categories of human difference in order to really matter. For a time, this made sense. The gene-for model of associating genetic variants with established diseases and traits was much-hyped in 1991, when

Abby Lippman coined the term *geneticization*: the idea that many categories of human difference would be "reduced to their DNA codes, with most disorders, behaviors and physiological variations defined, at least in part, as genetic in origin" (Lippman 1991a:19; see also 1991b, 1998). The prospect of widespread genetic reductionism raised important questions about medical practice, stigma, the experience of illness, and our capacity to situate health outcomes in social environments.

When it comes to actual genetics research, however, it turns out that human differences can only very rarely be reduced to changes in our DNA. With a handful of notable exceptions, the characteristics of our genomes do *not* line up neatly with the sorts of conditions and traits that Lippman and others had in mind. In response, important sociological work has focused precisely on the *failure* of the genes-for conditions, such as cystic fibrosis, to correspond perfectly to clinical diagnostic criteria as well as the liminal cases produced by this discrepancy (Hedgecoe 1998, 2000; Kerr 2000, 2004; Miller et al. 2006; Timmermans and Buchbinder 2011). But social scientists have still tended to assume something like the gene-for model, even if our main focus becomes its failure to work out neatly and the sociotechnical work done to clean up the mess. Even Paul Rabinow's enormously influential formulation of "biosociality" only allowed for identity formation on the basis of genetic risk factors for existing conditions (Rabinow [1992] 1996), while Nikolas Rose's "molecular gaze" (2007b) does not consider the possibility that genomics could provide a new basis for classifying illness rather than a new terrain upon which to explore existing conditions. One way or another, the social studies of science and medicine remain beholden to this outdated gene-for framework. So, how else might the juggernaut that is human genetics transform the way we understand human difference?

Genomic Designation

The categories that we use to understand one another have a profound impact on our lives. Take Ian Hacking's notion of "kinds of people" or "human kinds": categories that interact, or "loop," with the people who are so classified in a way that dynamically transforms the categories, expert practices, and the people themselves (Hacking 1995, [1995] 1998b, 2007). Instead of reductionism, I argue, we need to start paying close attention to the way knowledge about genetic mutations can give rise to *new* kinds of people.

Increasingly, biomedical researchers are following the US National

Human Genome Research Institute's "Grand Challenge II-3" in its call for "a new molecular taxonomy of illness [to] replace our present, largely empirical, classification schemes" (Collins et al. 2003:841; see also Check Hayden 2008; Insel 2013). In this vein, Loscalzo, Kohane, and Barabasi (2007:1) directly challenge the "contemporary classification of human disease [which] dates to the late 19th century, and derives from observational correlation between pathological analysis and clinical syndromes." They argue for nothing less than "redefining human disease in this postgenomic era." A genomic perspective can draw powerful distinctions between indistinguishable phenotypes and render previously unrelated ones deeply akin (see also Goh et al. 2007).

The turn to genomic classification is now firmly established in research fields that deal with developmental difference, where it briefly seemed to coalesce under the rubric of "genotype-first" discovery and diagnosis (Cody 2009; Ledbetter 2008, 2009a, 2009b; Saul and Moeschler 2009). A growing movement in psychiatry, not least the leadership of the National Institute of Mental Health, has called for their diagnostic system to be revised in accordance with biological etiology and genetics in particular (Insel 2013; Regier et al. 2009; Whooley and Horwitz 2013). In these and many other fields, the failure of the gene-for model has led researchers to reclassify illness in a way that *starts* with genetic mutations and works from there. But how does this work when the mutation is more or less clear, yet its effects are anything but? How does a category shape clinical practice, social action, and personal identity when the people who have the mutation in question could never have been grouped together on the basis of what they are actually like?

These are not hypothetical questions. Many biomedical experts, clinicians, patients, and health activists have already moved beyond a reductionist version of geneticization. They have adopted a radical strategy for mobilizing mutations that I propose we call *genomic designation*. Rather than relying on correlations with existing categories, they discover, delineate, and diagnose disease strictly according to observations of the genome. Sometimes, genomic designation takes place in the face of enormous phenotypic heterogeneity. To be clear, genomically designated conditions are *not* clinically diagnosable. Yet under certain conditions, they can give rise to specialist clinics and vibrant patient advocacy organizations. Furthermore, genomically designated conditions can be used to pry open far-reaching questions about human difference or, in other settings, to realign clinical judgment.

I discuss the concept of genomic designation in far greater detail in chapter 1. For now, a few important points of clarification: First, genomic designation can reclassify disease in many different ways. I devote the most attention to striking cases like 22q11.2DS, Fragile X syndrome and XYY syndrome, where knowledge about a mutation had a radical impact on medical classification. However, it is important to keep in mind that genomically designated conditions can have complex relationships to more long-standing clinical categories. Genomic designation can be used to lump, split, and recalibrate disease categories as well as create entirely new ones. Insofar as a mutation comes to be necessary and sufficient for a diagnosis, we are dealing with a genomically designated condition.

Second, genomic designation can be seen very powerfully in the classification of cancer (e.g., Venkitaraman 2002; for sociological studies on genomic oncology, see Bourret, Keating, and Cambrosio 2011; Nelson, Keating, and Cambrosio 2013), and even the delineation of species of bacteria (e.g., Rowan and Powers 1991; Zeaiter, Liang, and Raoult 2002). It also plays a central role in the classification of metabolic disorders: a recent *Genetics in Medicine* paper presented a nosology of 1,015 inborn errors of metabolism (and counting), all of them tied to mutations in specific genes. The authors were crystal clear: "The involvement of different gene products is considered sufficient for separation into different entries, even if the phenotype is similar" (Ferreira et al. 2018:table 1). However, I mostly ignore the way genetics has given us new categories of malignant growth, inabilities to metabolize food, or novel species of bacteria. Instead, I focus on the way mutations have been used to carve out new categories of human disease that almost always involve childhood developmental difference.

Finally, genomic designation simply refers to the practice of classifying human difference on the basis of genetic mutations. In the large majority of cases, it amounts to little more than a few papers on a new mutation and the "syndrome" it causes. I focus on the less common but more sociologically interesting cases where a mutation comes to mean far more than that. Whether, when, and how a mutation truly shapes people's lives is always an empirical question—the central question that I grapple with throughout this book.

A Brief Note on Methods

Throughout this book I shamelessly focus on sites that embody the transformative potential of genomic designation. The point is not to mislead the reader: I freely acknowledge genomic designation is *not* the reigning mode of medical classification, and—despite major gains in just the last few years—it is unlikely to become dominant anytime soon. Rather, my aim is to examine the conditions, organizations, and people who exemplify genomic designation in order to show something new and important emerging at the intersection of genetics, medicine, and patient advocacy.

My primary method is qualitative, comparative-historical research. Using the record of published biomedical research, along with a variety of publicly available resources, archival materials, and oral histories, I outline the varied history of genomic designation as a way of classifying people over the last sixty years. My framework for comparing the way mutations have been mobilized across cases, places, and historical periods is discussed in detail in the next section. In addition, I use bibliometric analysis of the Institute for Scientific Information's (ISI) Web of Science database at several points throughout the book in order to model the impact of genetics on nosology and assess the status of mutations in pertinent medical literatures.

The entire book also draws on IRB-approved fieldwork conducted at conferences and events for genetic disorders, primarily 22q11.2DS but also Fragile X syndrome and 22q13DS. During these conferences, I attended hundreds of presentations and breakout sessions by researchers, clinicians, patients, parents, and others, as well social events where they all mingled as a single community united by their mutation of interest. I conducted dozens of interviews with biomedical researchers, clinicians, advocates, and parents and visited carefully targeted sites where genomic designation is playing out, such as Elwyn Services, the Geisinger Autism and Developmental Medicine Institute, the MIND Institute at UC Davis, Children's Hospital of Philadelphia, and a meeting of the US Department of Health and Human Services' Secretary's Advisory Committee on Heritable Disorders in Newborns and Children on newborn screening. Finally, I was also fortunate enough to have many illuminating, informal conversations with patients, parents, and allied experts during the course of this fieldwork that, while I cannot quote them directly, shaped this book in innumerable ways. All of these methods are discussed in further detail in the relevant chapters.

Writing the History of Mutations

What do I mean by a comparative-historical analysis of genomically designated conditions? In the simplest sense, it is the history of the genetic mutations that have been cast as novel disease entities in the human genetics literature. Dozens upon dozens of new medical conditions have been reported in the literature since 1959 according to the logic of genomic designation. However, the fate of those novel genetic conditions is radically uneven both within and across cases. Some never amount to much more than a case report or two, while others have become powerful categories of human difference underwritten by complex networks of research, treatment and social mobilization.

To be sure, mutations do not simply appear as distinct, fully formed abnormalities when researchers scrutinize people's genomes (see Rabeharisoa and Bourret 2009; Hogan 2016; Timmermans 2017). Oftentimes, the mutations themselves start out as what Rheinberger (1997) calls "epistemic things"—objects that have no clear referent outside of the "experimental system" in which they first come into view and have the capacity to surprise researchers and redirect their work. Over time though, they are often largely stabilized or "black-boxed" (à la Latour 1988; Rheinberger 1997:30) and thereby turned into technical things that can be studied across labs and even different testing platforms. In this way, a mutation itself may cease to be an epistemic thing in the world of genetic testing. But that is only the end of the beginning. As Rheinberger argues (1997:30), science studies scholars tend to overlook black-boxing's "impact on a new generation of emerging epistemic things." Once they are rendered more or less stable as genetic test results, mutations can begin new and incredibly generative careers in many other fields ranging from molecular biology, neuroscience, and pharmaceutical development through medicine, clinical psychology, and special education. That is the sort of history I want to tell.

Simply knowing that a mutation exists does not get us very far. It is only after years of painstaking work and cooperation spanning an array of biomedical fields and stakeholders that a mutation comes to index a new kind of person. That is why even the same genetic mutations can mean very different things over time. A sociological analysis of genomic designation must therefore go beyond the fact that mutations can be stabilized as objects of knowledge, or even the fact that they can give rise to new syndromes in the literature. We need to examine how it is that those new categories *matter* to the way we understand and act on human difference. It must go beyond the field of human genetics, for which genetic classification came as an unproblematic turn once they were able to observe abnormal chromosomes. Instead, we need to examine how genomic designation has been taken up by researchers in other fields, clinical practitioners, commercial enterprises, media, advocates, and the diagnosed themselves. This section therefore outlines my framework for analyzing the historical conditions of possibility, processes of network formation, and forms of collective action that can turn a genetic mutation into a new kind of person, with all that means for the diagnosed and their families.

Reiterated Fact-Making

How can we explain the contrasting fates of mutations over time? For our purposes, the traditional comparative-historical logic is fatally undermined by the fact that even our comparisons *between* cases are far from independent or equivalent (Sewell 1996): many researchers and advocates are very much aware of and can often be found working with multiple genomically designated conditions, while the physiological implications of the different mutations themselves are often far from equivalent. Furthermore, when we are analyzing the shifting meanings of the *same* mutations over time, a conventional comparative logic is clearly a nonstarter.

In order to overcome these obstacles, I adopt a comparative approach that draws on what Jeffrey Haydu (1998) calls "reiterated problem solving"—a way to gain explanatory leverage by "rethinking sequences of events across periods." Haydu offered reiterated problem solving as a comparative-historical tool that incorporates key insights from narrative and path-dependency approaches, but departs from them by examining how actors respond to similar problems or crises in different historical periods. He deftly applied it to the example of successive industrial-relations regimes in the twentieth-century United States. "Rethinking the connections between events in different time periods as reiterated problem solving," Haydu explains, helps us to "mak[e] use of continuities across periods, and [avoid] certain pitfalls of variable-based comparisons by putting historical particulars to explanatory work" (341). This approach allows for the study of social action in different historical settings, the explanation of different outcomes, and careful attention to the way that settlements in one period constrain and enable actors working to solve a recurrent problem later on. Reiterated problem solving therefore holds great promise for a comparative study of genomic designation over the last half century.

However, we cannot really say that we are "connecting events between periods through sequences of problem solving" (Haydu 1998: 349). Why not? Haydu rightly insists that in defining and delimiting "recurring problems," "one criterion must be the social actors' own understandings" (355). At this point, it seems as though we have reached something of an impasse. It is simply not the case that human geneticists in the 1960s and a parent advocate today would "recognize a common dilemma," as Haydu put it,[2] even if their interest is in precisely the same genetic mutation. Even today, we find incommensurable formulations of the matter at hand. Mobilizing mutations was not a "problem" that competing groups fought over or that geneticists failed to solve, but an entirely new project or "problematization" (see Foucault 1990a:257) that had to be taken up by actors with very different orientations and expertise. Forging alliances with new groups of actors and *rethinking* the very matter at hand—that is, the problem to be solved—is central to the rise of genomically designated conditions.

What did remain constant across different times and places—or at least constant enough for a comparative analysis—were the mutations themselves. They are the unifying thread that allows for a comparative-historical analysis of genomic designation, not the actors and their conceptions of what to do with them. The shifting ways in which we understand and use knowledge about those mutations is largely *explained* by changes in the networks of actors assembled around them. As much as the fields of human and medical genetics exhibit significant continuity over the half century covered in this book, we cannot remain focused on geneticists if we want to understand how conditions like 22q11.2DS, 5p– or Triple X syndrome became so powerful.[3] Nor can we assume that geneticists were really, in the mid-twentieth century, aiming to create anything like the kind of clinically and socially salient categories of difference we see today. To foreshadow, many of these mutations were well established in the genetics literature for decades before they began to gain real traction elsewhere. It is not that no one knew about these mutations; rather, no one had figured out how to do all that much with our knowledge about them. As we will see, mutations cannot be effectively mobilized by geneticists alone. So, while reiterated problem solving "puts social actors at center stage" (Haydu 1998:357), my approach casts objects of knowledge as the main attraction and allows human actors to enter and exit over the course of the play.

How then should we think about mutations as objects of knowledge and practice? Consider Ludwik Fleck's seminal work on scientific *facts* ([1935] 1981). Fleck is most cited for his insight that "thought styles" decisively shape knowledge production (see especially Rose 2007a, 2007b)—a concept that is often compared to Foucault's "episteme" or Kuhn's "paradigm."[4] The bulk of Fleck's magnum opus, however, charts the long scientific and cultural history leading to the biochemical delineation of syphilis according to the Wassermann reaction. He recounts how his work in the venereal section of a large hospital convinced him "that it would never occur even to a modern researcher, equipped with a complete intellectual and material armory" to isolate the disease entity "syphilis" from the totality of her cases (22). Fleck goes on to masterfully explain the way changing thought styles, research cul-de-sacs, evolving disciplinary boundaries, and evolving cultural imperatives shaped the history of syphilis as a disease entity. Fleck may be most known for his ideas about thought styles, but his real focus—as evidenced in the very title of his book—is the dynamic way they shaped "the genesis and development of a scientific fact."

Fleck explains why "the development of the disease phenomena requires decades" ([1935] 1981:22).[5] He discusses the arduous path a fact must take from "journal science" to "vademecum," or atlas science, and eventually all the way to "popular knowledge." Although Fleck acknowledged that "popular exoteric knowledge stems from specialized esoteric knowledge" (113), he was adamant that there is not a simple, unidirectional relationship between the two: *Certainty, simplicity, vividness originate in popular knowledge. That is where the expert obtains his faith in this triad as the ideal of knowledge*" (115; emphasis in original).[6] It is only once it achieves traction at the level of popular knowledge, Fleck writes, that a "fact becomes incarnated as an immediately perceptible object of reality" (125). For a disease to be full-fledged fact, it has to be something that a doctor can relay to patients or their caregivers.

I want to draw on this insight from Fleck and explore the way that genomically designated conditions emerge as tentative facts in human genetics research but then go on to take very different paths. Why do most remain halting, insecure findings that never make it past the pages of esoteric journals, while others have gone on to gain traction far beyond the vanguard of geneticists who discovered them? Above all, how do mutations get transformed as objects of knowledge and practice when they are taken up by what Fleck calls "exoteric" fields and publics (1981:113)? To answer these questions, I trace mutations as facts across cases, places, and historical periods. I want to combine the original English usage of the word *fact*—a thing that is done, performed or achieved—with the capital-M Modern notion of facts as out there, independent of our investigation or our will, and waiting to be discovered. On the one hand, I want to take it mostly for granted that these mutations are real and that they have most likely wrought various forms of difference and illness on human beings for thousands of years. On the other, I show how what Hacking calls "looping processes" have made and remade mutations as facts in the few decades that we have been able to observe them. In so doing, we see how mutations are transformed as facts.

I call this approach "reiterated fact-making." By combining Fleck and Haydu's different approaches, reiterated fact-making helps us trace facts across time periods, study the changing networks built up around them, and wrestle with the contrasting forms of knowledge and practice they give rise to.[7] In short, reiterated fact-making allows for a comparative-historical analysis of genetic mutations as facts over time. More broadly, it is a tool that can bring the kind of causal explanation advocated by Haydu to bear on topics traditionally addressed in the history of science and medicine. Indeed, some of the most illuminating work in the history of medicine implicitly adopts this style of analysis.[8] This approach will guide my analysis of genomic designation over the last sixty years, but I also hope that it will prove useful to scholars interested in the way that scientific facts are held stable even as they undergo radical change across different times and places.

How Mutations Can Loop

There is, of course, a prehistory to this book. For many thousands of years, genetic mutations have undoubtedly existed in human populations without being recognized as such.[9] I call this a prehistory because, working with Hacking's framework of "dynamic nominalism" (2007, 1998b, 2006b, 1995), we see how important the act of labeling a group of people can be. To be sure, people with the genetic mutations discussed in this book have been subject to many different sorts of labeling for hundreds and thousands of years. Our story, however, begins when people began to be labeled as having this or that genetic mutation in 1959.

Hacking draws our attention to the "looping" processes that cause categories of human difference and expert practices to recursively change one another over time, sometimes quite dramatically. Crucially, looping processes actually change the people who are classified. Sometimes, Hacking explains, "People classified in a certain way tend to conform to or grow into the ways that they are described." At other times, however, they "evolve in their own ways, so that the classifications and descriptions have to be constantly revised" (Hacking 1998b:21). The argument has two key steps. The first, familiar to sociologists at least since "labeling" theory (Becker 1963), is that classifications shape the identities and behavior of the people to whom they are applied. These classifications can bring what Hacking calls a new "human kind" (1995), or "kind of person" (2007) into being.[10] The second and more innovative part of the argument is that what these kinds of people are like, not to mention what they do, often defies experts' expectations. As researchers wrestle with new findings, these unanticipated characteristics and behaviors can reshape the original classification. In this way, the downstream effects of labeling a group of people can actually loop back and force experts to reconsider the category itself, what we think we know about it, and the sorts of treatment and practice associated with it. These looping processes therefore bring experts, categories, classified people, and other stakeholders into a dynamic interaction that can unfold over the course of years and decades. The constant back-and-forth between the category and the population it is applied to renders kinds of people into "moving targets" (Hacking 2007).

At first glance, it might seem as though this argument only applies to the looser "psy" categories (Rose 1998a), such as multiple personality disorder or autism (Hacking's most fully fleshed-out examples [1995, 2006b]). Perhaps, one could plausibly argue, classifications that are affixed to biomarkers and especially genetic mutations do not loop in the same way. Indeed, Hacking once wrote that "quarks, probably genes, possibly cystic fibrosis" are natural kinds; labeling them as such does not affect their behavior. At the same time, Hacking (1995:372) also argued that "biologizing human kinds does not thereby make them immune to looping effects." A genetic mutation might be a natural kind, but a type of person indexed by a mutation is a human kind; while the gene may work the same way before and after being labeled, telling people that they have the "gene for" cystic fibrosis, 22q11.2DS, or some other condition is another matter entirely.

So, could a person have 22q11.2DS in 1975 or 1848? Yes and no. It is inarguable that there were people who, were they alive today, could have been found to bear microdeletions at 11.2 on the long arm of the twenty-second chromosome.[11] Most of them probably experienced ailments associated with 22q11.2DS. However, being categorized as a particular kind of person actually changes a human being. This was perhaps the key distinction between human and natural kinds in Hacking's original formulation (1995): calling some wet dirt "mud" does not change it, but calling a person who habitually drinks to excess an "alcoholic" brings with it a host of expert, moral, and personal expectations and practices. As Hacking explained, there surely were people who, had they lived today, would have been diagnosable with autism or multiple personality disorder long before either became available as diagnostic categories. Nevertheless, the creation of those diagnoses and the myriad forms of action undertaken on their basis have real effects on the people who are so classified. Hacking's key point is that the classification of people is dynamic: kinds of people may be "constructions," but they make and remake both themselves and the people whom they designate.

The same is true for categories of human difference that are fixed to genetic mutations. To have 22q11.2DS in the fullest sense of the term, you have to be diagnosed with it. The diagnostic criteria may be unusually clear and rigid, but that does not change the fact that the category shapes people's lives and experience of difference. Nor does it make 22q11.2DS somehow immune to looping processes. The act of naming, diagnosing, studying, or treating a condition like 22q11.2DS still sets processes of development and revision into motion, even though the category is fixed to a genetic mutation. To paraphrase Hacking (1995), a "biologized" kind of person can still loop, even if its biological fixity changes the looping dynamics involved.

There is clearly less scope for looping in terms of *who* can be diagnosed with genomically designated syndromes. However, there is plenty when it comes to their phenotypic profiles and the implications of a diagnosis. The very meaning of genetic mutation grows and morphs when experts and advocates mobilize it. The arc of this book shows how genetic mutations were first used to delineate esoteric "syndromes" in human genetics almost as soon as they came into view under the microscope in 1959, but also how that was just the very beginning of the story. Only much later, and in a small minority of cases, were those syndromes assembled into robust facts that could be considered kinds of people in the full sense of Hacking's term.

Bringing a community of patients, advocates, clinicians, and researchers together around a mutation generates a wealth of new knowledge. Sometimes, this means discovering a broader-than-expected range of IQs and developmental outcomes or a series of unanticipated medical symptoms. Indeed, with sufficient caseloads and enough lay feedback, researchers often uncover highly specific features of genomically designated conditions—the "spasmodic upper-body squeeze" in Smith-Magenis syndrome, the verbal-performance IQ split in 22q11.2DS, the aversion to eye contact in Fragile X, or the inability to cry in *NGLY1* being key examples we will encounter in this book. Features like these then loop to become part of the underlying mutation's phenotype, shaping expectations and treatment strategies for the people in whom it is detected. They also create ascertainment biases that guide who gets tested for the mutation in the first place and therefore who gets diagnosed. Above all, finding a mutation can profoundly reshape expectations and treatment programs, triggering new loops that reverberate between the classification and the classified. Thinking through reiterated fact-making therefore helps us explain how a genetic mutation can become the essential referent of a new kind of person and a locus of novel looping processes.

Classification and Networks of Expertise

The insight that classification—the ways in which we divide up the world into categories—is a product of collective, social processes goes back at least to Durkheim ([1912] 2001). In recent years, considerable social scientific attention has been devoted to the importance of standardization in general (see Timmermans and Epstein 2010 for a review) and medical classification in particular (Armstrong 2011; Bowker and Star 2000; Timmermans and Berg 1997). The observations we privilege in the classification of disease—symptoms, anatomical observation, psychiatric characteristics, or genetic test results, to name a few—have shifted repeatedly throughout the history of medicine. As Armstrong wrote, "Underlying classificatory principles . . . both constitute and reflect the very nature of identity" (2011:802). When a system of classification (of disease or whatever else) is at its most powerful, there is a prima facie acceptance, or "taken-for-grantedness" about the way it organizes experience. It has become "apodictic," as Fleck put it. That is how classificatory systems can withstand the constant "effacement" or resistance discussed by Foucault (1973:9; see also Armstrong 2011) when a doctor is dealing with an actual patient who can never quite fit the mold that has been cast for them.

Genomic designation therefore depends, in part, on prevailing ideas about illness and identity (see Taussig, Rapp, and Heath 2003:59). As Duana Fullwiley (2011:20–21) would put it, human mutations cannot become salient without also being "encultured" by the world around them. However, it also depends on the agentive work of actors seeking to establish genomically designated conditions in institutions that are not geared toward genetics. At every given site where a parent may seek to bring a genomically designated condition to bear—a hospital, a general practitioner's examination room, a school, the psychologist's office, and so forth—she may find actors and institutional structures that are resistant or even hostile to genetic classification. Genomically designated conditions therefore need to be assembled as networks of expertise (Eyal 2013) one journal article, doctor, advocate, clinic, testing kit, treatment protocol, and individualized education plan at a time, often in the face of considerable resistance. These are the sorts of resources that parents can deploy when they are faced with a skeptical doctor who is unwilling to let knowledge about a genetic mutation shape a child's clinical treatment. Without such a network, a genomically designated condition will remain a sociologically thin fact with no hope of withstanding the discordances and obstacles that inevitably plague any attempt to classify human difference. As we will see, these networks have to be assembled using parts that were designed for clinical categories, not genomically designated ones. To abuse a classic formulation: people do not classify human difference just as they please, under self-selected circumstances, but under circumstances existing already, given and transmitted from the past. To mobilize a mutation, actors have to work within prevailing institutions, norms, and systems of classification even as they seek to transform them.

From Illness to Disease and on to Etiology

To understand the history of genomic designation, we need to go deeper than the experience of illness, or even the classification of disease. The sociology of science and medicine has already made the highly productive turn away from a prescribed focus on the experience of *illness* and the social factors associated with it—the focus of medical sociology from Parsons's 1951 conceptualization of illness as deviance (1991:288–322) onward. Today, there is a growing engagement with the enactment of *disease* itself (see especially Mol 2002; Timmermans and Haas 2008). However, the frequency,[12] ascertainment, and construction of *etiological* findings—genetic mutations in this case—are also powerfully shaped by social forces. We therefore need to delve even further into what is perhaps uncomfortable biomedical terrain and grapple with issues related to biological etiology.

The point is not that the "lesions" that cause disease are "social constructions." Far from it. Some genetic mutations, for example, do have consistent clinical outcomes, and even more consistently have some kind of phenotypic effect. However, genetic mutations intersect with different technological capabilities, systems of classification, and institutional structures, or what Foucault would call the "surfaces of emergence" (Foucault 2002:41) for genomic designation. Only certain populations are likely to be referred for genetic testing. As those populations, the ways in which we classify and treat them, and the institutions through which we do so change, so too does the meaning of mutations themselves. I show how the same genetic mutation can be associated with divergent symptomatologies and comorbid conditions, take on strikingly different meanings, and lead to different forms of treatment, prospect horizons, and social action in different times and places. In short, affixing a disease entity to a genetic mutation does not magically bypass the social processes that shape the way that medical classifications are understood and acted upon. We are still left with the question, "Etiology for what?" The prevailing nosological systems— that is, the kinds of people we care about enough to diagnose and investigate—decisively shape the meaning of genetic mutations and the projects they are enrolled in. By extending the reach of medical sociology not just from illness to disease but all the way to etiology, we therefore get a fuller account of the way social structures and cultural schemas mediate even the most seemingly clear-cut categories of biological abnormality.

Overview

The rest of this book explains how some genetic mutations have become powerful facts that can transform our approach to human difference, while others languish as sociologically flat objects in genetics journals and databases. I argue that certain forms of social mobilization can radically change the status of a genetic mutation as a fact— both what we know about it and what it means to have it. Genomic designation is therefore as much a question of collective action, repertoires of mobilization, and institutional infrastructures as it is one of genes, proteins, and physiological pathways.

This book can be broken down into four sections. In chapters 1 and 2, I explain what genomic designation is and outline its early history in human genetics. Chapter 1 defines genomic designation and puts it into dialogue with some of the most important concepts in the social studies of genetics and medicine. Drawing heavily on two conditions—the 22q13 and 22q11.2 Deletion Syndromes—it provides a typology of the various ways knowledge about mutations is being used to reshape medical classification. Chapter 2 charts the emergence of genomic designation in the biomedical literature from 1959, with the delineation of conditions like Triple X and 5p– syndrome. However, I show how these novel disorders, and the mutations that they were fixed to, did not amount to much outside of esoteric human genetics. During the 1960s and 1970s, the historical conditions and repertoires of collective action that would one day turn those very same mutations into powerful categories of difference were just not yet in place. Even the spectacular but fleeting attention garnered by XYY, or "Super Male" syndrome, and especially its infamous association with aggression and crime, ended up being what I call the exception that proves the rule. These mutations and genomically designated conditions were important facts in the genetics literature, but not further afield.

The middle section, chapters 3 and 4, examines the all-important relationship between genomically designated conditions and more common categories of human difference. In chapter 3 I look at the way genomically designated conditions are often used to get at bigger, otherwise intractable questions—a process I call "leveraging mutations." When a rare mutation is strongly associated with a common trait or medical condition, the population with that mutation becomes a tantalizingly powerful biological model for more general gene-protein-physiological processes. I draw on a trio of case studies to show how researchers have leveraged rare mutations to get at big questions in human biology: aggression and crime, sociability and language, and psychiatric disorders such as autism. Indeed, the leveraging alliance between the Fragile X syndrome and autism patient movements was so successful it became a beacon for advocates dedicated to other genetic disorders. Yet, as chapter 4 illustrates, *autism* had to become a broader and more encompassing kind of person before it could be strongly tied to the sort of genetic mutations discussed in this book. This only happened after a decades-long looping process that was itself shaped by ideas and evidence about the genetics of autism. By studying the rates of autism in genomically designated conditions over time, a very clear picture comes into view: looping changed the genetic makeup of the autism population by bringing a host of new mutations like 22q11.2, XYY, and Fragile X into the fold. In this way, we see how changes in clinical medicine and psychiatry shape the conditions of possibility for genomic designation—they determine what it means to have a genetic mutation at the level of symptomatology. At the end of chapter 4, I delve into the alliances, or "trading zones," between genomically designated conditions like 22q13DS and psychiatric disorders like autism to show how the two sides manage to work together despite divergent goals and ideas about disease, cause, and symptom.

In the penultimate section, chapters 5 and 6, I explore the cutting edge of genomic designation. In chapter 5, I examine the networks of experts and advocates who have turned conditions like Fragile X, XYY, and 22q11.2DS into increasingly powerful kinds of people. Over time, they have developed innovate repertoires of collective action for mobilizing mutations. More and more people are being diagnosed with conditions like 22q11.2DS. Once diagnosed, they now find an array of resources at their disposal—a medical literature and management guidelines, a network of specialist clinics, pharmaceutical trials, activist foundations and support groups, a dedicated summer camp, and a wealth of information about what a 22q11.2 microdeletion is likely to mean for them and their future. In this way, knowing that someone has a genetic mutation can transform their life. Chapter 6 then takes a deeper dive into the many different ways a diagnosis like 22q11.2DS can affect treatment and care. Even in a highly developed country like the United States, most people do not have easy access to genetic testing, never mind the sorts of health insurance and "cultural health capital" (Shim 2010) it takes to get all the extra tests and treatments recommended by 22q11.2DS experts. Still, we will see how more and more people are able to draw upon the networks built up around rare mutations to reframe ideas about illness, reorient expectations for development, and reshape practice in medicine, psychology, and education.

Whether genomic designation will fade into obscurity, lead to improved health outcomes for millions, or become what we might call, borrowing from Troy Duster ([1990] 2003), a "backdoor to eugenics" remains to be seen. A full-blown futurology would doubtless be a fool's errand. Still, the final section of this book turns a cautious eye toward the emergent future for genomic designation. In chapter 7, we see how the knowledge that someone has a genetic mutation can remake the distinction between the normal and the pathological. For example, when someone with a 16p11.2 or 22q11.2 microdeletion has an IQ of 87—well above the clinical threshold of ≤ 70 necessary for an intellectual disability diagnosis—they may still be seen as being affected by their genetic mutation. More and more, experts and advocates argue that a patient should not be denied care just because their phenotype does not reach some arbitrary clinical cutoff. Even some "carrier" genes are now being recast as mild genetic disorders in their own right.

Chapter 8 sketches out some of the factors that are likely to shape the way genetic mutations are mobilized in the coming years. I show how next-generation sequencing, new genomics databases, and social media have allowed researchers and advocates to discover, report, and mobilize mutations with unprecedented rapidity. I also look to some of the broader trends that seem to point to the continued growth of genomic designation as a feature of modern health care and personal identity formation. But that is not the only emergent future for genomic designation. Although it may seem as though the book paints an unwavering arc toward the formation of networks of care and support for people with genomically designated conditions, there is no teleology that makes their newfound status secure or others certain to follow in their footsteps.

I therefore address a second trajectory that has come into view in the last few years: the dramatically increased *prenatal* ascertainment of genomically designated conditions. Most of the mutations included in the new wave of noninvasive testing kits that are revolutionizing prenatal genetic testing are the very ones discussed in this book. This is bound to create vexed dilemmas for would-be parents: not only is there huge uncertainty about the phenotypes of these mutations, but what we even think we know is severely limited by ascertainment bias. Furthermore, with so many would-be parents finding out about 22q11.2 microdeletions, extra sex chromosomes, and so on just nine or ten weeks into pregnancy, noninvasive prenatal testing promises to reduce the prevalence and remake the socioeconomic demographics of a growing number of genetic mutations. In short, these extraordinarily personal decisions about genetic abnormality and abortion may end up having eugenic consequences at the population level. For as much as groups dedicated to conditions like 22q11.2DS and XYY syndrome have come a long way in recent decades, they still remain dependent upon broader biomedical trends and social forces whose impact they can only hope to partly control.

It is time for the social studies of science and medicine to go beyond geneticization. Just as geneticists leverage rare mutations to get at more general questions about human biology and disease, we can use them to gain new perspective on the way genetics and patient advocacy are changing what it means to be different today. We need to think about the emergence of *new* kinds of people, forged at the interface of biomedicine and collective action, and carved out at the level of the human genome. We also need to grapple with the way knowledge about biological abnormality is shaped by social forces, even when the underlying genetics is rendered stable and thereby held constant. The discovery of a genetic mutation may indeed precipitate "biosociality," but social action can also reshape the meaning of the mutation itself. Mobilization can make a profound difference—the difference between a genetic test result that can perhaps explain some kind of medical or developmental issue, and one that can radically change the way a person is understood, how she is treated, and the social world she is part of. The rest of this book therefore explores the many varied ways genetic mutations have been mobilized and transformed in the sixty years since it became possible to see abnormal human genomes. In other words, I try to explain how a missing stretch of DNA on an image of stained chromosomes can mean so much.

ONE

Genomic Designation: How Genetics Creates New Medical Conditions

But this order of the solid, visible body is only one way—in all likelihood neither the first, nor the most fundamental—in which one spatializes disease. *There have been, and will be, other distributions of illness.*
MICHEL FOUCAULT, *THE BIRTH OF THE CLINIC*

From the clinical standpoint, [22q13 deletion] syndrome may be under-diagnosed because of the *lack of a recognizable phenotype that would lead the clinician to request studies to rule out this specific chromosome 22 deletion.*
PHELAN ET AL., "22Q13 DELETION SYNDROME"

For sixty years now, we have been delineating medical conditions that are united not by observations of patients' bodies, evaluations of their psyches, or predictions of their fate, but by specific genetic mutations. Finding a mutation can lead experts to report a completely new category of human disease and difference. In other cases, it can result in the lumping together, splitting up, or recalibration of existing disease categories. This chapter introduces and defines this practice, which I call the *genomic designation* of medical conditions.

Genomic designation is the delineation and diagnosis of medical conditions strictly according to observations of abnormal genomes, be it whole chromosome duplications, tiny point mutations, or anything in between.[1] When a newly discovered mutation does *not* line up with an existing condition and instead comes to designate a new disorder, we have a case of genomic designation. Most genomically designated conditions lack the phenotypic coherence or distinctiveness to be clinically diagnosable at all. Instead, the genome itself is the locus of classification.

Ever since 1959, genomic designation has been endemic to genetics research. As we explore in chapter 2, the ability to see, count, and distinguish between chromosomes under a microscope led almost immediately to the first cases of genomic designation. In the decades that followed, innovations in genetic testing quickly led to the discovery of new genomically designated conditions. Meanwhile, long-standing mutations have been rendered visible and more or less stable across different genetic testing platforms—from karyotype analysis to whole genome sequencing. Hundreds of conditions have now been discovered or reshaped through genomic designation. So far, however, only a much smaller number have become the sorts of categories that can truly transform people's lives. Beginning in this chapter, we are going to explore the varied history of carving up human difference through genomic designation.

For people with a genomically designated condition, having a genetic mutation means something that is at once crystal clear and deeply uncertain. Take one of our main case studies in this chapter: the microdeletion of genetic material at site 13.3 on the long arm of the twenty-second chromosome. Having this 22q13.3 chromosomal deletion means someone has 22q13 Deletion Syndrome (22q13DS—not to be confused with 22q11.2DS). Yet had the 22q13 deletion never been discovered, 22q13DS would be unthinkable. Even the researchers most responsible for establishing 22q13DS in the medical literature noted the "lack of a recognizable phenotype" that could even indicate genetic testing (Phelan et al. 2001:98).

This makes 22q13DS quite unlike most well-known genetic disorders—Huntington's disease, cystic fibrosis, Down syndrome, and so on—or genomic risk factors like the *BRCA* variants. In all of those cases, established medical conditions were found to have a significant relationship with genetic mutations. By contrast, 22q13DS reverses this sequence of genotype-phenotype association. This syndrome is actually one of the most consistently severe conditions discussed in this book. Even so, it could never have been conceived of until *after* the identification of the 22q13 (pronounced twenty-two-q-one-three) chromosomal deletion. Hence, the 22q13 deletion became a subject of scientific investigation around 1988, some thirteen years before the syndrome named after it was proclaimed and the 22q13 Deletion Syndrome Foundation was formed. The patient population and its clinical profile depend entirely on the people found to carry a 22q13 deletion and what they are like. Today, knowledge about 22q13DS—now known as Phelan-McDermid syndrome (PMS)—and the work of the renamed Phelan-McDermid Syndrome Foundation have a powerful impact on the lives of patients and their families. This very clear process of discovery, delineation, and mobilization captures the essence of genomic designation.

A New Front in the Social Studies of Genetics and Medicine

While genomic designation establishes an unusual level of certainty at the level of etiology, it often does so at the expense of clinical specificity. In most cases it is unlikely that diagnosis could, even in principle, take place on the basis of what someone is actually like (i.e., their phenotype). Conditions like 22q13DS therefore go beyond the matter of social action undertaken on the basis of reductionism or risk, which in one form or another has been the focus of most of the social scientific literature on genetics and medicine (e.g., Callon and Rabeharisoa 2003; Hacking 2006a; Hedgecoe 2001; Lippman 1991b; Rabinow 1996; Rose 2007b). In this way, genomic designation builds upon but also powerfully subverts the "clinical gaze" (Foucault 1973; Rose 1998b)— the nosological relationship between the observed and the unobserved that privileges localized anatomo-clinical observation—which has dominated medical classification since the nineteenth century. In conditions like 22q13DS, genetic mutations take on great meaning, not as a proxy in the form of a predisposition or an essentializing explanation, but as the core referent of a new category of human difference. The sociological interest in genomic designation therefore goes beyond the study of a bunch of new disease entities, or what Hacking called "human kinds." Instead, it extends to the emergence of a *new kind of human kind* that can reconfigure the way we understand and act on difference, illness, and disability.

Grappling with genomic designation forces us to rethink the relationship between genetics, medical classification, and human difference. Existing research has shown how discovering explanatory mutations may or may not reshape diagnostic protocols for conditions like Huntington's and Cystic Fibrosis, how finding a mutation in a seemingly normal patient can create a "patient in waiting," and how it takes a network of experts to simultaneously understand the clinical and biological significance of mutations.[2] Looking at genomic designation, however, shows us how knowledge about genetic mutations can be used to carve out novel medical conditions and communities, not just refine, destabilize, or help us understand old ones.

Genomic designation therefore both challenges and extends three seminal concepts in social studies of genetics: *biosociality*, *geneticization*, and the *molecular gaze*. Abby Lippman's work on geneticization helped spark an explosion of interest in the "ongoing process by which differences between individuals are reduced to their DNA codes, with most disorders, behaviors and psychological variations defined, at least in part, as genetic in origin" (1991a:19). Scholars have paid particular attention to the way this process of geneticization essentializes differences between persons, sometimes in ways that contribute to stigmatization (see Phelan 2005; see also Hedgecoe 2001 on "enlightened geneticization").

So, genomic designation could be understood as a radical form of geneticization: it is, if nothing else, built on the premise that we should parse human difference according to genetic abnormality. Many of the concerns Lippman raised when she introduced geneticization to the social sciences—the power of genetics to define abnormality and disability, the social implications of prenatal testing, and the resurgent specter of eugenics—may even be more likely to emerge through genomic designation than the gene-for model. And yet, genomic designation does not simply reduce existing categories to genetic mutations: it *produces* new categories of disease and difference.

Paul Rabinow's (1996) discussion of biosociality was a similarly formative moment in the social sciences' engagement with genomics (Hacking 2006a). Rabinow foresaw biosociality playing out on two dimensions. First, there was the potential for altering human DNA in pursuit of socially derived ends—hardly a novel topic. Second, and far more innovative, was the idea that social action and network formation might occur on the basis of a perceived genetic predisposition or risk for developing a clinical disorder. As Rabinow ([1992] 1996:102) presciently argued, "It is not hard to imagine groups formed around the chromosome 17, locus 16,256, site 654,376 allele variant with a guanine substitution." He even predicted these groups "will have medical specialists, laboratories, narratives, traditions, and a heavy panoply of pastoral keepers to help them experience, share, intervene, and 'understand' their fate." In this way, he explained, "Older cultural classifications will be joined by a vast array of new ones, which will crosscut, partially supersede, and eventually redefine the older categories"

(103). However, Rabinow's discussion of this new biosociality was clear that the social power of genomic difference would remain limited to questions of risk for something else. Observations of the genome, he averred, "carry with [them] no depth; . . . it has no meaning" (102).

Cases like 22q13.3 deletion allow us to extend the incredibly productive concept of biosociality. Mutations *can* acquire meaning when networks of knowledge production and social mobilization are assembled around them. Knowledge about genetic mutations can give rise to entirely new categories of human difference and therefore forms of identity that go far beyond mere risk factors. Furthermore, I show how these networks powerfully shape the course of biomedical research and the very knowledge produced about genetic mutations. Knowledge about the genome can set new forms of biosociality in motion, as Rabinow presciently recognized, but biosociality can also transform the way we understand the mutations themselves.

Genomic designation also represents a clear realization of what Nikolas Rose has called the "molecular gaze" (2007b, 2007a). Rose outlined the transformation of contemporary biomedicine's "style of thought" (Ludwik Fleck, cited in Rose 2007a:12) via an array of techniques aimed at understanding the body at the molecular level. By turning to molecular processes, Rose argues, contemporary biomedicine has begun to supplement the "clinical gaze" famously documented by Foucault (1973), with its focus on localized bodily observation as the basis for medical classification (Rose 2007b:11–15). To take just a couple of examples, previously indistinguishable forms of breast cancer have been differentiated on genetic grounds, and disjunct diseases have been found to share a genetic etiology, leading researchers to draw distinctions and see underlying unities that would not have been possible on a clinical basis (see Loscalzo, Kohane, and Barabasi 2007). In sum, the hegemony of anatomo-clinical classification is facing a serious assault from researchers armed with new molecular technologies.

Still, it is genomic designation that represents a molecular gaze in the true Foucauldian sense. Rather than *localized* anatomo-clinical observation (Foucault 1973:3–4), disease is increasingly classified according to genetic mutations that are usually found in every cell of the body. Knowledge about these mutations is being used to carve out medical categories, bringing about what Foucault (1973:195) called a "syntactical reorganization of disease in which the limits of the visible and the invisible follow a new pattern," and bringing previously unthinkable categories of illness into view. To be clear, I argue that genomic designation thrives when it enters into a productive interface with the prevailing clinical modes of classification. Anatomo-clinical medicine may have achieved a rapid and decisive victory over its predecessor, at least as told in Foucault's forthright account in *Birth of the Clinic* (1973; see Armstrong 2011 for a more circumspect account). By contrast, there is no foreseeable prospect of genomic designation quickly or straightforwardly supplanting what came before.

Way back in 1935, Ludwik Fleck presciently explained how "the modern concept of disease entity . . . [is] by no means the only logical possibility. As history shows, it is feasible to introduce *completely different classifications of diseases*" (Fleck [1935] 1981:21; my emphasis). Likewise, Foucault insisted (1973:3) that "this order of the solid, visible body is only one way—in all likelihood neither the first, nor the most fundamental—in which one spatializes disease. There have been, and will be, other distributions of illness." Genomic designation is precisely such a new way of locating and classifying disease. When genetic mutations such as the microdeletion at 22q13.3 come to serve as more than explanations for disease categories like hypotonia or autism and instead become the essential referents of new medical conditions like Phelan-McDermid syndrome, we begin to see geneticization, biosociality, and the molecular gaze writ large.

Clarifying Genomic Designation

What exactly do I mean by *genomic designation*? It is not a concept that one finds in the genetics literature, some recent discussion of "genotype-first" disease discovery notwithstanding (see chapter 8). So, because genomic designation has not previously been recognized as a distinct form of human classification, conditions have to be identified on a case-by-case basis. My criteria are straightforward: a condition is genomically designated if it is delineated and diagnosed strictly according to a genetic mutation. In other words, the observation of a specific genetic mutation is necessary and sufficient for diagnosis. The phenotype of the condition is then tabulated post factum by studying people if and only if they have the mutation in question.

In the clearest cases of genomic designation, like Triple X syndrome, 22q13DS, or *ADNP* syndrome, the mutation is discovered, and a brand-new condition is delineated on its basis. In less straightforward cases, a mutation that is strongly associated with an established clinical disorder ends up radically reshaping medical classification by lumping, splitting, and/or recalibrating more long-standing categories. We will return to the different varieties of genomic designation later in this chapter after exploring a couple of case studies.

Many hundreds, perhaps even thousands, of genomically designated conditions have been reported in the genetics literature. As a sociologist, however, I am especially interested in the cases where a genomically designated condition becomes a category of practice and social action—where it gives rise to the kind of clinical guidelines, specialist centers, advocacy organizations, and support groups that make it a bona fide medical and social category.

There are at least twenty-five clear-cut genomically designated conditions that match this ideal type, ranging in size from a mere handful to many thousands of diagnosed patients. They are all radically different from any preexisting clinical diagnosis, and they all have some sort of registered foundation or formal advocacy group established in their name (see table 1.2 below).

A key question for genomic designation moving forward is this: How many of the countless mutations and genomically designated conditions reported in the literature—a list that grows with every passing week—will join that vanguard? Countless other syndromes do not fulfill all these conditions perfectly, but, as we will see below with the 16p11.2 Deletion Syndrome and Williams syndrome, they should be understood in terms of genomic designation nevertheless. Once we recognize its clearest cases, genomic designation becomes useful as a broader conceptual tool for investigating the impact of contemporary genetics research. Indeed, *thousands* of genetic mutations are best thought of in these terms: they do not line up with preexisting clinical categories, and the extent to which they give rise to new disease entities in the medical literature, inform clinical practice, or become objects of social mobilization is an empirically open question. A typology of genomic designation is outlined below. First, where did genomic designation come from?

Origins

Down syndrome serves as both a useful point of reference and an important precursor to genomic designation. It is often diagnosed through karyotype analysis—the visual inspection of the chromosomes of a cell—and underwrites a substantial social and clinical network. However, the Down syndrome phenotype was first characterized on the basis of hospital observations in England by Dr. John Langdon Down in publications in 1862 and, more prominently, in 1866.[3] The latter article, "Observations on an Ethnic Classification of Idiots" (Down 1866), described Down's clinical observations and delineation of what was called Mongolian Idiocy. He sought to establish that, among the "large number of idiots and imbeciles" he observed, "a considerable portion can be fairly referred to one of the great divisions of the human race other than the class from which they have sprung." Down had discovered and delineated a syndrome on the basis of a clinically observed phenotype even as he posited a hereditary explanation (of sorts) for Mongolian Idiocy.

Perhaps the idea that Mongolian Idiocy represented some kind of error of inheritance inspired Jérôme Lejeune and his colleagues to look at people with Down syndrome as they sought to establish cytogenetics' relevance to medicine. Indeed, a chromosomal explanation for Mongolian Idiocy had been advanced years earlier (see chapter 2). Still, even though Down syndrome is now identified with trisomy of the twenty-first chromosome, it is clearly *not* all that useful to think about it in terms of genomic designation: a characteristic of the genome was not necessary for its discovery and delineation as a disease category, nor is it necessary for a Down syndrome diagnosis today. As a review of the early cytogenetic findings in the *Journal of Pediatrics* put it at the time: "Exceptions to the association of an extra chromosome 21 and Mongolism have been recorded, indicating that from a cytogenetic point of view, there are at least two forms of Mongolism" (Rappoport and Kaplan 1961:428; see also Polani et al. 1960).[4] Down had employed the clinical gaze, not genomic designation, and mongolism continued to be diagnosed on the basis of its phenotype even once the association with trisomy 21 had been established.

As I discuss in chapter 2, the identification of Down syndrome with chromosome 21 trisomy was nevertheless a landmark achievement in cytogenetics. It made it clear that an observation at the level of the chromosomes (more fine-grained observations of the genome were not yet possible) could be correlated directly with a medical condition. Within months, Turner syndrome (Ford et al. 1959) and Klinefelter syndrome (Jacobs and Strong 1959) were also associated with missing or extra chromosomes.

Crucially, further aneuploidies were quickly found in people who were *not* diagnosable with a shared clinical condition. These abnormal chromosome complements were therefore used to delineate new syndromes. First came "Super Female," or Trisomy X syndrome (Jacobs, Baikie, et al. 1959), in September 1959, closely followed by trisomy 18, or Edwards syndrome (Edwards et al. 1960), and trisomy 13, or Patau syndrome (Patau et al. 1960) in back-to-back papers in the *Lancet* in April 1960.[5] In other words, genomic designation began as soon as cytogenetics became capable of drawing distinctions between human genomes. More genomically designated syndromes would be delineated over the following few years, including ones fixed to chromosomal abnormalities much smaller than full aneuploidies. However, genomic designation had very little impact on clinical practice and social action during its first few decades—a history that I take up in the next chapter. For now, let's fast-forward to a recent, clear-cut case in order to clarify what makes genomic designation a distinct form of classification.

22q13 Deletion Syndrome

On the end of the long arm of the twenty-second chromosome, at locus q13.3, a deletion that includes the *SHANK3* gene can occur.[6] This 22q13.3 deletion has been observed in more than a thousand people worldwide, though its true incidence is thought to be at least one in twenty thousand. The resulting haploinsufficiency—or decreased protein production from the missing genes—is associated with a complex set of physical and psychological symptoms ranging from autistic behavior and delayed speech to fleshy hands and poorly formed ears (Manning et al. 2004; Phelan 2008).

Initial studies reported a deletion at 22q13 alongside features like developmental delay and hypotonia (see Gustavson et al. 1986; Hinkel et al. 1997; Phelan et al. 1992; Phelan, Rogers, and Stevenson 1988). By 1997, a paper that included David Ledbetter and Helen McDermid as coauthors was specifically discussing the "22q13.3 deletion syndrome" (Wong et al. 1997). In 2001, 22q13DS was delineated in a paper by Phelan et al. (2001). The 22q13 Deletion Syndrome Foundation was founded shortly thereafter.

For years prior to that 2001 paper, Mary C. Phelan (today known as Katy) had been conducting research on the 22q13 deletion and working with affected families. She published one of the first studies on the deletion, "A De Novo Terminal Deletion of 22q" (Phelan, Rogers, and Stevenson 1988), in a quarter-page report in the *American Journal of Human Genetics* that reported "physical features, [including] a central notch in the maxillary alveolar ridge, an abnormal palmer flexion crease on the left, four digital arches, minimal proximal cutaneous syndactyly of toes 2 and 3 bilaterally, and generalized hypotonia" (A118).

The Phelan-McDermid Syndrome Foundation notes that Phelan was a "telephone buddy" to the fifteen original families affected by

22q13DS diagnoses.[7] Then an ongoing series of semiannual 22q13 conferences began in 1998, when twenty of the twenty-three families with diagnosed children at that time met in Greenville, South Carolina, near the genetics lab where Phelan worked. In other words, by the time the syndrome was delineated in Phelan et al.'s 2001 paper, an active network of a couple dozen families was already in place. At the third conference, in 2002, the families founded the 22q13 Deletion Syndrome Foundation. The executive board met in 2003, agreeing to use the name Phelan-McDermid syndrome, or PMS, mainly because it made the syndrome easier to relate to outsiders.

The renamed Phelan-McDermid Syndrome Foundation (PMSF) now includes more than 1,400 diagnosed people and their families worldwide. It holds an annual conference that brings together hundreds of researchers and families; hosts support groups, scientific conferences, regional and international subgroups and parent forums; sells merchandise; and coordinates with relevant scientists and clinicians.[8] They are hiring staff and increasingly working to facilitate and redirect biomedical research on 22q13. In chapter 4, we will see how the foundation is thriving as never before now that 22q13DS is strongly associated with autism.

Meanwhile, PMSF advocates have made progress in their fight for PMS research and care. For example, a 2016 PMSF press release reported a "campaign [which] shows the power of parent advocacy." "Florida Gov. Rick Scott recently signed into law a bill whose inspiration was an online petition launched by the father of a child diagnosed with Phelan-McDermid Syndrome." They explain how the "bill requires the state to provide non-waitlisted Medicaid waiver services to individuals with Phelan-McDermid Syndrome, also known as 22q13 Deletion Syndrome. More than 100,000 Floridians signed the Change.org petition started by Greg Creese, father to Avery." PMSF President Susan Lomas weighed in on the achievement: "So many single acts snowball into collective action. . . . Working together is powerful." The same press release explained that "Lomas worked with their staffs as well as the Agency for Persons with Disabilities (APD), which manages Florida's Medicaid programs, to finalize the bill's PMS and 22q13 Deletion Syndrome language" (Shattles 2016). With the PMSF winning victories like these, the 22q13.3 microdeletion is becoming an ever-more-salient clinical finding.

In October 2016, the PMSF announced its intention to hire a professional executive director—a major milestone for a rare disease advocacy movement—summing up the moment as follows:

Since its founding 14 years ago, the Foundation has grown immensely in the number of families it serves and the worldwide connections it has made to raise awareness of PMS. We are eager to continue that growth and feel this is a critical time to move your Foundation forward. [Our new strategic plan] will aggressively move the PMS Foundation to the next level, with a focus on family support, advocacy, a higher-profile Web presence, worldwide engagement and expanded research initiatives. Once finalized, we'll share it with our families and community. "We feel these moves will help the Foundation to achieve new heights, ones we could not begin to imagine when 23 families met for the first time in Greenville, South Carolina in 1998," said Nick Assendelft, Vice President of the Board of Directors. "Today, we firmly believe the Foundation is in a strong, unique position to make even greater impacts on the everyday lives of our families."[9]

In less than fifteen years, the 22q13 group had blossomed from a handful of genetics experts and a small group of families into an increasingly professionalized, ambitious foundation. What it means to have a 22q13.3 microdeletion has been utterly transformed in the process.

Our understanding of the 22q13 deletion's phenotype has been transformed as well. The support group's characterization of PMS stands in stark contrast to the very limited phenotype reported by Phelan, Rogers, and Stevenson in 1988 (above). For example, the foundation's website gives the following account of PMS's behavioral phenotype:

There is not as much specific data on the behavioral aspects of individuals with deletion 22q13 as there is in other areas. Many of the behaviors listed below were brought up in parent sharing sessions. One parent would explain a particular behavior and many others would say they have observed it with their child too. Due to this, there is only one behavior with a known percentage showing what portion of the deletion population exhibit it.

Some behavioral characteristics:

· Chewing on nonfood items (clothing, bedding, toys)—70%
· Teeth grinding
· Tongue thrusting
· Hair pulling
· Aversion to clothes

Dr. Desmond Kelly compiled this list of attributes also, saying many children outgrow the behaviors.

Avoidance Strategies:

· Show anxiety in social situations
· Sometimes flap arms and hands/repetitive movements

- Scream when excited
- Self-stimulatory behavior, rocking
- Bite and/or hit themselves
- Sleep problems (many require fewer than normal hours of sleep, many don't sleep through the night)
- Enjoy TV, music, movies that are repetitive

Many children fall somewhere in the autism spectrum in terms of their behavior. There is debate as to whether these children are autistic and have a chromosome abnormality or if having deletion 22q13 negates an autistic diagnosis. "Autistic-like" traits that the deletion population may exhibit are poor eye contact, tactile sensitivity, and communications issues, as well as some listed above and others . . .

Finally, individuals with deletion 22q13 are able to express a wide range of emotions, including joy, happiness, and love.[10]

In addition, they report that all children with PMS have developmental delays, in varying degrees of severity, and almost all have absent or delayed speech.

Similar, though better-quantified, results are reported for physical characteristics. Most children suffer from hypotonia and display an increased tolerance to pain. Common visible features include "Thin, flaky toenails" (78%); "Large, fleshy hands" (68%); "Prominent, poorly formed ears" (65%); "Pointed chin" (62%); "Dolicocephaly (elongated head)" (57%); and "Ptosis (droopy eyelids)" (57%). Meanwhile, many have visible features like long eyelashes, "syndactyly (webbing) between 2nd and 3rd toes," fair skin, puffy eyelids, deep set eyes, "epicanthal folds (fold over inner corner of eye)," full cheeks, a wide nasal bridge, full eyebrows, and "minor anomalies of head, ears, hands, feet, and face." Finally, fewer than half, or an unknown percentage, suffer from seizures, strabismus (lazy eye), spinal anomalies, and difficulties with vision. With new projects of "deep phenotyping" underway, we can expect the 22q13.3 microdeletion's phenotype—that is, the characteristics of Phelan-McDermid syndrome—to become increasingly detailed over the coming years.

Thus, what it means to have a 22q13.3 microdeletion is determined by interaction and dialogue between biomedical experts on the one hand and subjects and parents, who are in many ways uniquely knowledgeable about the condition, on the other. In this way, genomically designated syndromes' phenotypic profiles can change considerably over time as new studies are undertaken and new cases are identified. When biomedical experts, patients, and their parents work together, often through organizations like PMSF, they can produce a wealth of new knowledge and care strategies. Other genomically designated syndromes have followed a similar trajectory, and several are actually far more developed in this regard.

In sum, the history of 22q13DS exemplifies the path that a growing number of genomically designated syndromes have taken en route to real salience: a genetic mutation was discovered and established in the literature, and *then* started to become the focus of dedicated clinical practice and social action. All of this takes place even as the core scientists note, as we saw in this chapter's epigraph, "the *lack of a recognizable phenotype.*"

What's in a Name?

To capture what is new and important about cases like 22q13DS, it is useful to consider the *meaning* of syndrome names. A syndrome is an association of features or symptoms that tend to afflict subjects simultaneously, or in some combination, where the clinical identification of certain symptoms can therefore point toward others. Indeed, it is precisely this variability in clinical syndromes that led so many to turn toward biomarkers, particularly genetic mutations, as a more objective and efficient basis for diagnosis (e.g., Collins et al. 2003). However, when biomarkers are identified and enrolled in screening programs, they often turn up in people who do not seem to have the associated disease. This may push frontline medical professionals to engage in "bridging work" to reconcile the marker, the people who have it, and the medical condition in question (Timmermans and Buchbinder 2012).

In genomic designation, however, the incongruence between genetic test results and existing categories of illness is resolved by simply delineating entirely new categories of illness at the level of the genome. The resulting phenotypic profiles are usually too nonspecific to even resemble the diagnostic criteria for a medical condition. Genetic mutations can therefore serve as the essential referent of terms like "*x* syndrome" rather than just a biological *explanation* for what those people are like. Hence a qualitatively new form of human classification comes into view that marries staggering phenotypic complexity and rigid genomic designation.

Phelan-McDermid syndrome, for example, refers precisely to the effects of deletions at q13.3 on the twenty-second chromosome that include the *SHANK3* gene, not a phenotypic profile. There is a "rigid designation" (Kripke 1980) binding the genetic mutation to the syndrome (see Navon 2011:216–19). In other words, genomic designation creates a logically necessary relationship between a disease name as "signifier" and the population of people with a genetic mutation, who are the "signified" (de Saussure 2011). Nevertheless, what it means to be diagnosed with a genomically designated condition is still subject to change and wide variability.

This juxtaposition of rigidity and fluidity raises two of this book's central questions: How does a condition develop or "loop" when it is rigidly fixed to a genetic mutation, yet simultaneously deeply uncertain and highly mobile when it comes to what that means for the people who are actually diagnosed with it? How does genomic designation therefore change what it means to be diagnosed with a medical condition at all?

Consider the contrast with Down syndrome. While the discovery of people with the Down syndrome phenotype but without chromosome 21 trisomy would create a nosological conundrum with an uncertain outcome,[11] discovering people with the paradigmatic characteristics of PMS but without a deletion at 22q13.3, would not be problematic in the slightest: they are not diagnosed with PMS or admitted into its community. Conversely, the (unlikely) discovery of a person with chromosome 21 trisomy but without the Down phenotype would probably not lead to a diagnosis of Down syndrome, while discovering a person with a 22q13.3 microdeletion and an atypical 22q13DS profile simply expands the phenotype of the mutation and therefore the clinical profile of the syndrome. In the case of 22q11.2DS, one of the most prevalent genomically designated conditions, parents lacking any of the main phenotypic characteristics have been diagnosed when they have tested positive for the microdeletion through follow-up testing; the profile of the syndrome thus changes accordingly to include "mild phenotypic presentations" (e.g., Bales et al. 2010). The scope for phenotypic variation in genomically designated conditions (particularly findings in "control" populations) remains an open question. Still, in chapter 7 we explore how subclinical traits are being reframed as symptoms, and carrier genes are being recast as mild genetic disorders.

The vast majority of medical conditions are associated with a phenotype—the outcome of interactions between genetic, epigenetic, metabolomic, environmental, social, developmental, and many other factors. Researchers may draw distinctions and make connections between phenotypes based on genetic mutations—a process that can sometimes lead to genomic designation. However, the conditions themselves usually remain intact as diagnostic categories. Even if there is a gene for a condition, like Rett syndrome, when someone meeting the clinical diagnostic criteria comes along, they may still be diagnosed even if they do not have the mutation in question. Hence most conditions are "genetically complex."

In genomic designation, by contrast, the condition or syndrome refers to the effects of a particular genetic mutation, whatever they are. The population is delineated strictly according to the mutation: you are diagnosed if and only if you are found to have the mutation in question. The mutation provides a clear and strict criterion for diagnosis, even if the phenotype associated with it is vague or variable. Finally, a genomically designated condition's clinical profile is determined by the post hoc observation of the phenotypes observed in people with the mutation. One could summarize the distinction like this:

- For a *clinical condition*: You have condition *Y* if and only if you have a particular phenotype: that is, you present with a set of symptoms or signs that matches, closely enough, some diagnostic criteria or developed clinical acumen. The genetic variants associated with the condition may be of great interest, but they do not constitute a basis for diagnosis.
- For a *genomically designated condition*: You have condition *X* if and only if you have a particular genetic mutation.[12] The phenotypic features observed in people with the condition may be of great interest, but they do not constitute a basis for diagnosis.

Consider table 1.1, which places PMS alongside previous syndromes that have been ascribed a genetic etiology.

Down syndrome, a condition that was first delineated in the 1860s, was associated with trisomy 21 almost a century later. Today, Down syndrome is considered to be nearly coextensive with trisomy 21. Autism was first reported much later, in 1943, and began to be associated with *multiple* genetic mutations in the 1970s. There are now hundreds of mutations and variants associated with autism spectrum disorders, with each accounting for a fraction of the autism population (see chapter 4). Still, despite their many differences, Down syndrome and autism came to be associated with genetic mutations via an intuitive sequence: a condition that is based on some set of observable features or impairments is later shown to have some sort of genetic etiology. A single genetic mutation might be found to be virtually coextensive with a syndrome and therefore ascribed causality, as with Down, or multiple mutations and variants may combine to create genetic complexity, as with autism. Either way though, the condition came first,

Table 1.1 Genotype-phenotype relations in five genetic conditions

Genetic mutation	Trisomy 21	Multiple	MTOR mutations (at 1p36)	16p11.2 microdeletion	22q13.3 microdeletion
Syndrome name	Down syndrome	Autism	Smith-Kingsmore syndrome	16p11.2 Deletion Syndrome	22q13 Deletion/ Phelan-McDermid syndrome
Year of first publication naming syndrome	1866 (Down)	1943 (Kanner)	2016 (Moosa et al.)	2007 (Ballif et al.)	1997 (Wong et al.; see also Phelan et al. 2001)
Year of first publication on mutation and its phenotype	1959 (Lejeune, Gautier, and Turpin)	1970s	2013 (Smith et al.; see also Lee et al. 2012)	1992 (Buiting et al.)	1986 (Gustavson et al.; see also Phelan, Rogers, and Stevenson 1988)
Relationship between mutation and syndrome's phenotype	Nearly coextensive; genetic explanation of an established syndrome	Complex; many mutations that confer various risk factors	Coextensive: diagnosis if and only if mutation is found; phenotype is delineated post factum	Coextensive; arguably found in "control" populations	Coextensive; syndrome's phenotype is delineated post factum
Clinical/social networks?	Yes	Yes	No	Minimal	Yes

and its genetic etiology came much later when mutations were found in people who had already been diagnosed.

Genomic designation reverses that process of discovery and association. Take Smith-Kingsmore syndrome. In 2013, a missense mutation in the *MTOR* gene at p36 on chromosome 1 was reported in a girl with seizures and megalencephaly, or an abnormally large brain (Smith et al. 2013). By 2016, "Smith-Kingsmore syndrome" was explicitly discussed in a paper, while dysmorphic facial features and developmental delay had been added to the phenotype (Moosa et al. 2016). By now, several other clinical associations have been added as well.[13] Only a handful of Smith-Kingsmore syndrome cases have been reported to date, but not because its symptoms are especially rare. A person is diagnosed with Smith-Kingsmore syndrome if and only if they have an *MTOR* mutation. That is what makes it a genomically designated condition.

However, Smith-Kingsmore syndrome has *not* yet formed the basis of any significant clinical programs or patient organizations. The same applies to hundreds of mutations that have been cast as novel genetic syndromes in the literature—conditions like "proximal 3q microdeletion syndrome," the 19p13.13 microdeletion syndrome (Dolan et al. 2010; Jorge et al. 2015), or the *PPM1D* syndrome (Jansen et al. 2017).

The 16p11.2 microdeletion represents a borderline case, in that it has given rise to limited levels of clinical research and social mobilization. It remains to be seen whether a 16p11.2DS foundation akin to the organizations dedicated to 22q11.2DS, 22q13DS, Fragile X, or other genomically designated conditions will ever be established.[14] Perhaps studies finding the 16p11.2 microdeletion in control populations make its consolidation as an independent clinical entity less likely (Weiss et al. 2008). However, when we return to the fascinating case of mildly affected 16p11.2 bearers in chapter 7 we will see that they are *not* seen as normal nor even as mere carriers. The 16p11.2 microdeletion seems to be at a crossroads in its social career. It would not be surprising to see it catapulted into clinical and social salience in the next few years. Mutations like the 16p11.2 microdeletion or *MTOR* missense mutation, and conditions like 16p11.2DS and Smith-Kingsmore syndrome, are reported all the time. They represent the great bulk of genomically designated conditions. Only time will tell how many of them will become bona fide objects of medical practice or social mobilization.

The 22q13 Deletion Syndrome is unique in table 1.1: As with the 16p11.2 microdeletion and *MTOR* missense mutation, it was first delineated in a paper a few years after the relevant mutation was reported. However, 22q13.3DS families and experts have built a powerful network of support and advocacy headlined by a registered foundation. I focus on these kinds of conditions throughout most of this book.

There are at least a couple of dozen such genomically designated conditions (see the 25 conditions listed in table 1.2). In each case, a mutation was used to delineate a radically new condition that, in turn, has become the focus of considerable social mobilization. Many of the networks of clinical practice and social action referenced and discussed below are far *more* developed than the ones dedicated to 22q13DS. The prevalence estimates for these conditions are as high as ~1 in 1,000 in the cases of 22q11.2DS (Dupont et al. 2015; see also Bales, Zaleski, and McPherson 2010), and 1 in 1,000 females and males respectively for the XXX and XYY syndromes. Furthermore, many genomically designated conditions' prevalence estimates exhibit clear upward trajectories as ascertainment expands beyond the most severely affected cases. They

Table 1.2 Genomically designated conditions with established advocacy organizations (as of late 2017)

Syndrome name/locus	Key/illustrative papers	Notable foundation or organization
1p36 Deletion Syndrome	D'Angelo et al. 2010; Gajecka, Mackay, and Shaffer 2007; Shapira et al. 1997	1p36 Deletion Support & Awareness
5p Deletion/Cri du Chat syndrome	Lejeune et al. 1963; Overhauser et al. 1994; Fang et al. 2008	5p– Society (https://fivepminus.org/)
9p–/Alfi's syndrome	Alfi et al. 1973; Hauge et al. 2008; Barbaro et al. 2009	Chromosome 9p– Network
distal trisomy 10q	Aglan, Kamel, and Helmy 2008; Davies, Jaffé, and Bush 1998; Yunis and Sanchez 1974	Distal Trisomy 10q Families
13q Deletion Syndrome	Allderdice et al. 1969; Brown, Chitayat, and Warburton 1995; Quelin et al. 2009	World Wide Chromosome Deletion 13q Support Network
15q Duplication Syndrome	Rineer, Finucane, and Simon 1998; Moeschler et al. 2002; Hogart et al. 2009	IsoDicentric 15 Exchange, Advocacy & Support (IDEAS)
Smith-Magenis/17p11.2 Deletion Syndrome	Smith et al. 1986; Potocki et al. 2003; Gropman, Duncan, and Smith 2006	Parents & Researchers Interested in Smith-Magenis Syndrome (PRISMS)
Potocki-Lupski/17p11.2 Duplication Syndrome	Brown et al. 1996; Potocki et al. 2000, 2007	Potocki-Lupski Syndrome Outreach Foundation, Inc.
17q21.31 Deletion/ Koolen-de Vries syndrome	Koolen et al. 2006, 2008; Grisart et al. 2009	Supporting Families with Koolen-de Vries Syndrome (https://supportingkdvs.org/)
Edwards syndrome/ trisomy 18	Edwards et al. 1960; Boghosiansell et al. 1994	Trisomy 18 Foundation
18p–/de Grouchy syndrome	de Grouchy, Bonnette, and Salmon 1966; Turleau 2008	Chromosome 18 Registry & Research Society
18q– syndrome/ leukodystrophy	Feenstra et al. 2007; Kline et al. 1993	http://ulf.org/18q-syndrome; C18 Registry & Research Society
ring chromosome 20 syndrome	Alpman et al. 2005; Elghezal et al. 2007; Herva, Saarinen, and Leikkonen 1977	Ring Chromosome 20 Foundation
22q11.2 Deletion Syndrome	Bassett et al. 2011; Driscoll et al. 1992; Hall 1993; Scambler et al. 1991	International 22q11.2 Deletion Syndrome Foundation (http://www.22q.org/)
Phelan-McDermid/ 22q13 Deletion Syndrome	Dhar et al. 2010; Phelan et al. 2001; Phelan, Rogers, and Stevenson 1988	Phelan-McDermid Syndrome Foundation (https://www.pmsf.org/)

Syndrome name/locus	Key/illustrative papers	Notable foundation or organization
MECP2 Duplication Syndrome	Kirk et al. 2009; Ramocki et al. 2009; Ramocki, Tavyev, and Peters 2010	http://www.mecp2duplication.com/
Fragile X syndrome	Hagerman et al. 1986; Lubs 1969; McLennan et al. 2011; Verkerk et al. 1991	National Fragile X Foundation; FRAXA Research Foundation
XXX	Jacobs, Baikie, et al. 1959; Johnston et al. 1961; Tartaglia et al. 2010	Association for X and Y Chromosome Variations (AXYS), formerly KS&A (https://genetic.org/)
XXYY	Ellis et al. 1961; Parker et al. 1970; Tartaglia et al. 2008	AXYS and the XXYY Project (https://genetic.org/variations/about-xxyy/)
XYY	Jacobs et al. 1965; Lancet 1966; Ross et al. 2012; Sandberg et al. 1961	Association for X and Y Chromosome Variations (AXYS) (https://genetic.org/)
Patau syndrome/ trisomy 13	Baty, Blackburn, and Carey 2005; Patau et al. 1960; Smith et al. 1960	Trisomy 13 Support & Resources
22q11.2 Duplication Syndrome	Ensenauer et al. 2003; Mukaddes and Herguner 2007; Portnoï 2009	International 22q11.2 Foundation
NGLY1	Need et al. 2012; Enns et al. 2014; Lam et al. 2017	NGLY1.org
ADCY5 mutation	Chen et al. 2012, 2014, 2015; Mencacci et al. 2015	ADCY5.org
ADNP syndrome	Gozes et al. 2015; Helsmoortel et al. 2014; Huynh et al. 2018	ADNP Kids Research Foundation (https://www.adnpkids.com/)

all combine an otherwise untenable lack of phenotypic specificity with rigid designation according to a genetic mutation, and all have become objects of clinical practice and some kind of formal social/advocacy organization. This list has grown considerably over just the past decade.

Multiple Pathways to Genomic Designation

With 22q13DS, it was almost as though a new kind of person emerged from nothing—or *de novo*, to borrow a term from genetics—upon the discovery of a newly observed genetic mutation. 22q13DS helped us see genomic designation in stark relief and to begin to grapple with some of its implications for the social studies of science and medicine.

But we cannot equate genomic designation with limit cases like 22q13DS. To do so would obscure the many other ways in which mutations can be used to carve out new categories of human difference. Many other conditions are useful to think about in terms of genomic designation, even though their relationships to clinical nosology are more complex than those of 22q13DS. To reiterate, genomic designation is about the delineation and diagnosis of conditions according to genetic mutations. To the extent that genetic mutations supplant older clinical diagnostic criteria and go on to radically *reconfigure* long-standing nosological categories, it is useful to think about them as cases of genomic designation as well. We therefore need to take stock of the multiple pathways to genomic designation.

The 22q11.2 Microdeletion and the Unification of Medical Conditions

The very names of the 22q13 and 22q11.2 Deletion Syndromes point toward an important commonality—both are tied to microdeletions on the long arm of the twenty-second chromosome. However, there are profound differences between 22q11.2DS and our initial case study of genomic designation, 22q13DS. For one thing, 22q11.2DS is far more variable, usually considerably less severe, and much more common than 22q13DS. For another, 22q11.2DS has a much more complex history as a medical category—a history to which we now turn.

22q13DS was never thought to have anything approaching a one-to-one relationship with an existing disorder. 22q11.2DS, by contrast, was not cut from whole cloth. Rather, the 22q11 deletion was initially posited as an etiology for DiGeorge syndrome and then several other rare clinical conditions. Over time, however, research on the 22q11.2 microdeletion led to a complex reconfiguration of biomedical subfields, nosology, and medical populations. The case of the 22q11.2 microdeletion therefore suggests that we should pay close attention to the multiple pathways leading to genomic designation.

Reading the biomedical literature, one is struck by the way 22q11.2DS is often treated as synonymous with two other diagnoses: DiGeorge syndrome and Velocardiofacial syndrome (VCFS, also known as Shprintzen syndrome). Other syndromes, like Opitz G/BBB syndrome, conotruncal anomaly face syndrome, and Sedlakova syndrome, similarly predate 22q11.2DS and are often considered to have been subsumed by it. As a set of clinical guidelines for 22q11.2DS published in the *Journal of Pediatrics* put it, "22q11.2 deletions have been identified in most patients with DiGeorge syndrome, velocardiofacial syndrome, and conotruncal anomaly face syndrome and in a subset with autosomal dominant Opitz G/BBB syndrome and Cayler cardiofacial syndrome. Although this list of associated disorders may appear quite perplexing, it is understandable because the diagnoses were originally described by clinicians concentrating on their particular areas of interest. After the widespread use of FISH, however, patients with a deletion became collectively referred to by their chromosomal etiology: the 22q11.2DS" (Bassett et al. 2011:2). Similarly, a review in *Newborn and Infant Nursing Reviews* (Miller 2008:e11) tells us that 22q11.2DS "encompasses" what "were once thought to be different conditions with different diagnoses." One could cite many similar passages. Indeed, since Wulfsberg et al.'s 1996 paper, "What's in a Name?" (Wulfsberg, Leana-Cox, and Neri 1996; see also Wulfsberg, Leana-Cox, and Neri 1997), the situation has often been likened to the parable of the blind men studying different parts of an elephant, sometimes even with a cartoon "22" elephant to illustrate the point (McDonald-McGinn, Zackai, and Low 1997:247; McDonald-McGinn 2018:2056).

What are we to make of this? Does 22q11.2DS "encompass" these older syndromes because the deletion simply helped biomedical experts to see a clinical syndrome that they were previously blind to? The situation is far more complex. First, the proportion of people who are diagnosable with the clinical syndromes listed above who also have a 22q11.2 microdeletion varies, but never approaches 100%. Unlike Down syndrome, this is anything but a straightforward case of a genetic etiology being discovered for an extant diagnostic category. Second, 22q11.2DS's clinical profile consists of more than two hundred phenotypes, many of which were not part of the profile of the clinical conditions with which the 22q11.2 deletion came to be associated. Finally, it is *not* necessary for a subject to be diagnosable with one of those longer-standing syndromes, or indeed with any clinically diagnosable condition, for them to be diagnosed with 22q11.2DS.

Even though 22q11.2DS has strong relationships with the older clinical disorders that it has mostly subsumed, it is actually far more clinically variable than 22q13DS. It brings together patients with serious heart malformations, cleft palate, intellectual disability, ear infections, schizophrenia, anxiety disorder, constipation, autism, and around two hundred other symptoms and traits, along with incidentally ascertained people with few serious symptoms or none. As Donna

McDonald-McGinn, one of the leading biomedical experts and advocates for 22q11.2DS, put it to me in an interview in Philadelphia (2011) when discussing its nosological status, "22q *is* 22q; . . . it's a spectrum from no symptoms to every malformation under the sun."

Consider this passage from a review in *Genetics in Medicine*, which follows a discussion of the multiple syndromes now associated with 22q11.2 deletions: "Although the deletion is identical in most patients studied, the phenotype varies greatly. Goodship et al. report a case of monozygotic twins with 22q11DS where one twin's phenotype is more severe, showing that genotype alone does not account for the presence or absence of various features of 22q11DS. More than 180 clinical findings have been associated with 22q11DS. . . . Both the number of organ systems involved and severity of involvement vary. Severe cases may result in neonatal death, whereas mildly affected individuals may remain undiagnosed, even as adults" (Bales et al. 2010:135). Observing a microdeletion at 22q11.2 is both necessary and sufficient for a diagnosis of 22q11.2DS,[15] even though the population of persons with the deletion varies greatly. What's more, patients with the paradigmatic phenotype of, say, DiGeorge syndrome do *not* necessarily have 22q11.2DS, while "patients" lacking any of the associated clinical symptoms *can* have 22q11.2DS. As caseloads increase, and existing patients age, 22q11.2DS's already expansive phenotypic profile is likely to grow larger still.

Saying 22q11.2DS "encompasses" or "explains" the older clinical diagnoses therefore obfuscates a deeper shift in the relation between genotype, phenotype, and medical classification. How then did 22q11.2DS emerge as a distinct condition in the biomedical literature?

To understand 22q11.2DS, we need to attend to the development of three closely related but analytically distinct kinds of biomedical phenomena: clinical disorders, genetic mutations, and genomically designated conditions. The current case starts with a number of fairly rare *clinical* disorders, primarily DiGeorge syndrome, VCFS, and Opitz G/BBB syndrome, with their own symptomatologies and independent origins as medical conditions. Then there is the genetic mutation that came to be associated with those clinical conditions: a missing stretch of DNA from site 11.2 on the long arm of the twenty-second chromosome. Rather than embrace the idea of a complex relationship between genetic mutations and medical classification, however, some people began to think of the 22q11.2 deletion as delineating a syndrome that did not line up with existing diagnostic categories. Eventually, a new category emerged that subsumed the above clinical conditions—what is now called 22q11.2 Deletion *Syndrome*. Instead of seeing just geneticization and the reduction of human difference, we therefore need to examine how research on the 22q11.2 microdeletion was productive of a new medical condition. By analyzing the nosological career of the 22q11.2 microdeletion, we see how genetic mutations can be mobilized to restructure fields of clinical research and then reconfigure medical classification. In other words, it points toward a more complex pathway to genomic designation. The 22q11.2 deletion was far more than just an etiological finding: it was the object around which a hybrid subfield of research formed and then carved out 22q11.2*DS* as a qualitatively new medical condition.

Now, it is true that the 22q11.2 microdeletion *began* its career as a case of what the social studies of science and medicine would probably call "geneticization"—Lippman's idea that categories of human difference would be "reduced to their DNA codes" (Lippman 1991a:19, 1991b). It first came to medical relevance in the early 1980s as a genetic explanation for the rare disorder, DiGeorge syndrome (de la Chapelle et al. 1981; Greenberg et al. 1984), which dates back to the clinical work of Antonio DiGeorge in the late 1960s (DiGeorge 1968). However, even though it may have been first mobilized in the 1980s as a reductive explanation for an existing clinical disorder, the 22q11.2 deletion did not behave itself in the years that followed. Instead, some people diagnosable with DiGeorge syndrome had a full twenty-second chromosome, even as the deletion began to crop up in *other*, previously unrelated conditions.

Most notably, beginning in the early 1990s, 22q11.2 deletions began to be observed in people with Velocardiofacial syndrome (VCFS)—another clinically delineated disorder with separate origins in the late 1970s (Shprintzen et al. 1978) and its own distinct literature. During this period fluorescence in situ hybridization (FISH) testing was refined and widely disseminated, making the detection of 22q11.2 deletions far more practicable (Larson and Butler 1995). A pair of 1992 papers, most notably one by Peter Scambler and his colleagues in the *Lancet* (1992; see also Driscoll et al. 1992) reported that the deletion at 22q11 was found in many cases of VCFS. Meanwhile, the same research program at Children's Hospital of Philadelphia identified a series of patients with 22q11 deletions whose symptoms, while related, were far too mild to have been considered for a DiGeorge or VCFS diagnosis (see Hogan 2016:166–67). An interview I conducted with Peter Scambler (2011), one of the medical geneticists who established the association between the 22q11 deletion and VCFS, confirmed that some degree of clinical overlap with DiGeorge syndrome informed the initial studies on 22q11 and VCFS. However, he also tested a number of other rare conditions for similar reasons, and, when 22q11 deletions were not observed, they remained unaffected by the new field of research. In short, it was 22q11 research that bridged the VCFS and DiGeorge syndrome communities.[16] In the years that followed, the subfields dedicated to these two syndromes were increasingly unified as research on the 22q11.2 microdeletion began to undermine the idea that they were distinct conditions at all.

Indeed, the discovery that 22q11 microdeletions caused most cases of VCFS had almost immediate nosological consequences. In 1993 an editorial by pediatrician Judith Hall introducing a special issue of the *Journal of Medical Genetics* on 22q11 recounted its initial association with DiGeorge syndrome before remarking, "To everyone's surprise and delight what had been thought to be a *very separate disorder*, the Shprintzen or Velocardiofacial syndrome, has been found also frequently to have a 22q11 deletion" (Hall 1993:801; my emphasis). She noted further associations with nonsyndromal conotruncal anomalies and advocated a shift toward the new, all-encompassing term, "CATCH 22," after which the editorial was named:

The acronym CATCH 22 . . . not only helps to remember the features of concern (Cardiac, Abnormal facies, Thymic hypoplasia, Cleft palate, and Hypocalcaemia) and the 22nd chromosome but also suggests the complexity which exists in 1993 with regard to defining the clinical features and understanding the genetic ramifications of a deletion from a specific area of a specific chromosome. What fun it is to find that *what were thought to be separate syndromes are now merging into one group, CATCH 22, while other patients who were thought to belong to those same previously separated syndromes are being excluded from that catchy acronymous group because they must have different mechanisms. . . . CATCH 22 is a wonderful model for what is to come over the next 10 years of human genome work.* (801–2; my emphasis)

In short, knowledge about a genetic mutation did not just change the way existing conditions were understood: it rapidly and radically reconfigured nosology and united all the people with the mutation, and only the people with that mutation, into a single disease category, while simultaneously excluding those with normal twenty-second chromosomes.

The name "CATCH 22," however, would be short-lived. A letter in response the following year (Lipson et al. 1994) noted that the range of outcomes was such that "the unifying feature appears to be the presence of a 22q microdeletion" (741), not some combination of the acronymous CATCH phenotypes (indeed, some 22q11.2DS patients have none of the five "CATCH" issues). Having a name that referenced symptomatology had already proven unfeasible for the 22q11 population. Meanwhile, patients, parents, and others objected to the derogatory implication of a "no-win" situation described in Joseph Heller's satirical novel about World War II airmen. As a result, the geneticist who first proposed the term *CATCH 22* eventually wrote an article (Burn 1999) named after Heller's less well-known sequel, *Closing Time*, in which he sought to remove the term from circulation.

In 1995, "22q11.2 Deletion *Syndrome*" first appeared in the literature (Lynch et al. 1995). Several of that paper's authors were involved in seminal work on 22q11.2 in the early 1990s and have since gone on to establish specialist centers and become leading figures in the International 22q11.2 Foundation. While it would be some time before "22q11.2 Deletion Syndrome" attained predominance, the old clinical fields were increasingly giving way to a unified, coherent field of research on a new genomically designated condition. People with other clinical diagnoses were eventually brought into the fold too, with conditions like Opitz G/BBB syndrome being integrated after the discovery that it too was strongly associated with the 22q11.2 deletion (Lacassie and Arriaza 1996; McDonald-McGinn et al. 1995; Robin et al. 1995).

In sum, several disconnected subfields of research on rare clinical conditions were brought together by findings about the 22q11 microdeletion. As that literature grew, and the deletion was observed in a growing variety of patients, a new kind of condition emerged: the genomically designated 22q11.2 Deletion Syndrome.

Increasingly, 22q11.2DS is supplanting its phenotypically delineated predecessors in the biomedical literature. Figure 1.1 shows the frequency of "DiGeorge syndrome" and "VCFS" (by far the most prominent such syndromes) and their synonyms alongside "22q11.2DS" in the titles of pertinent biomedical publications. Within a decade of its first appearance in the title of a biomedical paper in 1995, the name "22q11.2 Deletion Syndrome" had overtaken its two major predecessors. Ten years after that, it had gone on to dominate the field.

Attending an International 22q11.2 Foundation conference or visiting its website and the page devoted to their "Same Name Campaign,"[17] one is struck by the efforts to both explain and move beyond the old, lingering syndrome names. We return to this issue, and the social mobilization around 22q11.2DS more generally, in chapters 5 and 6. For

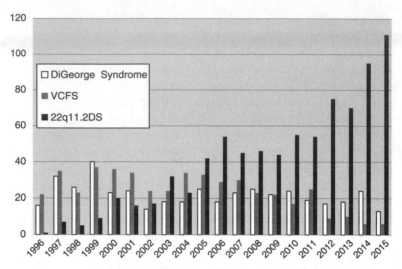

FIGURE 1.1. Every paper with "22q11.2DS," "DiGeorge syndrome," and "VCFS" (including synonyms) in their titles by year (1996–2015). (From Thompson Reuter's ISI Web of Science database; https://www.webofknowledge.com/)

now, the key point is this: although a dwindling minority remain committed to the VCFS label—a source of considerable acrimony between some advocates and experts—even they now consider it to be coextensive with the 22q11.2 microdeletion, its clinical origins notwithstanding (see the VCFS Educational Foundation; Shprintzen's 1998 paper, "The Name Game"). The relative ease with which the 22q11.2 microdeletion unified the field and led to a new "causal" diagnosis, even in the face of so much clinical variability, is suggestive of the privileged status often afforded to genetics.

In general, despite considerable and often heated debate about the *name* for the condition delineated by the 22q11.2 microdeletion (see, e.g., Wulfsberg et al. 1996), there was remarkably little debate about the move to delineate a syndrome on that basis. As Peter Scambler told me in an interview in London (2011), while some biomedical experts are careful to distinguish between VCFS, DiGeorge, and so forth as clinical diagnoses and 22q11.2DS as an overlapping genetic one, most now treat them as synonymous. My fieldwork confirmed that, at least for many in the field, the shift to a genomic diagnosis is taken to be self-evident. The continued disagreement about nomenclature therefore belies a consensus about the *nosological* significance of the 22q11.2 microdeletion.

Rethinking Genetics and Medical Classification

Taken together, the histories of our two "22q" syndromes help us rethink the way genetics can reconfigure medical research and classification. Research on the 22q11.2 microdeletion unified several small clinical subfields and went on to bring a host of new fields and stakeholders into the fold as well. The mutation is the epistemic thread that ties those fields together. The 22q11.2 microdeletion served as the "actant," or nonhuman actor (Latour 1988; Law 1992) that allowed researchers to see a new, hybrid subfield, uncover a population of patients that was invisible to clinical research, and eventually delineate a novel medical condition. At the same time, this actant also performs an exclusionary sort of "boundary work."[18] Patients who had been diagnosed with the pertinent clinical syndromes, but did not carry the 22q11.2 microdeletion, were now excluded. From the perspective of the post-22q nosology, they had been misdiagnosed.

We are challenged by 22q11.2DS to extend the concept of genomic designation to include cases where extant conditions are transformed in order to ensure that they correspond to specific genetic mutations. Although the 22q11.2 microdeletion entered the biomedical literature in what we might call an attempt to "geneticize" DiGeorge syndrome, its ultimate nosological impact was something else entirely. Nor did the 22q11.2 deletion simply help researchers and clinicians tinker with the diagnostic boundaries of DiGeorge syndrome or help to "rule in or rule out" borderline cases (Miller et al. 2005). Rather, as with the 22q13 deletion and PMS, knowledge about the 22q11.2 microdeletion served to create a qualitatively new biomedical subfield, carve out a novel population of people, and then delineate a new kind of medical condition.

So, the path of declaring a new syndrome cut from whole cloth is just one of the "ideal typical" ways in which genetics can remake nosology in its image. But what are the others? Following Weber (2011), I use the term *ideal type* to indicate that these pathways are intended as useful abstractions to guide sociological analysis, rather than distinct phenomena that are found in reality. Any given case of genomic designation will likely instantiate *several* of these ideal types in different ways and to varying degrees. Nevertheless, they represent the conceptual toolkit for a thorough understanding of the way genetics intersects with and realigns existing systems of human classification.

Here then, is our fivefold typology of ideal typical paths to genomic designation:

First, we have our old friend *geneticization*—the much-discussed but exceedingly rare finding of a near one-to-one match between a mutation and a medical condition with established clinical diagnostic criteria (e.g., Down syndrome).[19] We do not really need the concept of genomic designation to grasp this sort of genotype-phenotype correlation. Still, the "near" is crucial here: in almost every instance, the mutation in question fails to perfectly correspond to the clinical diagnostic criteria that predate its discovery. To the extent that the mutation is given primacy in the diagnosis and delineation of the condition, we have a weak case of genomic designation. Hence there is no clear-cut line between geneticization and our second ideal typical path.

Second, we have a kind of genomically designated *recalibration*. This is akin to geneticization, except that the process of affixing the condition to a mutation causes its population and clinical profile to undergo a considerable transformation. In some ways, many cases of "geneticization" in the literature more closely match this model of genomically designated recalibration. As Miller et al. (2005) have shown, changing a condition to fit a mutation is one nosological solution among several when the mutation, or "gene for," turns out to be a less than perfect fit with the clinical disease it is supposed to explain.[20] This kind of recalibration can depart quite radically from the "reduction" represented by geneticization. When a genetic mutation becomes both necessary and sufficient for diagnosis of a condition, we are often left with a *very* different population than the one picked out by clinical nosology. The name of the old clinical diagnosis may endure, even when genomic designation has rendered it a very different condition.

Take the case of Williams syndrome, to which we return in greater detail in chapters 3 and 4. When it was first delineated in the 1960s, Williams syndrome was associated with a very distinctive phenotypic profile—"elfin" facial features, developmental delay, and heart defects, alongside strikingly strong relative verbal, social, and musical abilities. However, when Williams syndrome was affixed to a 7q11.23 microdeletion in the mid-1990s, some who matched the clinical criteria were excluded and others were brought into the fold. After the landmark study that identified a deletion at 7q11.23 in around 90% of Williams syndrome cases (Nickerson et al. 1995), a follow-up paper found the deletion in 96% of 114 "classic" cases but only 8% of 39 "uncertain" cases and 60% of the 42 cases where clinical information was not available (Lowery et al. 1995). In sum, a small minority of "classic" Williams syndrome patients did *not* have the mutation, and neither did a large proportion of "uncertain WS patients."

Nevertheless, the 7q11.23 microdeletion served to genomically designate Williams syndrome, redrawing its population in the process. As the Williams Syndrome Association itself puts it, "It is important to stress that WS is a genetic diagnosis and an individual who does not have the gene deletion does not have Williams syndrome (i.e., a person who was clinically diagnosed with WS but was later found not [to] have a deletion in fact, does NOT have WS)."[21] So even while Williams syndrome is considered to have one of the most consistent and distinctive phenotypes among the disorders discussed in this book, tying it to a genetic mutation still required nosological boundary work in both directions: not only were some clinically diagnosed cases excluded, as seen above, but atypical cases in which a clinical diagnosis could not be made have been diagnosed when they tested positive for a 7q11.23 deletion (see Borg, Delhanty, and Baraitser 1995, esp. 694–95, for an early attempt to use genetic testing to adjudicate clinically ambiguous cases). In short, genomic designation can transform even the most phenotypically distinctive of disorders.

Third, conditions can undergo a process of *unification* or *lumping*. This is not just a question of creating blanket categories comprising related entities, but of actually collapsing multiple disease categories into one. This is in many respects the most radical and counterintuitive reconfiguration of nosology in this list, which is why I paid special attention to the case of DiGeorge syndrome, VCFS, and others, and how they gave way to the new genomically designated condition, 22q11.2DS.

Fourth, conditions can be *split* or *fragmented* according to genetic subtypes. This is well understood when it comes to cancers, and especially the role of mutations in the *BRCA* genes (e.g., Venkitaraman 2002; see Bourret, Keating, and Cambrosio 2011), but less well understood when it comes to broader surveillance categories like intellectual disability and autism. As we will see, when people with X-linked intellectual disability are found to have a duplicated *MECP2* gene or a sufficiently long trinucleotide CGG repeat in the *FMR1* gene at Xq27.3, new conditions known as *MECP2* Duplication Syndrome and Fragile X syndrome are diagnosed. Each comes complete with its own clinical profile and biosocial network (see table 1.2). Similarly, chapter 4 shows how Fragile X and many other genomically designated conditions are often thought of and mobilized as genetically specific subtypes of autism.

Finally, we have the clear-cut cases of genomic designation like Phelan-McDermid syndrome, XXX syndrome, 5p– syndrome and many others, where new conditions are delineated "de novo." The mutations in question were never thought to line up with established disorders. Instead, they were used to delineate totally new conditions whose features can only be determined by observing people known to have the relevant mutations.

Again, these ideal typical pathways are not mutually exclusive. From the perspective of autism or intellectual disability, Williams syndrome, 22q11.2DS, and Phelan-McDermid syndrome all represent cases of splitting, even though I explained how their nosological histories are perhaps most usefully framed according to the second, third, and fifth types discussed above. Nor are they ever perfectly instantiated: even Down syndrome has undergone a degree of recalibration as testing for trisomy 21 is used to arbitrate clinically questionable cases; meanwhile, one could plausibly argue that knowledge about the 22q11.2 microdeletion has also radically recalibrated the diagnoses of DiGeorge syndrome and VCFS for those who still use those terms. In short, this conceptual toolkit is precisely that: a set of tools for making sense of genomic designation, not a hard-and-fast schema for parsing the impact of genetics on the often messy reality of human classification.

Conclusion

Conditions like PMS and 22q11.2DS compel us to go beyond our existing social scientific toolkit and grapple with the oftentimes radical impact of genetics on nosology. This chapter uncovered and defined genomic designation, and then outlined the multiple ways genetic mutations can be mobilized to reconfigure medical classification.

But this just scratches the surface of genomic designation as a sociological phenomenon. After all, thousands of mutations have been reported in the human genetics literature over the last sixty years, and perhaps a few hundred have been cast in that literature as novel syndromes. Yet, it is only in the last couple of decades that genomically designated conditions have started to gain real clinical or social traction.

How then are these paths from the discovery of genetic mutations to novel "syndromes" in the literature, and then on to real medical and biosocial categories actually taken? Just because 22q11.2DS exists in biomedical journals does not mean that it automatically becomes an object of clinical practice, never mind a new kind of person. To put it more bluntly, so what if some geneticists talk about new syndromes in their journals if no one does the painstaking work necessary to imbue them with clinical and social salience?

Consider again for a moment Phelan-McDermid (i.e., 22q13 Deletion) syndrome. In 1993 Phelan reported another chromosomal deletion—2q37 (Phelan, Rogers, and Byrd 1993; see also Phelan et al. 1995)—that has only recently been subject to genomic designation (see Galasso et al. 2008) and has yet to achieve anything approaching the medical and social significance of 22q13. But why? During my interview with Phelan in New York in 2011, I asked her about the divergent outcomes of the 22q13 and 2q37 microdeletions. She paused, and said that it had very little to do with the physiological implications of the mutations. Instead, she felt it had far more to do with the fact that the parents of the first few 2q37 kids were satisfied with their existing clinical diagnoses. By contrast, the 22q13 parents began to communicate and organize.

Whether a mutation comes to truly matter depends on the work done, or not done, to mobilize it as a new kind of person. The simple fact that genomic designation is alive and well in the genetics literature raises a series of more sociologically complex questions that I tackle throughout the rest of this book: How do some mutations gain traction, while others languish at the level of squarely esoteric research? How are productive points of interface and exchange established between genomically designated conditions and categories based on other forms of classification? How do they reshape treatment and care, or realign our basic understanding of human illness and difference? Finally, what can the uneven history of genomic designation teach us about the broader intersection of bioscience, medicine, and society? To begin to answer these questions, let's turn to the early history of genomic designation.

TWO

Immobile Mutations: Nowhere to Go in the 1960s and 1970s (and the Exception That Proves the Rule)

During 1968 a special branch of the science of genetics was drawn from the quietude of laboratories and professional journals and exposed to the glare of courtrooms and newspaper headlines.
SALEEM ALAM SHAH, *REPORT ON THE XYY CHROMOSOMAL ABNORMALITY*

Almost as soon as it became possible to see, count, and label chromosomes in the late 1950s, human geneticists began to find people with chromosome abnormalities and delineate syndromes on their basis. However, save for one striking exception, genomic designation did not have much of an impact beyond genetics labs and biomedical journals during its first few decades. Genetic mutations were not yet very powerful facts. Even as we developed the technological capacity to observe more and more mutations, little changed for the people who had them. The meaning of those mutations depended on the networks of expertise and social mobilization formed, or not, around them. This chapter charts that early history, delves especially into the case of XYY or "Super Male" syndrome as the exception that proves the rule, and sets up a diachronic comparison with genomic designation today.

The First Cases of Genomic Designation

Once the number of chromosomes in a normal human was established, it did not take long for geneticists to discover people with abnormal chromosome complements. After some debate throughout the 1950s, as early cytogeneticists strained to observe, tally, and distinguish chromosomes under the microscope, it was in 1956 that a definitive study, "The Chromosome Number of Man" (Tjio and Levan 1956), established the number as forty-six. By 1960, a meeting in Denver had established an international system for numbering the twenty-two autosome pairs and identifying each sex chromosome (Lejeune et al. 1960). This required the standardization of the multiple numbering systems in use at that time (see Lejeune et al. 1960:1064). This was no easy task—the participants were apparently only able to reconcile the six competing nomenclatures after a Chinese system of classification was proposed (Harper 2006:142–46; see also Lindee 2008). From Denver on, human geneticists would be able to refer to chromosomes and aneuploidies (whole chromosome deletions or duplications) according to a single, standardized system.

The 1959 discovery that Mongolian Idiocy or mongolism, now known as Down syndrome, is strongly associated with chromosome 21 trisomy was a seminal moment in the nascent field of medical genetics.[1] As a review of "Chromosomal Aberrations in Man" in the *Journal of Pediatrics* in 1961 put it, "For the pediatrician, the association of an extra chromosome with most cases of Mongolism has been one of the most dramatic medical discoveries in recent years" (Rappoport and Kaplan 1961:428). T. C. Hsu, an important researcher in the field, even wrote (1979:39): "If it were not for Jérôme Lejeune's discovery of a trisomic condition associated with mongolism, human cytogenetics would probably have died soon after the correct diploid number was determined, and the chromosomes characterized. Lejeune's report created a new field of medicine—medical cytogenetics." To be clear, this is something of an exaggeration. Lejeune was far from the only one pursuing research on the cytogenetics of disease, or even Mongolian Idiocy itself. Other teams actually reported more systematic results on trisomy 21 later that same year (Harper 2006; Jacobs, Court Brown, et al. 1959). In fact, the idea that mongolism was likely due to a chromosome abnormality was floated in the literature at least as early as 1932 (Waardenburg, cited in Hsu 1979). More broadly, as Aryn Martin points out (2004:933–34), the very research that led to Tjio and Levan's seminal count of forty-six chromosomes in the normal human genome was animated by the hope that *ab*normal counts could explain conditions like Mongolian Idiocy and especially cancer. Still, the association between Mongolian Idiocy and trisomy 21 gave human cytogenetics unprecedented traction in medical research and diagnosis.

Even with this very first gene for (or "aneuploidy for") a major condition, human geneticists were attuned to the idea that a mutation might reshape medical classification. Josef Warkany summarized a 1959 National Association for Retarded Citizens conference on the etiology of mongolism for the *Journal of Pediatrics*: "Only a few months had passed since the first publication reporting the existence of an extra chromosome in Mongols. It is clear that this required a reorientation of medical thinking" (1960:417). He discussed the potential "diagnostic value of chromosome studies" for adjudicating clinically contested cases (415). His hope was that with "an exact cytologic diagnosis [rather than] the evaluation of a constellation of physical traits, . . . perhaps the nosologic concept of Mongolism will be extended to include forms of mental retardation heretofore eluding classification." In short, genetics might "solve the old problem of the 'formes frustes' of the disease" (417). Ultimately, genetic testing would mostly be used to adjudicate ambiguous Down syndrome cases,[2] but this is only because of the unusually close alignment of mutation and clinical syndrome. Subsequent findings would indeed require considerable "nosologic" innovation.

The Mongolian Idiocy finding also helped to direct the attention of human geneticists as their field began the transition to what we now call medical genetics. Hsu notes (1979:41) how the trisomy 21 finding "hit the scientific community like a storm" and led others to pursue similar research on people with congenital disorders, especially those characterized by multiple anomalies, developmental delay, and unusual craniofacial features. In other words, "'funny looking' kids became the prime targets of inquiry" (41). We will see below that they are still major objects of medical genetics research today.

Almost as soon as Mongolian Idiocy was associated with chromosome 21 trisomy in 1959, researchers started reporting people with other aneuploidies. Ford et al.'s identification of a missing sex chromosome, or "monosomy X," in cases of Turner syndrome (Ford et al. 1959) and Jacobs et al.'s identification of an XXY sex chromosome composition in Klinefelter syndrome came later that same year (Jacobs and Strong 1959).[3] The search was on for people with novel chromosome abnormalities.

Genomic designation can be traced all the way back to this heady moment in human genetics. As we saw at the very beginning of this book, researchers quickly began to discover chromosomal abnormalities that did *not* line up with extant medical categories. First came Jacobs, Baikie, et al.'s (1959) identification of a "super female" with three X chromosomes. Then, just months later in early 1960, the *Lancet* published back-to-back reports on cases of 18 trisomy by Edwards et al. (1960) and 13 trisomy by Patau et al. (1960; see also Smith et al. 1960). Triple X syndrome, Edwards syndrome, and Patau syndrome had suddenly come into view as newly recognized disorders that could only be diagnosed in the presence of the associated trisomy. They were the very first genomically designated conditions.

This was immediately recognized as an important opportunity for genetics to contribute to the world of medicine. There was some uncertainty as to how many such conditions would be discovered in living people: it was correctly hypothesized that many chromosomal aneuploidies would be incompatible with life (e.g., Patau et al. 1960:792), and the examination of spontaneously aborted fetuses soon became an important site for medical cytogenetics. A lead article in the *Lancet* nevertheless concluded, "Every one of the twelve chromosome pairs of that old friend of the materia medica, *Datura stramomium* [a common weed], can exist in trisomic form, and every one has its characteristic phenotype, or, as one calls it in medicine, its characteristic clinical syndrome. *Perhaps we will soon recognize equally characteristic syndromes for each of our own twenty-two autosome pairs*" ("Mongol Chromosome" 1960:1069; my emphasis). By 1961 Lejeune and Turpin would write in a review of "Chromosomal Aberrations in Man" that, in the twenty-two months since they published their "discovery of the mongolian Trisomy," "the number of observations obtained in many laboratories is so vast that at least 23 different aberrations have been collected, . . . [a] rate of about a syndrome a month" (Lejeune and Turpin 1961:175). Crucially, they observe that "the other trisomics actually described concern clinical entities less well defined than mongolism, for the very reason that in these, *individualization has resulted from the chromosomal findings*" (176; my emphasis). Clearly then, genomic designation was visible at the very outset of endeavors to link human difference to genetic mutations.

But genomic designation would not remain confined to whole chromosome changes for very long. As cytogenetic techniques improved, meetings in London (1963), Chicago (1966), and Paris (1971 and 1975) would establish conventions for banding chromosomes.[4] This allowed for smaller mutations to be observed, labeled, circulated, and compared in and between labs around the world (Shaffer 2009). Beginning in 1963, a series of reports by de Grouchy et al. focused on deletions on the short arm of the eighteenth chromosome, or 18p (de Grouchy et al. 1963; de Grouchy, Rossier, and Joab 1967). Meanwhile, a team led by Lejeune discovered several probands with a deletion at 5p (Lejeune et al. 1963). In 1967, de Grouchy and colleagues claimed that "the deletion on the short arm of chromosome 18 is the first autosomal deletion described in humans" (221; my translation). It would not be long before these mutations began to be treated as syndromes in the medical genetics literature: 5p deletion, Lejeune's or Cri du Chat syndrome (Dumars, Gaskill, and Kitzmiller 1964) and de Grouchy, 18p– or 18p Deletion Syndrome (de Grouchy 1963, 1967) respectively. Lejeune and de Grouchy were pursuing the logic inherent in the *Lancet* editorial quoted above: if we have the technical capacity to identify genetic mutations, then we should seek to delineate new diseases on their basis. This trajectory would allow for a proliferation of new genomically designated syndromes with every advance in genetic testing technology (Ledbetter 2008).

For as much as human genetics has been revolutionized in the decades since chromosomal abnormalities like 18 trisomy and 5p– were first observed under the microscope, the mutations themselves have been maintained as consistent objects of knowledge. They have been one of the few constants amid the myriad technical and conceptual changes it took to go from gazing at our genome's few dozen chromosomes to annotating its three billion DNA base pairs. Today, these early studies of chromosomal mutations and the new syndromes they unearthed are widely considered to represent the opening salvo of modern clinical genetics. It is no coincidence that genomic designation was there at the outset.

Stalled at Vademecum Science

In 1966, Victor McKusick—widely regarded as the "founding father" of medical genetics—began publishing his authoritative catalogs of genetic conditions, *Mendelian Inheritance in Man*. Those catalogs grew precipitously over the years (see the twelfth and final edition: McKusick 1998) as more and more mutations and disorders were reported. Nowadays, the catalog lives on as the *Online Mendelian Inheritance in Man* or *OMIM* database—perhaps the world's leading resource for information about genes, mutations, and genetic disorders. Already by 1966, McKusick was forcefully advocating the turn to genomic designation: "In medical genetics there is little place for expressions such as 'spectrum of disease,' 'disease A is a mild form, or a variant, of disease B,' and so on. They are either the same disease, if they are based on the same mutation, or they are *different* diseases. Phenotypic overlap is not necessarily any basis for considering them fundamentally the same or closely related" (McKusick 1966:x). Meanwhile, new studies, review pieces in major journals, and a host of textbooks and atlases of chromosomal mutations and associated genetic disorders were published throughout the 1960s and 1970s (e.g., Borgaonkar 1975; Court Brown et al. 1964; de Grouchy and Turleau 1977; Hamerton 1963, 1971; Lamy and de Grouchy 1967; Turpin and Lejeune 1969; Yunis 1977).

In these texts, we see how genomic designation was going beyond the esoteric sciences of specialist journals and entering the sphere of what Fleck called "*Vademecum* science" (1981:118–20): the solidification of the provisional knowledge produced by a "vanguard" of researchers (124), into the impersonal, certain knowledge of the textbook, atlas, and expert review. Genomic designation was employed in hundreds of journal articles during the 1960s and 1970s, ranging from case studies to systematic reviews. Over time, those findings were integrated into vademecum texts via what Fleck called (119) "the migration of ideas throughout the collective."[5] This process submits the tentative claims of journal science to the collective scrutiny of the field and creates the sort of certain, objective knowledge that is suitable for broader consumption. Without question, a plethora of genomically designated conditions had reached this level of collective significance by the late 1960s.

For geneticists then, carving out new disease entities on the basis of mutations came quite quickly and unproblematically. Being able to *see* an extra or a missing chromosome under the microscope required years of sociotechnical groundwork and made for a major finding. Delineating a new "syndrome" on the basis of a mutation, by contrast, was unproblematic for human geneticists. We see this very clearly in McKusick's strident declaration quoted above, not to mention the plethora of articles and textbooks on these new, mutation-specific disorders.

However, the syndromes they discovered were not taken up beyond the field of human genetics. They failed to gain traction as objects of clinical research and practice, never mind sustained social mobilization. As Ilana Löwy put it (2014), "In the early 1960s, studies of chromosomes was [sic] seen by some of the actors mainly as an academic topic." She quotes a 1962 letter from Klaus Patau responding to a request from a colleague who had "advised a mother of a mongoloid boy to ask Patau to perform a 'chromosome test.'" In the letter, Patau explained that his and other laboratories were focused on "fundamental research" rather than medicine per se: "I believe, the present lack of a service institution for chromosome analyses is not too much of a deficiency, as the cases in which there is any kind of practical need for a chromosome analysis are usually also of some research interest" (156). For the most part, finding abnormal chromosome complements was only really useful for genetics researchers. It did not yet have much to offer physicians, families, or patients.

Indeed, one finds no records of advocacy organizations, specialist clinics, or even clinical guidelines for genomically designated conditions. Very few people were actually being diagnosed. In a way, this is hardly surprising: Triple X syndrome tends to be mild phenotypically,[6] while Edwards syndrome is so severe that it almost always leads to in utero or infant death. Meanwhile, 18p Deletion and 5p– syndromes are extremely rare. And yet, we will see that all of these genomically designated conditions have become objects of sustained patient advocacy and clinical practice in recent years. Why did precisely the same disorders—defined, after all, according to the same genetic mutations—fail to gain traction in the early 1960s when they represented groundbreaking scientific discoveries, only to do so decades later? There was certainly no lack of scientific interest: finding after finding appeared in venues like the *Lancet*, *Science*, *Nature*, and the *New England Journal of Medicine*, not to mention all the leading genetics journals. Nevertheless, none of these important new biomedical conditions grew into robust clinical or biosocial categories during this period.

Historian Susan Lindee (2005: esp. 92–119) has outlined the early successes and the sociotechnical work done to make medical cytogenetics possible, particularly with the standardization of chromosomal terminology. Hers is just about the only work in the human sciences to notice what I am calling genomic designation. Before going on to cite the Lejeune et al. (1961) article discussed above, Lindee notes (but does not develop) that reports of chromosomal aberrations in these years "included links between chromosomal aberrations and some poorly defined clinical entities that the chromosomal condition basically defined: the chromosomal difference permitted some conditions to be extracted from the *undifferentiated mass of things causing mental retardation*" (Lindee 2005:103; my emphasis).

It is hardly surprising that Lindee does not pursue this observation. In the period she studied, no one other than medical geneticists found this differentiation to be very practicable. There simply was not much to be done with genomically designated difference. Most of the ascertained cases were institutionalized with mental retardation, and in those settings a chromosomal abnormality mattered little to the patient, caregiver, or the usually absent families. Asylums and institutions for people with developmental delays may have once pioneered modern heritability research (Porter 2018), but in the post–World War II period they wanted little to do with the field of genetics. Geneticists eagerly took to institutions for the mentally retarded and the like in search of mutations. However, we will see how it is only very recently that institutions for people with developmental disorders began to take an interest in geneticists' findings and adopt genomically designated syndromes as objects of practice.

Some researchers did see great public health potential in this new wave of findings. In 1964, for example, London's *Eugenics Review* reprinted the annual Galton lecture entitled "Some Mechanisms of Chromosome Variations and Their Relation to Human Malformations." The lecture dealt almost exclusively with the first years of medical cytogenetics—trisomy 21, Cri du Chat, and so on, as well as a series of translocations with unclear pathological implications. The author, Jan A. Böök, explained the significance of these developments as follows (1964:151; my emphasis):

In medical genetics we are concerned with genetical material that can be transmitted from parents to children and cause individual deviations of development, differentiation and function of such a significance that conventionally we would call them diseases or defects. This common denominator in basic etiology, very broadly speaking, exerts its important influence on the *individual as well as on the population*. Phrased differently, the two foci of interest and concern are the patient with his personal medical problem and the population with its epidemiological problems presented as a broad spectrum of genetical diseases or defects.

In passages like this we see how genomic designation might have become an important object of early twentieth-century eugenics research and policy if karyotyping had been developed a few decades earlier. However, medical genetics did not become an important tool of post–

World War II biopower, despite Böök's emphasis on the "two foci" of medical genetics—individual and population health (Foucault 1990b, 2003). Indeed, the very association with eugenics made such a broad deployment of medical genetics unpalatable (Ramsden 2009).[7]

Even though they could be reliably observed and described, genetic mutations did not find the "surfaces of emergence" (Foucault 2002) or a social-institutional circuitry in which they mattered all that much. No matter how much they captivated the field of esoteric human genetics, chromosomal anomalies could not truly speak to or "translate" the interests of clinicians, teachers, patients, and their families. Genomic designation gave rise to numerous "syndromes" in the human genetics literature, but it was not well-suited to the broader social and institutional currents of the time. Rates of diagnosis were low, and there was just very little scope for mobilizing genetic mutations to inform treatment, self-understanding, or social mobilization.

XYY Syndrome

There was one very notable exception to genomic designation's social and clinical impotence: males who have an extra Y chromosome, or XYY syndrome. I argue that XYY is, in fact, the exception that proves the rule.

When I quoted Hsu (1979) on the central role of "funny looking kids" in early cytogenetic research, I omitted the rest of the sentence and the two immediately following: "but inmates of mental institutions and criminal institutions also contributed heavily to our knowledge of human cytogenetics. Because of their association with abnormalities with sex chromatin, several kinds of congenital maladies received early attention. As a result, the relationships between the abnormalities in sex chromatin and sex chromosomes were clarified" (41). Children with congenital disorders proved the most fecund terrain for early cytogeneticists, but already we saw how people with sex disorders like Turner and Klinefelter syndromes were a close second. Yet the transition between Hsu's first and second sentences is almost cryptic. The reason is likely that, as he was writing his review in the late 1970s, cytogenetics was in the midst of a major controversy that grew out of precisely this pairing of research subjects drawn from prisons and psychiatric institutions with the analysis of sex chromosome abnormalities. Tracing the history of that controversy and the way XYY became perhaps the most famous, and certainly the most infamous, of the new chromosomal abnormalities helps us grasp the limited scope for genomic designation outside of human genetics in the 1960s and 1970s.

XYY had innocuous beginnings in the field. Shortly after the association of sex chromosome aneuploidies with Turner and Klinefelter syndromes, Jacobs, Baikie, et al. (1959) reported cases of women with an extra X chromosome and delineated a new "Super Female," or XXX syndrome. Only two years later, the equivalent extra Y chromosome syndrome was reported by Sandberg et al. in a *Lancet* letter to the editor (1961). Simply titled "An XYY Human Male," Sandberg et al.'s letter described (489) a "forty-four-year-old white man of average intelligence and without physical defects, despite the 47 chromosomes found in his marrow and blood, started work at seventeen after two years of high school." The XYY subject "claim[ed] to have a normal libido, and results of examination were unremarkable." In other words, he was not sexually abnormal despite the extra Y chromosome.[8] They continued, "He has somewhat large facial features, is obese and weighs 287 lb., and has a neurodermatitis, an umbilical hernia, and, in the left mandible, has had a cystic lesion for many years. The buccal-mucosa cells were chromatin-negative." Finally, the authors discussed the appearance of the extra chromosome, arguing that it looked more like the Y chromosome than the similar-looking 21 and 22 autosomes, while also pointing to the "absences of the severe mental and physical stigmata" associated with autosomal trisomies. "This case," they concluded, "may therefore be considered as an XYY male" (489). Other reports of XYY males with a variety of abnormalities appeared in leading journals over the next few years (e.g., Hauschka et al. 1962; Ricci and Malacarne 1964; Sandberg et al. 1963), but the clinical findings were scattered, and only a handful of cases were identified in total.

The "Criminal Chromosome"

XYY started to gain significant scientific and popular attention when a leading human geneticist, Patricia Jacobs, published a paper in *Nature* reporting a remarkably high prevalence of XYY males in Scottish prison and asylum populations in 1965 (Jacobs et al. 1965). The study was the result of a hunch (interview with Patricia Jacobs, in Harper 2006). Previous studies had found that around 1% of males in institutions for the "mentally sub-normal" were chromatin-positive, indicating the presence of an extra X chromosome. However, a study of *criminal* and difficult-to-manage men of low intelligence in Sweden had found a rate of 2%, while an unpublished study in England communicated to the authors had found a rate of 2.2% in 942 men tested in similar institutions. Crucially, 7 of these 21 chromatin-positive men had an XXYY chromosome complement. By contrast, a study of 2,607 "ordinary mentally sub-normal males" found that only 2 of 28 chromatin-positive cases were XXYY. This strange finding led Jacobs et al. "to wonder whether an extra Y chromosome predisposes its carriers to unusually aggressive behavior."

Jacobs et al. therefore set out to survey XYY rates in a "survey of mentally sub-normal male patients with dangerous, violent or criminal propensities in an institution where they are treated under conditions of special security" (1965:1351) near Edinburgh. Of the 197 samples taken, 12 had a chromosome abnormality, including 7 cases of XYY and one case of XXYY. By contrast, only 1 out of almost 2,000 males tested in other settings had "an XYY sex chromosome constitution." This finding led Jacobs et al. to suggest that "the finding that 3.5 per cent of the population we studied were XYY males must represent a marked increase in frequency by comparison with the frequency of such males at birth" (1352). Furthermore, the 7 cases of XYY in the Edinburgh penal institution were, on average, more than 6 inches taller than their XY counterparts (means of 73.1 and 67.0 inches, respectively), with men more than 73 inches tall having "an approximately 1 in 2 chance of having an XYY constitution." It was these associations—institutionalization in mental-penal settings and above-average height—that would drive both research on and ascertainment of XYY during the following decade (see Richardson 2013:84–90).

As similar reports quickly followed (Jacobs et al. 1968; Price et al. 1966; Price and Whatmore 1967; Telfer et al. 1968), XYY syndrome came to be increasingly associated with the profile of a "super male," characterized by acne, increased stature, aggression, criminality, sexual deviance, and mental subnormality. Its prevalence was estimated to be around one in every two thousand men. Unsurprisingly, there was intense interest from geneticists over the following decade. However, unlike other genomically designated syndromes in the 1960s and 1970s, XYY also gained traction in psychology, psychiatry, criminology, medical-penal institutions, courts, popular culture, and major media outlets.

Already by 1966 a leading article in the *Lancet* lauded the discovery of this "new and very interesting syndrome" ("YY Syndrome" 1966:583) they called "The YY Syndrome." They enthusiastically repeat Jacobs et al.'s 1965 findings alongside a new paper published in that issue of the *Lancet* that appeared to confirm the overrepresentation of

XYY males in penal institutions (Price et al. 1966). The *Lancet* summarized: "No new diagnostic features emerge. 8 of the 9 are high-grade mental defectives. Their type of delinquency was not clearly different from that of other patients in the hospital, though most were aggressive and violent" (583). Physically, above-average height was the only notable feature (six of nine were more than six feet tall), prompting the *Lancet* to proclaim, "The height is so striking a feature that it has been said that half of all men over 6 feet in special-security institutions are YY—probably an exaggeration, but unlikely to be a very gross one." In contrast to other chromosome anomalies, which are characterized by "largely non-specific mental defect," in XYY "we seem to have a fairly specific mental disorder associated with a highly specific lesion—a matter of *considerable psychiatric importance*" (583; my emphasis). This condition, they explained, was of immense "chromosomological" interest, joining as it did the "testis-evoking gene" and the "Indian hairy-ears gene"[9] as exceptions to the idea that the Y chromosome is genetically inert (583). Not only was this chromosomal lesion seen to have a distinctive psychiatric phenotype—a finding that held the promise of making medical genetics highly relevant to what Rose has called the "psy-disciplines" (Rose 1998a)—but that phenotype meant that "XYY must make its small but significant contribution to the country's delinquent population" (Price et al. 1966:583). The implications for legal and penal systems were plain to see.[10]

XYY also began to be invoked by defense teams in criminal trials, though with mixed results. One man standing trial for murder in Australia was acquitted in 1968, with mixed reports as to whether his XYY karyotype was a factor in the court's decision (Fox 1969; "Chromosome Precedent" 1969). That same year, a jury in France rejected the XYY defense in the trial of Daniel Hugon. The *New York Times* noted that a prominent French biologist suggested that people with chromosome imbalances should have to carry cards naming their defect—a proposal met by opposition from the leading communist newspaper, *L'Humanité*, which argued that it would stigmatize thousands of people as criminals in waiting and amount to a form of racism. Jérôme Lejeune, who established the association between mongolism and trisomy 21, was one of two medical experts to testify. He said that "the born criminal does not exist," but that people with chromosome abnormalities have a 30% greater chance of becoming criminals. Hugon, Lejeune said, had been doomed to be a sick man with a hereditary inability to exercise normal responsibility. The prosecution simply countered that many XYY men lived normal lives and that an extra Y chromosome could therefore be no more than a contributing factor. In the end, the jury delivered a guilty verdict in less than forty minutes (Garrison 1968), though it appears that the XYY diagnosis gained Hugon a significantly diminished sentence of seven years ("XYY Chromosome Defense" 1968:892).

In the first such case in the United States, Sean Farley of Brooklyn sought immunity from prosecution for the brutal rape and murder of a forty-nine-year-old woman in Queens in 1968. The case was covered extensively in the *New York Times*. Although psychiatrists had declared him competent to stand trial, a cytogenetic examination was undertaken (possibly because Farley was extraordinarily tall). Sure enough, he was found to be XYY (*New York Times* 1968a:18). However, a geneticist giving expert testimony argued that XYY alone could not cause criminal behavior (*New York Times* 1969a:53), and in April 1969 Farley was convicted on the charges of rape and murder and given a twenty-five-years-to-life sentence the following July (*New York Times* 1969b:42). A number of similar cases followed, but it is not clear if an XYY-based defense was ever successful in winning an acquittal in the United States.

However, the trials did bring plenty of attention to XYY. One 1968 article about XYY, entitled "Genetic Abnormality Is Linked to Crime," even appeared on the front page of the *New York Times* (see fig. 2.1; Lyons 1968a). Coverage reached new heights when it was reported that the notorious Chicago serial killer, Richard Speck, had XYY syndrome. Stories appeared in a host of leading newspapers and magazines ("Criminal Law" 1968; "Genetics: Of Chromosomes & Crime" 1968; *New York Times* 1968b; Lyons 1968b; Stock 1968). When Mary Telfer, perhaps the leading XYY researcher in the United States, was asked about the case, she said, "If I had to pick anyone who fit the XYY pattern, I would have chosen Mr. Speck." His features and record, she averred, were good evidence that he was XYY. A leading human geneticist, Hideo Sato, and Speck's head lawyer agreed that he almost certainly carried an XYY chromosome complement. When they actually examined Speck's chromosomes, however, it turned out they were all wrong: Speck had a normal 46, XY karyotype. Nevertheless, the Speck case was a vital episode in the XYY story that helps explain why XYY left a lasting imprint on popular culture.

A *New York Times* editorial published that same month addressed some of the dilemmas raised by XYY and the way it "reviv[ed] the old argument as to whether it is nature or nurture that creates a criminal" (*New York Times* 1968b:46) After reviewing the state of knowledge about XYY, the *Times* wrote, "Should such persons be held responsible

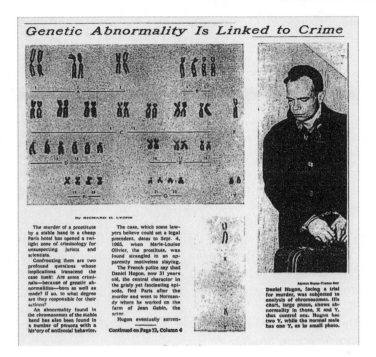

Continued on Page 72, Column 4

FIGURE 2.1. XYY story on the front page of the *New York Times*, April 21, 1968. (© 1968 The New York Times. All rights reserved. Used by permission and protected by the copyright laws of the United States. The printing, copying, redistribution, or retransmission of this content without express written permission is prohibited.)

for their crimes, or treated as victims of conditions for which they are not responsible, on a par with the criminally insane?" They cautioned against hasty conclusions, noting that "many XYY males are neither criminals nor mental defectives," and speculated that people with XYY may have problems in sexual development during adolescence, exacerbating the challenge of growing up and therefore engendering deviance. Finally, they suggested that a "fruitful line of research may stem from early identification, . . . which perhaps would enable preventive measures" to help people with XYY (46). However, while early identification and intervention may be the gold standard when it comes to genetic disorders today, we will see that precisely such a line of research would be the undoing of XYY as a major topic of inquiry and criminal management.

A 1968 letter by Patricia Jacobs and her boss, William Court Brown (Court Brown, Price, and Jacobs 1968:513) expressed their mixed feel-ings about the use of XYY in criminal trials as well as the coverage it was beginning to receive in the popular press:

> The defence in both cases might have been different had it not been for the discovery in 1965 and 1966 of the high incidence of XYY males in the British maximum security hospitals, an incidence so high that it was clearly not due to chance, nor were there any grounds for suspecting it due to biased sampling. This discovery has led to a world-wide search for these males in maximum security institutions, in prisons, among juvenile delinquents, and among the psychiatrically disturbed. At the same time the discovery has itself been discovered by the popular news media, and a good deal of nonsense has been written and broadcast about the "born criminal" and about the "criminal" chromosome.

Jacobs, like seemingly everyone else in the field, had little doubt that the XYY-criminality link was real. At the same time, questions were being raised regarding the strength of that association and its implications for treatment, prognosis, and criminal justice.

New Uncertainties and the Move toward a Newborn Screening Study

Jacobs and Court Brown pointed out two "disturbing features" of knowledge about XYY in 1968. First, "the bulk of our information on XYY's [sic] is based on the examination of adults found from the surveying of groups of men which by definition consist of men the great majority of whom, if not all, have criminal records." Second, there were no good estimates of the incidence of XYY either at birth or in the general population, making comparisons with the selected group impossible. In their own research, they had seen a great range of cases, "from the apparently normal through those with a mild personality defect to those who are severe psychopaths." They wanted to at once stand steadfastly by the significant overrepresentation of XYY caseloads in mental-penal institutions while pointing out the wrongheadedness of determinist ideas about a "criminal chromosome." What was called for, they argued, was large-scale research to determine the true prevalence and developmental implications of an XYY chromosome complement. As Court Brown put it in an extensive review of XYY that same year, "In the end there can be no substitute for an extensive and prolonged study of newborn children" (Court Brown 1968:357).

By decade's end the association between XYY and criminality was being called even further into question. Things came to a head in the summer of 1968 at the Bar Harbor genetics course—an annual event sponsored by the March of Dimes and run by Victor McKusick that brought together leading geneticists and interested parties from other disciplines, the media, and various stakeholders to promote the value of medical genetics. Researchers began to discuss the possibility that XYY may be far more common than previously thought. Evidence from Edinburgh, New Haven, Pittsburgh, and London, Ontario were presented that suggested a prevalence rate of as high as 1 in 300 men, based on examinations of 3,700 newborns (roughly half male). As Dr. Park S. Gerald of Harvard put it in a presentation to a group of science writers reported in the *New York Times*, the *Washington Post*, and elsewhere, this meant there could be one-third of a million XYY men in the United States as of the late 1960s. Gerald said it was unclear if XYY "doomed" its bearers to a life of crime and violence, but if so, "we have to deal with these people differently from the ordinary criminal. They should be restrained, not punished." He called for a long-term prospective study of 50,000 male infants and a 10–15-year follow-up of the XYYs. Such a study would cost around $750,000, he said, and was set to go ahead at Harvard "until the Vietnam war cut off our funds" (quoted in Brody 1968:34; see also Black 1968; Cohn 1968).

Just months later, Nobel Prize–winning biologist Joshua Lederberg took to the *Washington Post* to outline the "considerable discussion" generated by XYY at the 1968 meeting of the American Society of Human Genetics. He pointed to the now widely recognized need to obtain good population estimates for XYY, but also the wide variation in existing estimates from newborn studies. While he was clear that there "is enough evidence to support the concept that XYY males are abnormally predisposed to . . . the most serious difficulties in their social adjustment," he stressed that "we have no idea about the roots of the problem or just what fraction of XYYs will make such miserable failures of their own lives and inflict so much harm on others." However, Lederberg also foresaw some of the dilemmas that would confront newborn studies: Our lack of understanding of "the biology of violence" meant that it was "of the greatest importance to follow the development of [XYY] children through adulthood." At the same time, he argued that "it would be a tragic injustice to identify them," because doing so could both bias their development and the evidence gathered. Finally, he wrote, "One line of thought would lead naturally to the sacrifice of XYY newborns as a more humane disposition than allowing them to live out their predisposed fates. To say this is to reject it in favor of the alternative: to learn how to restore to them the possibility of membership in the human community." After all, Lederberg reminded us, "even a single Y chromosome already conveys a strong disposition to violence in our species" (1968:A15).

The following year it became even clearer that XYY's incidence was considerably higher than previously thought. A paper in the *New England Journal of Medicine* by Sergovich et al. (1969) conducted a karyotype analysis of 2,159 consecutive newborns, with 1,066 successful cultures from newborn males obtained. They found 4 XYY males, suggesting a prevalence of around 1 in 250. They acknowledged that this finding could be the product of statistical chance, but still argued that the prevalence of XYY "is far higher than the previous estimate of 1 in 2000 male births." Foreshadowing a line of thought that has gained favor today, they wrote, "It may be that chromosome anomalies contribute to a spectrum of neurologic deficit that may become manifest in some persons as overt mental handicap and in others determine a more subtle form of deviation." Amid so much uncertainty and with such high stakes, they argued, "In no other syndrome is the necessity for prospective study more evident than in the XYY genotype" (854). There could no longer be much doubt that there were many men with an extra Y chromosome who had not come to the attention of the criminal justice system or psychiatric institutions.

The paper was covered in the *New York Times* under the title "Scientists Doubt 'Criminal' Genes" (April 18, 1969:59), noting that "there may be well-adjusted persons with an XYY make-up, casting doubt on its so-called predisposition to criminal tendencies." Sergovich is quoted saying that XYY "does influence behavior, but it probably isn't ann [*sic*] all-or-nothing phenomenon. There's too much diversity among the XYY's we have studied to say outright that an XYY man is inevitably going to have abnormal behavior." In reference to the ascertainment bias of previous studies, Sergovich said, "If you look only at abnormal populations, you will find only abnormal XYY's. But unless you study the population at large, you can't say how many XYY men may be functioning reasonably normally." An article in the *Times* the next month (May 6, 1969:93) reported that two hundred thousand men may have the XYY "genetic make-up." They quoted a speech from the American Psychiatric Association meeting that year: "There is growing evidence that many XYY individuals are stable, law-abiding citizens. . . . It appears that the XYY male has been falsely stigmatized." It now seemed undeniable that there were plenty of "normal" XYYs out there.

But even as these findings suggested that the XYY-criminality association was looser than previously thought, public, state, and biomedical interest in men with an extra Y chromosome continued unabated. *Newsweek* was about to publish its XYY piece entitled "Congenital Criminals?" (1970), and while the tenor of published work on XYY became more nuanced, the basic object of inquiry remained. For example, one review funded by the National Institutes of Health (NIH), published in the *American Psychologist* in 1973, noted that only a small (if wildly disproportionate) minority of violent crimes were likely committed by XYY males. Yet, they went on to write,

the XYY genotype may have importance exceeding by far its numerical impact in contributing to our understanding of aggressive behavior. As previously noted, the Y chromosome is the male determining chromosome; therefore, it should come as no surprise that an extra Y chromosome can produce an individual with heightened masculinity, evinced by characteristics such as unusual tallness, increased fertility (although most XYYs do not have children, some have produced as many as 10),[11] and powerful aggressive tendencies. *The XYY genotype may be seen as highlighting the association between maleness and violence.* (Jarvik, Klodin, and Matsuyama 1973:679–80; my emphasis)

Furthermore, they hoped that "with the XYY syndrome as a research tool, it is conceivable that advances can be made in our understanding of the complexity of factors that together tend to either produce or curb aggressive responses" (680–81). In an era concerned with overpopulation and rising rates of violent crime, this was no small matter. Jarvik et al. put the matter in stark terms: "as our population continues to spiral upward at an alarming rate and our planet becomes crowded to its very limits, . . . [d]isaster will follow if we do not make a concerted effort to understand ourselves now. Hopefully, the XYY genotype can contribute to such an understanding" (681).

In sum, the discovery that many XYY males were "normal," socially adapted people did not undermine the rationale for continuing research on XYY syndrome and criminality. To be sure, a more complex story about XYY was beginning to be widely accepted, as was the need for unbiased prevalence estimates. However, even the more liberal iteration of that story assumed that the increased "maleness" conferred by an extra Y chromosome brought significant risks to both its bearer and to society.

Against this backdrop, a two-day conference was convened by the National Institute of Mental Health's (NIMH) Center for Studies of Crime and Delinquency in June 1969. In attendance were thirteen researchers from leading American universities, along with less-specialized researchers, heads of several other NIMH centers, and representatives from the Department of Justice and the NIH. At least two of those attendees, Park Gerald and Stanley Walzer, went on to lead major NIMH-funded studies into the incidence and development of boys with sex chromosome abnormalities that I discuss at length below. Little did they know that they were about to be embroiled in a major episode of public contention that would forever alter the field of XYY research.

The resulting report, written by the Center for Studies of Crime and Delinquency's "chief," Saleem Shah, was intended for a general audience, as well as researchers and professionals. However, it was "especially addressed to persons who are most likely to be confronted with important questions and decisions pertaining to the topic discussed, e.g., lawyers, judges, administrators of correctional, mental health and related programs, research administrators, legislators and policy makers" (1970:1). Shah captured the exceptionality of XYY as a genomically designated condition well (3; my emphasis): "During 1968 a special branch of the science of *genetics was drawn from the quietude of laboratories and professional journals and exposed to the glare of courtrooms and newspaper headlines.*" Given the existing knowledge about XYY, the aforementioned legal issues and the "many press and broadcast stories [that] have appeared about the allegedly antisocial propensities of persons with the XYY chromosome abnormality," Shah argued that there were "some important medical-legal-ethical questions" that urgently needed to be addressed (4).

However, there remained a huge gap in knowledge about XYY's behavioral implications. Researchers could not point to biologically proven pathways that led from the YY aneuploidy to abnormal behavior, nor unbiased population data to ground comparisons with institutionalized caseloads. Thus a "pervasive note struck throughout the conference was the need for more knowledge obtained through extensive and meticulous research" (Shah 1970:34). Amid the newly recognized uncertainty of outcomes, there was an emerging consensus among both critics of the XYY-criminality nexus like Sergovich and promoters like Gerald and Jacobs (above): prospective studies were the only way to get to the bottom of the XYY conundrum. Participants at the NIMH conference emphasized the need to balance the "scientific as well as societal need to conduct further research" on XYY with the "important social values which require that the rights, welfare, confidentiality and privacy of research subjects be safeguarded in such research endeavors" (4). It would prove an impossible circle to square.

The Undoing of the XYY-Criminology Nexus

Following the 1969 conference, the NIMH funded at least two significant XYY studies that Shah hoped would yield better prevalence and incidence data (Shah, quoted in Bauer et al. 1980:3). Both studies, however, would attract the ire of activists concerned about children's rights and the lingering specter of eugenics—a backlash from which the XYY-criminality nexus would never recover.

The first major study was led by Shah's frequent collaborator, Digamber Borgaonkar of Johns Hopkins University, and received $300,000 over three years. The project, approved by Maryland's Departments of Health and Juvenile Services and federal agencies, planned to test some fifteen thousand boys for XYY—around six thousand from juvenile jails and seventy-five hundred drawn overwhelmingly from poor black families enrolled in a free medical program at Johns Hopkins. The initial protocol did not include obtaining consent from parents, on the grounds that the XYY tests were to be conducted on the same blood samples used for routine anemia checks, nor did it include informing them of results unless requested. However, they did plan to give the results to the juvenile correctional institutions involved. According to the director of Juvenile Services, those would "probably be passed on to the courts for whatever use they can make of [them]" (quoted in Bauer 1972:342).

Groups like the American Civil Liberties Union, as well as concerned parents, doctors, and lawyers, rose up in opposition to the study. They vehemently objected to its total lack of an informed consent procedure and the potential abuse of knowledge about the XYY status of juvenile detainees, who might be given harsh sentences even for minor offences on the grounds that they were genetically predisposed to criminality. By February of 1970 a lawsuit was filed against both the NIMH and Johns Hopkins, and Shah temporarily suspended the study pending the revision of consent procedures.

By May 1970, XYY testing was resumed. Consent was now sought from parents, but without any information about XYY or even which abnormalities were being tested for. The form simply noted, "The chromosome study ordinarily costs about $100, . . . [but] no fees will be charged to you" (cited in Bauer 1972). While Borgaonkar and his colleagues continued to publish on XYY during the coming years, it is unclear whether they ever completed the full survey. At the 1972 annual meeting of the American Society of Human Genetics in Philadelphia, Borgaonkar (1972:13a) reported on progress "in an ongoing chromosome survey," along with the "socio-legal issues" related to consent and the results of "correspondence with approximately 15,000 parents." Chromosomal analysis was successfully performed on around 3,300 boys, and XYY results were as follows: 2 of "1,800 institutionalized juveniles"; 2 of "300 mentally disturbed institutionalized juveniles"; 1 in "200 boys in a private center for emotionally disturbed children"; none in "1,000 normal boys." However, Borgaonkar's subsequent papers on XYY strongly suggest that the survey of institutionalized Maryland boys did not obtain chromosome analyses or conduct follow-up research on anything approaching the proposed volume of cases (Money et al. 1974; Money, Franzke, and Borgaonkar 1975).

The other project the NIMH funded was led by two participants of the 1969 XYY conference, Stanley Walzer and Park Gerald. It was conducted at Harvard Medical School, Boston Children's Hospital, and the Boston Hospital for Women. Their goals were threefold. By screening a large, unbiased sample of newborn boys at Boston Hospital for Women (the plan was to screen every baby born at the hospital over several years), they hoped to provide a baseline incidence rate for XYY (and XXY) against which cases ascertained in institutional settings could be measured. They also planned to conduct a longitudinal examination of the subjects found to have a sex chromosome abnormality in order to provide a detailed evaluation of the developmental course of XYY from infancy through adolescence and into adulthood. Finally, they aimed to provide early diagnosis and intervention to avoid or mitigate the adverse outcomes associated with sex chromosome abnormalities, especially XYY. This research received an eight-year, $465,000 grant from the NIMH Center for the Study of Crime and Delinquency.

Not long after the study got underway, a group of professors at Harvard led by biologist Jonathan Beckwith raised grave concerns about the study, and especially what they called the "XYY myth." They charged that it was not possible to obtain fully informed consent in this case. Furthermore, they cautioned that with all the publicity about the "criminal chromosome," there was a serious risk of biasing expectations against boys found to have XYY, leading to a self-fulfilling prophecy. Finally, they argued that this kind of essentializing research represented nothing less than a return to the dangerous and discredited ideas of the eugenics movement and diverted attention and resources away from the real, socioeconomic causes of violence and crime (Bauer et al. 1980:197; Beckwith 1975; Beckwith and King 1974; Pyeritz, Beckwith, and Miller 1975; see Beckwith 2002 for a retrospective account).

When internal review procedures at Harvard failed to halt the study, Beckwith, MIT biologist Daniel King, and others embarked on a program of public opposition to the study under the banner of "Science for the People." They attracted extensive coverage in leading media outlets in the process (e.g., Brody 1974b; Knox 1974). Walzer agreed to have his work periodically reviewed and the study design potentially modified by a Harvard committee, calling it "a good and sensible request." "'If it appears that the vast majority of XYY's are developing normally, it may be better for them not to know, not to be identified at birth,' Dr. Walzer said. 'But right now we simply cannot answer this question. That's what this study is attempting to do'" (Brody 1974a:20). Beckwith called the committee a "whitewash" and criticized the lack of public involvement, which contravened Department of Health, Education and Welfare guidelines (20). Walzer, however, rejected criticism that the XYY "myth," as Beckwith and others described it, would have adverse outcomes for children. Instead, he argued, his careful counseling and the potential for early intervention and therapy if behavioral problems did arise far outweighed the risks (Brody 1974a).

Eventually, the study was discontinued. As the *New York Times* reported, this was due to "continued controversy over the study's ethics and potential scientific value. The chief investigator, Dr. Stanley Walzer, a psychiatrist at Harvard University, said in an interview that while he had originally intended to stop screening in any case 'sometime this year,' he was also worn down by harassment, unrelenting controversy and the threat of further opposition to his work by *groups supporting children's rights*. He said it was impossible to continue working in the atmosphere that had been created" (Brody 1975:6, my emphasis). The article explains that it was XYY and the issues raised by Science for the People that drove the controversy, despite reviews by five professional committees at various institutions that supported the study. In fact, the Children's Defense Fund was about to begin a campaign against the research before the announcement that it would be halted. Walzer reported receiving threatening phone calls at his home, and complained, "These groups could make a difference. They could help an investigator, make him change his mind in some cases. . . . I think more people should participate in decisions relevant to research, but not in the way it happened to me" (6; see also Culliton 1975; Weiss 1975). Beckwith and his colleagues were adamant, however, that the XYY study—and the entire XYY research program—

was a grave danger to men and boys found to have an extra Y chromosome and part of a broader, insipidly eugenicist failure to address the social causes of crime (Beckwith and King 1974; Pyeritz et al. 1977).

By 1977 the *New York Times* was discussing XYY in far more critical terms (Adams 1977:188). Following a brief discussion of Lombroso's late eighteenth-century theories about inherited criminality and the phrenological characteristics of criminals, the author reports that "a more recent biological theory linked violent criminality with the so-called XYY defect in men." She notes the findings from studies with criminal populations, and (re)quotes geneticist Fred Sergovich's statement, "If you look only at abnormal populations, you will find only abnormal XYY's." She discusses a study conducted in Denmark by a Princeton psychologist, which found no evidence that XYY offenders were more likely to commit violent crimes than XY offenders and even suggested that higher conviction rates among XYY men "may reflect a higher detection rate than a higher rate of commission."

Having been effectively tied to the specter of eugenics, XYY was truly receding as a legitimate explanation of violence and criminality. Hence when Stephen Jay Gould added an epilogue to the chapter entitled "Measuring Bodies" in his masterful 1981 critique of race science, phrenology, eugenics, and intelligence testing, *The Mismeasure of Man*, XYY would be his main piece of evidence for this important idea: "We live in a more subtle century, but the basic arguments never seem to change. . . . The signs of innate criminality are no longer sought in stigmata of gross anatomy, but in twentieth-century criteria: genes and fine structure of the brain" (1996:173). Gould dismissed the XYY program as "a myth" based on "elementary flaws of method" and "the singularly simplistic notion that since males are more aggressive than females and possess a Y that females lack, Y must be the seat of aggression and a double Y spells double trouble." He argued that we would do better to attend to the social ills and forms of oppression that engender criminality rather than "the determinist philosophy of blaming the victim" (174–75) if we want to understand modern crime and violence.

Even Walzer, Gerald, and Shah, the key XYY researchers at Harvard and the NIMH, conceded in a coauthored *Annual Review of Medicine* piece entitled "The XYY Genotype" that it may be "inappropriate to allude to an XYY syndrome. The term syndrome implies a degree of symptom consistency that is not supported by the data available at this time" (1978:568). They even acknowledged many of the criticisms from Science for the People, pointing to a study by Money, Franzke, and Borgaonkar (1975), which found that social class strongly mediated the type of treatment behaviorally disturbed XYY men were likely to receive—correctional facilities like jails and reformatories for lower-class and lower-middle-class subjects, and therapy or mental hospitals for the upper middle class. Still, Walzer, Gerald, and Shah were not about to give up on the idea that an XYY genotype did in fact confer behavioral traits like impulsivity, aggression, and outbursts. Summarizing another study, they wrote, "XYY individuals living apparently normal lives in the community could be distinguished from non-XYY men on the basis of formal psychological assessment" (1978:568).

Walzer, Gerald, and Shah still spoke of the need for longitudinal, prospective studies in order to explain the "epidemiological data pertaining to the XYY genotype, [which] suggest that there is a three- to fourfold overrepresentation of XYY individuals in mental and penal settings and a twentyfold overrepresentation in mental-penal (special security) settings." However, they quickly pointed out that the "reasons behind the risk for behavioral disability are not known at this time." In short, they found themselves back where they started: "Since much of the available information about the XYY sex chromosome complement is biased," they argued, "more data is required before definitive statements can be made about the personality characteristics or intelligence of the vast majority of XYY men not appearing in social settings oriented towards behavioral deviancy" (1978:569).

Nevertheless, it was clear that XYY syndrome was not going to be viable as a major topic of research or category of institutional practice in the aftermath of the intense controversy of the mid-1970s.[12] Articles and letters about the controversy itself were still common, and existing studies continued to get their results published over the next few years (though generally in far less prestigious venues). However, published research output on XYY declined dramatically from the early 1980s and never again approached its previous heights.[13]

XYY did linger on at the margins. One 1973 high school textbook, after discussing Down syndrome and the other sex chromosome conditions, turned to XYY: "Another abnormal condition results when a normal X-bearing egg is fertilized by a YY sperm, formed by nondisjunction during spermatogenesis. This produces an XYY male who is usually over six feet in height and very aggressive. Studies have revealed that a high percentage of inmates [in institutions] for the criminally insane have this chromosome abnormality" (Otto and Towle 1973:185). XYY also served as the premise for a popular British novel and TV series called *XYY Man* (1976; Royce 1973, 1977), and it has made appearances on shows like *Law and Order*. In David Fincher's *Alien 3*, Ellen Ripley crash-lands on a "Maximum Security Double Y Chromosome-Work Correctional Facility" where the prisoners have taken over. Described by their leader as "thieves, murderers, rapists and child molesters . . . all scum," our hero is therefore left to contend with both an alien killer and a group of genetically depraved criminals (Fincher 1992). Yet in the realm of nonfiction, XYY syndrome had become much like other genomically designated conditions in the late 1970s and 1980s: it had little relevance as a biosocial category.

Prenatal Testing for Mutations

The potential to prenatally diagnose and selectively terminate fetuses with chromosomal abnormalities was almost immediately recognized as the main medical affordance of the karyotype. Even before prenatal testing was technically possible, the ability to report recurrence risk was seen as one of the major accomplishments of the emerging field. For example, after recounting all of the chromosomal aberrations reported at the time, the early review of the new cytogenetics in *Pediatrics* cited above concluded, "For the pediatrician, the studies on Mongolism are of primary importance. The genetic aspects of the condition have been clarified and a basis for the familial occurrence emphasizes the necessity of chromosomal analysis in providing information in regard to future pregnancies in young mothers with affected children" (Rappoport and Kaplan 1961:434).

Once amniocentesis came into view in the mid-1960s (Steele and Breg 1966), Down syndrome and a host of genomically designated syndromes could be used for the selective termination of pregnancies (see Harper 2006:162; Reinhold 1968). Thus, when Bentley Glass delivered his presidential address to the American Academy of Arts and Sciences in 1970, published in *Science* the following year, he told the audience assembled in Chicago,

Human power is advancing with extraordinary rapidity in this realm of control over the genetic characteristics of the unborn. Perhaps, as Carl Becker so pregnantly stated, our race, far from having any aversion from power, will welcome this power too, will seek it, fashion it, and grasp it tenaciously. *Unlimited access to state-regulated abortion will combine with the now perfected techniques of determining chromosome abnormalities in the developing fetus to rid us of the several percentages of all births that today represent uncontrollable defects such as mongolism (Down's syndrome) and sex deviants such as the XYY type.* (1971:28; my emphasis)

Indeed, the literature on chromosomal trisomies like Down and Edwards syndromes makes it clear that prenatal detection was far and away the primary object of research on *medical* intervention for those conditions in the early decades of genomic designation.

But what about XYY? Did abortions of XYY fetuses cease once it became clear that most males with an extra Y chromosome have minor physical and psychiatric problems at most? The answer is simple: no. An editorial in the *British Medical Journal* entitled "What Is to Be Done with the XYY Fetus" (1979) observed (p. 1519) that "in the sex chromosome aneuploidies there may be a wide range from near normality to severe handicap," but that "in practice termination is usually requested. . . . 47XYY, is a clear example of this problem" (1519). They discuss the options, each of which were adopted by many clinicians, when XYY was found prenatally: do not tell the parents; tell the parents but emphasize the relatively small risks; tell the parents and explain "that the risks are high enough to justify abortion." As they put it, "the dilemma remains" (1520). In the 1980 retrospective conference on XYY discussed above, Stanley Walzer explained his approach in the frequent calls he received from women asking whether they should terminate a pregnancy on the basis of an XYY or XXY finding: "What I will do is sit down with the people, and I will go over with them in confidence the developmental data that I have available on my fourteen XYYs. I will show them photographs of these lovely children. I will talk to them about some of the problems the kids are having and how wonderful the other ones are doing. I will present the facts—all the facts that I have. And I will then tell them to go back home and make their own decision" (quoted in Bauer et al. 1980:10). In other words, even parents with the capital to "sit down" with one of the world's leading experts were still left with a deeply uncertain dilemma. As we will see in chapter 8, where I explore the topic of modern prenatal testing for genomically designated conditions, rates of termination, even for mild conditions like XXX and XYY syndrome, remain high. Meanwhile, recent technological advances are beginning to make the prenatal diagnosis of genomically designated conditions an extremely common phenomenon.

Mobilizing Mutations beneath the Specter of Eugenics

XYY turned out to be the exception that proves the rule. Ascertained in medical-penal institutions, mobilized beyond the lab as a tool of social control, and delegitimated through social activism, XYY demonstrates the very limited potential for genomic designation to achieve socio-cultural traction in the 1960s and 1970s.

The turn to genomic designation was an easy one for human geneticists. The pertinent question then is, Under what conditions do such mutations *matter*, and to whom? Following Fleck, we can trace genomically designated conditions as scientific facts from their initial, hesitant instantiation in a human genetics journal through their codification in review articles and databases, and on to significance at the level of institutional practice and identity formation. This framework helps us to see how genomic designation quickly achieved what Fleck would call esoteric and vademecum reality, but mostly failed to attain the kind of traction at the level of what he called "popular knowledge" that endows a scientific fact with certainty and power. So, what can we learn about the conditions of possibility for genomic designation from our study of its early years and the exceptional case of XYY syndrome?

One hypothesis is that XYY gained the traction it did, but then ultimately failed, because of the lingering but no longer legitimate imperatives of eugenics. There is much to be said for this hypothesis. Eugenics dominated early twentieth-century thinking and practice around genetics and human difference. There was no real difference between the two. Animated by concerns about the degradation of the human gene pool and utopian ideas about how we could wrest back control and scientifically manage our own evolution, eugenics gained favor across the political spectrum. Campaigns to promote better breeding and, above all, to protect both society and future generations from the feebleminded, criminal, and unfit, led to programs of forced sterilization, large institutions of mass confinement, and overtly racist immigration policies in the United States that remained in place until the 1960s (Stern 2005). Eugenic ideas and policies in the United States, not least California's program of forced sterilization, were a direct source of inspiration for Nazi leaders beginning in the 1930s (Kuhl 2002). Of course, eugenics reached its horrific nadir in Hitler's Germany, where it played a key role in Nazi ideology and helped motivate the systematic genocide against millions of Jews, gypsies, homosexuals, and people with mental or physical disabilities. The eugenics movement would never recover from its association with the very worst of European modernity (Kevles 1985; Paul 1995; Stern 2005).

Modern human genetics grew quite directly out of the field of eugenics (Kevles 1985). Genomic designation was no exception. Important early work on conditions like XYY and XXYY, not to mention Mongolian Idiocy/trisomy 21, was conducted at the Galton Institute in London and published in its *Annals of Human Genetics*, which had been the *Annals of Eugenics* until 1954 (see Kevles 1985:252). Geneticists still found their most interesting karyotypes and human subjects within the walls of institutions that were indelibly tied to the eugenics movements of a few decades prior. Indeed, Ted Porter (2018) has shown how modern heritability studies can be traced all the way back to eighteenth-century asylums and institutions for the feebleminded—a resource that eugenics researchers and medical geneticists alike drew upon with great zeal. In short, there were very direct ties between early cytogenetic research and eugenics. In both XYY-criminology research and the discourse around prenatal testing, we see how the imperatives of early twentieth-century eugenics, which had been present since the birth of both medical genetics (Kevles 1985) and molecular biology (Kay 1996), were very much active in genomic designation's early years. So, was it not a quintessentially eugenic impulse that drove scientific, state, and popular interest in XYY syndrome and criminality but, thankfully, also elicited the fatal backlash against it? Did genetics have to gain distance and fully break with eugenics before mutations could be meaningfully mobilized?

Unfortunately, this straightforward argument does not bear the weight of further scrutiny. It was not simply a lag time that undid the debilitating specter of eugenics and made genomic designation practicable in recent years. Despite vast differences, there are deep, enduring continuities that tie modern genomics to early twentieth-century eugenics. It took years of painstaking work by actors ranging from biomedical researchers and genetic counselors to parents and patient activists to rehabilitate the idea that genetics was a legitimate basis for shaping practice in fields like pediatric care and special education (Finucane, Haas-Givler, and Simon 2003; Kerr, Cunningham-Burley, and Amos 1998). Furthermore, one can still trace a direct lineage from early twentieth-century eugenics to contemporary medical genetics (Kevles 1985), and the charge of eugenicism still functions as a powerful rhetorical tool in scholarly and popular critiques of genetics and prenatal testing (e.g., Carlson 2012; Duster [1990] 2003; Shakespeare 1998).

Nor was it a fundamental change in practice that obviated the homology with eugenics. Phrenology is endemic to the clinical description of genomically designated conditions in all but name. We saw how "funny looking kids" became "the prime targets of inquiry" in the years after the trisomy 21/mongolism discovery. Medical geneticists continue to discuss "FLKs" to this day, often comparing photographs and discussing the facial features that remain the only clinical signs that point toward genomically designated diagnoses with any reliability whatsoever (though it is still generally poor) (Morelle 2007; Shaw et al. 2003). Genetics still focuses on the same sorts of populations— especially what eugenicists called the "feebleminded," "epileptics," the insane, and people thought to be prone to criminality.

Finally, the mutations discussed in this book remain leading targets of prenatal testing, and with the advent of noninvasive prenatal genetic testing this may well have eugenic consequences (see chapter 8). Although proposals for mandatory testing and elimination of people with mutations like XYY or trisomy 21 are thankfully no longer found in the literature, they were extremely rare in the 1960s and 1970s as well. In sum, we cannot simply say that the charge of eugenicism has lost its discursive force or that there is no longer any basis upon which to levy it.

What then of the XYY genotype? Was not that an unfortunate episode of eugenicist thinking that sought to use a mutation to manage a portion of the criminal population and perhaps gain insight into the remainder? It is true that the activists who mobilized against the XYY-criminality nexus tied it to eugenics, and with good reason. However, XYY research had moved on by the time that charge was mobilized. After all, Walzer, Gerald, Borgaonkar, and Shah were by no means a bunch of crass eugenicists. We saw how they came to hold quite circumspect views on the implications of an XYY karyotype, qualms about the more sensationalist reportage associated with it, concerns about the role of class in mediating outcomes for XYY males, and strongly held views *against* its hasty employment in criminal justice systems. Indeed, one of the findings of the Harvard study (Walzer and Gerald 1975) refuted the prevalent idea that there was a correlation between XYY and low socioeconomic status.

In fact, it seems none of Walzer's families left the XYY study at Harvard, despite their freedom to do so at any time and the intense controversy that surrounded it. We even see striking glimpses of the kind of parent-advocate discourse that drives genomically designated conditions today. While the Harvard controversy raged on, one mother explained in a letter to the *New England Journal of Medicine*,

I am the mother of a son who happens to be an XYY karyotypic male. Our son, now 21 years of age, is certainly not a criminal. He is a gentle, nice guy, somewhat inadequate occupationally and socially, but always doing his best to succeed. Since birth he has been developmentally atypical, and his behavior has been impulsive. He had behavioral, speech and learning problems in childhood. We were not aware of his genetic make-up until he was 16 years old. He was karyotyped at my request at Johns Hopkins Hospital, after I had learned about a possible behavioral effect of a supernumerary Y chromosome. In the Johns Hopkins XYY program, he has for the first time received informed and intelligent treatment for his condition. If we had known at an early age that he had the XYY genetic make-up we could have provided more adequate help for him instead of traveling through mazes of misdiagnoses and mistreatment for 16 years. (Franzke 1975:100–101)

This belief that a genetic *cause* provides the soundest basis for understanding and acting on developmental difference drives patient advocacy for genetic disorders to this day. Again, this idea was already available for parents like Franzke, who wrote that "the emotional damage of 'not knowing' has been enormous for the child and his family." She was adamant that one had to use knowledge about the causes of a child's problem in order to provide adequate help, arguing, "If the parents are denied the knowledge, and early treatment for XYY boys is thus not available, these boys may not have the chance for a normal life" (100). Franzke went on to ask, "Should this be taken from them just because of some person's theory?" before excoriating Beckwith "and his 'Science for the People'" for working to deny vital genetic information to troubled children and their families.

This mother had become something of a lay expert on XYY: "According to my own research and knowledge of the XYY literature, no XYY boys have been located who have not displayed noticeable developmental deviancy in childhood, regardless of when labeled XYY. Early diagnosis appears to offer more benefit to these boys and their families than lack of a possible stigmatizing label" (Franzke 1975:101). That is, at least some of the parents of XYY children enrolled in the very studies that attracted such devastating *oppositional* activism were invoking strikingly similar arguments to the ones that animate activism in *support* of genomically designated conditions today. Franzke's letter evokes key features of contemporary parent advocacy for genomically designated conditions: the deployment of lay expertise, the frustration with what is now often referred to as the "diagnostic odyssey," and the fervent belief that a genomically designated diagnosis would have provided both an explanation and the basis for sound treatment.

Walzer and Gerald had failed to build a broader alliance. They were supported by most of their colleagues at Harvard and in the academy more generally. They even had the ardent support of at least some XYY parents. However, they found themselves *confronted* by activist groups and advocacy organizations concerned with children's rights. Once those activists mobilized against XYY research, the network dissolved and left the XYY classification bereft of the power to really *matter* much to anyone. As a result, XYY syndrome fell into crushing disrepute as a biomedical category. While longitudinal studies in Canada, Scotland, and Denmark did continue for a time, the public controversy that had derailed the Harvard study was picked up in the United Kingdom by 1978, ensuring that XYY could give rise to little more than what Fleck called journal or esoteric science. Patricia Jacobs, whose 1965 study launched the XYY-criminality nexus, poignantly left Edinburgh for Hawaii to conduct research on spontaneously aborted fetuses—a population with extremely high rates of chromosomal abnormality but very little capacity to inform practice or attract controversy.

During this period, there was just very little scope for mobilizing mutations. To be sure, the more or less speculative *ascription* of genetic etiology for established disorders like phenylketonuria (PKU; see Lindee 2005:28–57), Tay-Sachs disease, or autism (see chapters 3–4) during the 1960s and 1970s could help spur social mobilization. Nevertheless, it is simply hard to see how newfangled conditions like XYY, XXX, and 5p– syndromes could have become powerful categories of clinical practice and social mobilization during this period. Genomic designation was stalled at vademecum science. Thankfully, what might have transpired if XYY and other mutations had been visible during the heyday of early twentieth-century eugenics remains little more than a disquieting counterfactual.

Coda

Conditions like Cri du Chat/5p– syndrome and de Grouchy/18p Deletion Syndrome have become objects of bona fide social action. Today, groups like the 5p– Society and the Chromosome 18 Registry & Research Society are providing support, raising funds, promoting awareness, facilitating research, and holding conferences for patients, parents, clinicians, and researchers.[14] These and other genomically designated conditions have been transformed as objects of knowledge and practice, even in cases where we are talking about precisely the same genetic mutations. When viewed through the lens of what I call "re-iterated fact-making," this trip through the 1960s and 1970s therefore provides crucial comparative-historical perspective on genomic designation as a form of human classification. It shows us how historical conditions and repertoires of collective action powerfully shape what it means to have a genetic mutation.

Even Edwards syndrome/trisomy 18 now has an active Trisomy 18 Foundation dedicated to support, advocacy, and research.[15] It is equipped with family, medical, and research advisory councils, fundraising operations, a board of directors, staff, and a network of volunteers. Consider a letter from their founder, Victoria Miller, who began working to establish a trisomy 18 community after losing her own son to the condition eleven days after he was born. "Since our beginnings," she explains, "over 10,000 mothers, fathers, grandparents, and family supporters have been served by our nationally recognized programs." This means that people "just learning about their child's Trisomy 18 diagnosis can immediately access diverse community support from peers who have walked the same path as theirs." The same passage then turns to directly address its constituency with a pledge to "provide you with the information, support and tools you need. . . . [W]e will be here, walking beside you, throughout you[r] and your child's journey with Trisomy 18."

The foundation works hard to interface with biomedical researchers and health care professionals. As the website explains, "Families need more than just comfort while they cope and endure. They need immediate solutions for themselves and their children who struggle and die too soon. The Foundation is busy crafting those solutions in collaborative efforts with health professionals groups, international research leaders, and public health agencies cutting across many different disciplines and medical specialties. Your help is needed to get there!"[16] Thus the first of their five goals is to "insure that all appropriate physicians and health care providers are aware of the full range of health outcomes, have ready access to the latest information . . . and can easily make use of the resources they need to provide access to effective medical treatments and psycho-social care for the entire family." They also advocate for greater funding from the NIH and the Centers for Disease Control and Prevention (CDC) and seek to emulate the success that other genetic disorders have had in this regard. As they point out, *"Many disorders effecting [sic] many fewer children per year than Trisomy 18 have this kind of public research support, but not Trisomy 18.* The difference is that these other disorders have had an effective patient advocacy organization lobbying to make this happen." If they can emulate these organizations and "lobby the key decision-makers," they urge, "we will be heard in the halls of Congress."[17] Trisomy 18 may have been one of the first genomically designated syndromes, but it was *not* the first one to benefit from a powerful new advocacy model. The foundation is, however, making a concerted effort to follow suit.

What then of XXX syndrome, the first genomically designated condition reported in the literature and one of the most consistently mild. Today, it too has been taken up as an object of research, care, and advocacy. Founded in 1989, the recently renamed Association for X and Y Chromosome Variations (AXYS)[18] is working to promote awareness and research on sex chromosome aneuploidies in collaboration with the eXtraordinarY Kids Clinic at Children's Hospital Colorado and the eXceptional Kids Clinic at EmorY. Triple X syndrome appears on popular health review pages like Mayo Clinic, WebMD, and Healthline,[19] as well as the bevy of new sites and databases dedicated to genetic disorders. Finally, local support groups are being established around the country, and they have held national conferences every other summer since 2011. They are explicitly trying to get sex chromosome aneuploidies like XXX and XYY recognized by general practitioners; a series of brochures designed for pediatricians is available for download from their website.

They have high hopes for these kinds of efforts:

Imagine handing your child's pediatrician the generic brochure and the brochure that describes your child and then having this conversation: "Doctor, did you know that 1 in 500 individuals has an X or Y chromosome variation? It's true. So, it [*sic*] you have 2000 patients in your practice, that means that there are probably 4 children that you care for who have this condition. Are they all diagnosed?" Let's start a movement to enlighten every professional you encounter and help them understand—and diagnose—every child who has X and Y chromosome variations![20]

In other words, we now see the parents of children with trisomies like XXX and XYY advocating for early and universal diagnosis, evaluation, and intervention. Today, finding a sex chromosome aneuploidy is considered to be a valuable and sometimes even empowering piece of clinical and self-knowledge, rather than a dangerous and stigmatizing label.

XYY Redux

After a couple of decades in the wilderness, XYY syndrome is making a comeback, but in a form appropriate for the times.[21] It receives the same kind of press as other genomically designated syndromes, such as a piece in the United Kingdom's second biggest newspaper, the *Daily*

Mail, about a former actress and the challenge of raising a son with learning difficulties (Giles 2008).[22] Networks of support and advocacy are emerging as part of the Association for X and Y Chromosome Variations and the Unique charity for children with chromosomal disorders in the United Kingdom (see Unique [2008]). New programs of research and specialized treatment are underway.[23] An AXYS-sponsored series of children's books—for example, *Jack and His Extra Y* (Colvin 2014)—is indicative of the way that the sex chromosome aneuploidies are becoming increasingly powerful categories of expectation and identity formation. Indeed, the AXYS XYY leaflet featured in figure 2.2 (KS&A was renamed AXYS a few years ago, when it merged with the main Klinefelter syndrome organization) captures just how much has changed in the way we understand what an extra Y chromosome means for a boy's development.

Clinical profiles and guidelines for XYY are appearing, but rather than deviance, criminality, and "mental subnormality," it is now characterized by increased risk of ADHD and autism, and an average

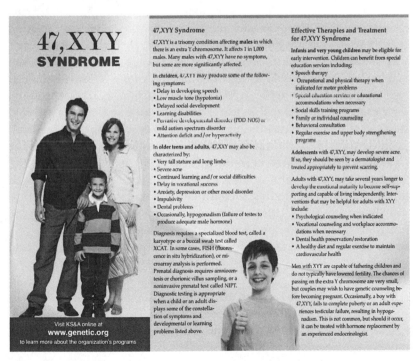

FIGURE 2.2. XYY brochure from KS&A, now known as the Association for X and Y Chromosome Variations (AXYS). (Reproduced by permission from AXYS)

of 10–15 IQ points lower than unaffected siblings (see, e.g., Ross et al. 2012; Bishop et al. 2011; Cordeiro et al. 2012; Geerts, Steyaert, and Fryns 2003; Hagerman 1999:185–92; Ratcliffe 1999; Tartaglia et al. 2006; Leggett et al. 2010).[24] There is a renewed emphasis on early detection and intervention, but the noxious link to criminology has been completely severed. In a 2015 interview in Cambridge, Massachusetts, Jonathan Beckwith—perhaps the single most important slayer of the XYY-criminology nexus—told me that he sees nothing wrong with these new programs of research, even as he stands 100% behind his oppositional activism from the 1970s. The very phenotype of XYY is dramatically different now that there are different conditions of possibility for using it as an object of knowledge and practice. In short, XYY is being made suitable for our age.

Conclusion

In the aftermath of the XYY controversy, the president of the American Society of Human Genetics bemoaned the "genetic McCarthyism" (Hamerton 1976:109) of groups like Science for the People and insisted that XYY research was both important and sound. The battle, however, was lost: when geneticists *confronted* activists, they came away bemused and beaten. But they did not stay down for very long. When Patricia Jacobs, perhaps the key figure in XYY research, gave a speech after receiving a career award at the American Society of Human Genetics in 1982, she too insisted that "the finding of an excess of XYY males in medical-penal settings . . . should have provided a useful, objective tool in the rational study of human behavior" (Jacobs 1982:693). Discussing the activism that halted almost all XYY research, she said, "Can we, with hindsight, try to insure that such an episode is never again allowed to sully human genetics?" Her answer in 1982 was not quite there yet: she just wanted the American Society of Human Genetics to be more of a public force and for geneticists to be wary of media misappropriation of their findings.

Even in 2004 she seemed incredulous that XYY research had attracted such a backlash. After describing the process that led her to suspect that an extra Y chromosome might contribute to aggressive behavior, Jacobs said, "If you stop and think about it, 98% or some such number of the prison population are males. So you can't say that the Y has got nothing to do with behavior" (quoted in Harper 2006:90). For Jacobs, it seems, Stephen Jay Gould's "singularly simplistic notion" was nothing less than prima facie correct: "And they try to tell me the Y has got nothing to do with it. Absurd!" (90). It does not take much imagination, however, to deduce that the "they" here is the early critics of XYY research, like Science for the People, who essentially obliterated the early programs of research and social management related to XYY syndrome.

In other words, Jacobs and her colleagues in medical genetics did not yet appreciate the alliances and sociotechnical work that would be required in order to make mutations really matter to the way we understand and act on human difference. But later in her speech (696) Jacobs pointed to a new syndrome she and others were working on, suggesting that "X-linked mental retardation associated with a marker at Xq28 will be to the 1980s what Down syndrome was to the 1960s." Jacobs was more prescient than she could have known at the time. She was talking about what we now call Fragile X syndrome, which has since gone on to pioneer a new model for mobilizing genetic mutations that every other group seeks to emulate.

That new model for mobilizing mutations is the subject of the following chapters. For now, we need to consider how it came to be that, nowadays, it is actually patient advocates who are calling for the sort of initiatives that attracted such ire from activists in the 1970s. They often call for newborn studies and even national newborn screening for genomically designated conditions. They also argue for programs of treatment and early intervention based on a child's genetic mutation. Even XYY has been recast as a mild developmental *syndrome*, albeit one suitable for this new social circuitry of research, care, and advocacy for children with genetic disorders.

So here we have proof that the impact of a genetic mutation is as much a sociological phenomenon as it is a biomedical one. Indeed, the distinction breaks down altogether when it comes to mutations like XYY, the 22q11.2 microdeletion and the kinds of people delineated on their basis. Through the perspective provided by reiterated fact-making, we see that genetic mutations have to be mobilized in order to really matter. This is how they attain their meaning as objects of knowledge and categories of practice. The general failure of genomically designated conditions in the decades after 1959 to catch on beyond esoteric journals, textbooks, and prenatal testing, as well as the spectacular but fleeting exception of XYY syndrome, therefore helps us better understand the resurgence of genomic designation in recent years. The standardization of chromosomal analysis was necessary, but far from sufficient. In order to really matter to lived experience, genomically designated "syndromes" must be able to translate the interests of actors outside of human genetics and achieve a degree of commensurability with other fields, be it criminology, clinical medicine, or special education. By tracing the shifting networks of actors formed around mutations, we can conduct a truly comparative-historical study of genomic designation and with it the meaning of genetic difference.

Before we turn to the new sorts of research, treatment, and advocacy that have animated genomic designation in recent years, it is important to examine another key condition of possibility: the variable ways in which genomically designated conditions intersect with and are used to get at more common categories of human difference. I take up that project over the course of the next two chapters.

THREE

Leveraging Mutations: Going from the Rare to the Common in Human Genetics

[A]nomaly appears called upon to explicate the formation of the normal, not because the normal is an attenuated form of the pathological, but because the pathological is the normal impeded or deviated. Remove the impediment and you obtain the norm.   GEORGES CANGUILHEM, *KNOWLEDGE OF LIFE*

Genetic disorders give us insight into the normal, . . . like photographic negatives from which a positive picture of man's genetic constitution can be made   VICTOR MCKUSICK, *MENDELIAN INHERITANCE IN MAN*

The gene-for model has proven chimerical for most salient traits and medical conditions. It has just been unexpectedly difficult to turn observations of the genome into meaningful and potentially actionable information (Check Hayden 2008; Kolata 2012b; Lock 2005; Wade 2009). In response, "postgenomic" researchers have adopted a series of innovative approaches that embrace genetic complexity. They have turned to the study of gene-environment interaction, epigenetics, bioinformatics, metabolomics, proteomics, and many other frameworks for turning seemingly opaque genomic data into knowledge about questions we care about.

This chapter discusses a more long-standing but mostly

overlooked strategy for making sense of our genomes: conducting research on people with rare mutations to get at more general, population-level variation. People with genomically designated conditions like 22q13 and 22q11.2DS are what several geneticists have described to me as "a low hanging fruit." When a disorder is fixed to a specific mutation, there is a particularly cogent rationale for studying it: the mutation allows biomedical researchers to "control" for genetic etiology and then use the population with that condition as a kind of a natural experiment. In this way, many of the mutations discussed throughout this book have been taken up with the goal of answering huge questions about genetics and human difference. I want to unpack the way that rare, genomically designated conditions can become privileged sites of biomedical knowledge production. Following the lead of many researchers, I refer to this research strategy as "leveraging" mutations.

Leveraging is not just a fascinating research strategy, but one with very real consequences for people with genetic disorders. What's more, it is a research strategy that inherits a long legacy of using the abnormal as a lens onto more general questions in biology and medicine. By leveraging mutations, human genetics research has raised a series of novel questions. Some pertain to the pathways that lead from genetic mutations to pathophysiology and eventually disease states, while some speak to core human faculties and population-level variation. Others are enigmatic, even bizarre: Are there genetically predisposed "warriors" among us? Did the elves and pixies of medieval lore have a microdeletion on the long arm of the seventh chromosome? In other words, genetic mutations and the people who have them are being leveraged to get at a wide array of topics in contemporary biomedical research, from cardiac defects, obesity, and psychiatric disorders to aggression, sociality, and the human capacity for language.

Patient advocacy organizations, however, are not simply brought along for the ride. Sometimes, they also seek to leverage their genomic specificity and the biomedical value it confers in order to shape the direction and organization of research. In so doing, they hope to attract the huge volumes of funding and attention that it takes to garner care and services and eventually develop pharmaceutical interventions, despite their small-n status as a population.

This chapter will therefore examine the different ways in which genetic mutations can serve as "boundary objects" (Star and Griesemer 1989) that unite diverse biomedical disciplines, funding agencies, commercial actors, and patient/parent activists, all with divergent interests and frameworks for grappling with genetics, disease, and difference. Rather than just note that genetic mutations can come to serve as boundary objects, however, this chapter repeatedly asks, "Boundary objects for whom?" In this way, we see how the very meaning of a genetic mutation can be transformed by the changing networks built up around it.

This chapter focuses on three rare genetic disorders that all share developmental delay as their most clear and consistent feature. And yet, they have all been leveraged as biological models for other symptoms and traits, and therefore swept up into very different worlds of knowledge production and social action. First, I discuss the extremely rare case of Brunner syndrome, caused by a mutation in the *MAOA* gene at p11.3 on the X chromosome. Beginning in the late-1990s, Brunner syndrome was used to identify a common, low-expression *MAOA* gene variant that has been widely publicized and commercialized as a "warrior gene" that can speak to our variable proclivities for violence and aggression. Second, I turn to Williams syndrome and research into the role of the 7q11.23 genetic microdeletion with respect to its key traits: sociability, strong relative language skills, and musicality alongside intellectual disability, physical dysmorphism, and an "elfin" facial structure. Finally, I discuss how Fragile X syndrome attracts enormous levels of biomedical interest in the hope that it can provide a genetic model for neurodevelopmental disorders like autism. By way of conclusion, I discuss the contrasting "biosocial" (Rabinow [1992] 1996) outcomes of these three instances of leveraging and discuss the implications of all this for the way we understand human genetics today. As we will see, the Fragile X network pioneered a new model for mobilizing mutations as privileged sites of biomedical research—a model that has become a beacon in the field that we return to repeatedly over the next few chapters.

Making Sense of Leveraging

The topic of identifying human subjects for biomedical research was recently taken up by Steven Epstein in his outstanding book, *Inclusion* (2007a). Epstein demonstrates how agitation by marginalized constituencies made the recruitment of representative subject populations a priority for the NIH and other major research organizations. He situates this shift, in part, as the result of contestation about generalizability: "Whenever one conducts a clinical trial on a set of individuals, the assumption is that knowledge gained from a few can be extended to the many. But what sorts of extrapolations are appropriate?" (23). Epstein's fascinating research question concerns a series of debates, struggles, and changes in accepted research practices for identifying a group of human subjects who are *representative* of a larger population and making the findings that result *generalizable*. This chapter, by contrast, examines the inverse: when an acutely *un*representative population's abnormality is extrapolated or leveraged to better understand far larger categories of people, and perhaps even the population as a whole. It attends to the way contemporary "politics of difference in medical research" (Epstein's subtitle) are reconfigured when the goal is to leverage abnormality rather than assemble representative subject populations.

Although a few contemporary studies have touched on the issue of leveraging mutations, most do so only very fleetingly.[1] The better place to begin our discussion is the much older literature on the use of abnormal people as models in biological research. Leveraging genetic mutations is a continuation of a long-standing strategy. Leveraging today, however, functions in the context of transformed social and epistemic frameworks for understanding and acting on human difference. As we will see, it also takes different forms that decisively impact the kinds of biomedical research and social action that a genetic mutation can give rise to.

Abnormality in Biological Research

Leveraging pathological states has a long lineage in biological research. Reading Georges Canguilhem's 1965 *Knowledge of Life* (2008), one cannot help but be struck by the pairing of the final two chapters—"The Normal and the Pathological" and "Monstrosity and the Monstrous." In the first and far more widely cited essay, Canguilhem argues that what makes an anomaly "pathological" is not just some isolated biological property, but whether it encumbers one's capacity to thrive and achieve his goals in a certain environment. The distinction between the normal and the pathological is therefore recast as both historically and environmentally embedded. Beginning in that essay and continuing into the next, Canguilhem discusses the role of what he calls "monsters" or "monstrosity" as a tool for biological research. Canguilhem argues that, in its stark deviation from normal development, "the monster bestows upon the repetition of species, upon morphological regularity, and upon successful structuration a value all the more eminent in that we can now grasp their contingency" (2008:135). Divergence from the usual course of development therefore provides a window onto the normal, such that "whether in embryology, classification, or physiology, the eighteenth century made the monster not only an object but an instrument of science" (142). In particular, the rise of teratology and teratogeny in the nineteenth century allowed for "the scientific explanation of monstrosity": "From then on, monstrosity appears to have revealed the secret of its causes and laws, while *anomaly appears called upon to explicate the formation of the normal*, not because the normal is an attenuated form of the pathological, but because *the pathological is the normal impeded or deviated*" (143; my emphasis). This "transparency," as he puts it, "cuts monstrosity off from any relation to the monstrous," and makes it an invaluable tool of biological research. In short, Canguilhem explained, "Remove the impediment and you obtain the norm" (143).

Nobel Prize–winning biologist François Jacob makes a similar point in his magisterial 1973 work, *The Logic of Life*. Take his discussion of late nineteenth-century embryology (Jacob 1993:122–29). "The study of developmental anomalies," Jacob argued, "acquired a new importance. . . . Experimentation in physiology had usually involved modifying the natural state of an organism in order to disturb one function or another. However, the same result can be obtained by observing certain pathological conditions. . . . In many cases no experiment can reproduce a departure from normality so precisely and selectively. If knowledge of the physiological state was obviously necessary for the interpretation of pathological conditions, *the study of pathological conditions also provided a precious instrument to study biological functions*" (1973:123; my emphasis). In other words, the study of discrete pathology has long served to pry open issues of normal biological development.

Much later in the book, when Jacob is discussing the twentieth-century turn toward the molecule as the primary site of biological research, he notes how monsters can be created almost at will by altering the "programme" (genome) inside the organism rather than disrupting its structure or function from without. "Molecular biology," Jacob explains, "provokes lesions from inside the organism as a result of mutations," and uses in vitro studies "to obtain almost at will monsters in which a chosen function is damaged by mutation." Studying mutations in this way had a profound impact on the organization of bioscience, according to Jacob: physiology/morphology and biochemistry—and in vivo and in vitro research more broadly—"are no longer two independent fields, but two aspects of the same investigation. What changes had been wrought in the attitude of biology!" (265–66).

I argue that mutations like the 22q13.3 microdeletion are once again bringing together previously disjunct fields working with different biological models. But more than that, leveraging today brings in many other fields and actors as well, not least the human beings who have been diagnosed with genomically designated conditions like 22q13DS.

Genetics has always required difference and abnormality to drive knowledge production. Since Thomas Hunt Morgan's seminal work with *Drosophila melanogaster*, which identified the chromosomes as the main locus of inheritance (1915), geneticists have long used model organisms in order to study the relationship between chromosomal material and phenotypes. In recent decades, mice have emerged as arguably the primary model system in neuro-, medical, and behavior genetics (see Nelson 2018; Davies 2010; Rader 2004).[2] For obvious ethical reasons, however, deleterious mutations cannot be induced in humans. As a result, the laboratory analysis of "monsters" focuses primarily on nonhuman animals and in vitro cultures, leaving researchers to draw connections between human genotype-phenotype correlations and their mostly murine homologs.

This is the context in which mutation-specific populations (i.e., people with genomically designated conditions) have become privileged sites of biomedical research. They provide a starting point from which to map the path from genetic anomaly to illness and disease, and they inform the creation of animal models with mutations linked to everything from obesity and autism to language and aggression. This book therefore adds a new, postgenomic chapter to the long history of using "monsters" in the life sciences.

Leveraging can actually be traced back to the earliest years of genomic designation. When Patau and his colleagues (1960) reported their discovery of chromosome 13 trisomy in the foundational paper on what is now often called Patau syndrome, their discussion also noted that

we may expect that an aetiologically unique group of a limited number of "autosomal trisomy syndromes" will become established. To the human geneticist these will be of continuing interest; he will in particular look forward to cases in which the presence of known genes in the parents can be related to peculiarities in the trisomic child. It seems likely that every component anomaly of a trisomy syndrome reflects, by way of a dose effect of gene action, the presence in the respective chromosomes of *at least one gene locus that plays a prominent role in the normal development of the afflicted organ.* (792–93; my emphasis)

The authors went beyond the identification of genes that play a role in normal development. They also argued that such a strategy could provide a research platform for more common pathologies: "We suspect that many of the trisomy anomalies can also be produced individually in euploid persons by the heterozygous or homozygous presence of a suitable mutated allele of the responsible gene." By way of example, they noted that "polydactyly and hare lip with cleft palate in the present patient may be cases in point." Their argument would prove to be highly prescient: "Trisomy may become instrumental in establishing for the first time autosomal linkage groups in man" (793). In short, chromosomal mutations were immediately recognized as a potentially vital resource in the broader project of understanding the role of the genome in normal human development and common disease.

Similarly, the very first editions of Victor McKusick's *Mendelian Inheritance in Man* (now reincarnated as the authoritative online database OMIM.org) explained a key part of the "Usefulness of the Catalogs" as follows: "*Genetic disorders give us insight into the normal.* These catalogs of hereditary traits are like photographic negatives from which a positive picture of man's genetic constitution can be made." McKusick went on to explain, "As complete knowledge as possible of the normal genetic constitution of man is bound to be useful in the long run. Physicians have a unique opportunity to contribute to the knowledge of what Richard Lewontin referred to as 'man's mutational repertoire'" (1966: xiii; my emphasis). This intertwining of the normal and the pathological has been at play ever since researchers began studying the human genome.

Contemporary Genetics, Advocacy, and Commerce

How, then, can we reconcile Epstein's important point about the politicization of subject recruitment in biomedical research with the long-standing use of abnormality, or "monsters," as a platform for studying the normal in biology?

There is by now a wealth of scholarship on the complex mix of actors—spanning experts, activists, patients, politicians, and highly capitalized biotech and pharmaceutical companies—involved in research and advocacy for genetic disorders. Some have gone so far as to argue that a new form of "genetic citizenship" has emerged (Heath, Rapp, and Taussig 2004; also see Rose and Novas 2007 on "biological citizenship"). In this vein of research, Panofsky (2011) identified five mechanisms discussed in the literature on advocacy organizations dedicated to rare genetic disorders: economic resources, social-movement-style mobilization, being an early mover, lay expertise, and organizational controls. To this list, Panofsky added a sixth: the generation and strategic manipulation of "sociability"—the social relationships established between advocates and researchers. We will see all six of these mechanisms at play throughout the remainder of this book. However, this chapter makes a distinct addition to Panofsky's list of strategies that such groups use to attract resource-intensive biomedical research: they can strategically leverage their rare genetic mutation to attract researchers, media, and pharmaceutical companies interested in common forms of human difference. In order to get a sense of how leveraging mutations can function, the different ends toward which it can be directed, and the implications for our larger study of genomic designation, let's turn to our three cases.

Our Genetic Elves

With an incidence of around 1 in 7,500 (Stromme, Bjornstad, and Ramstad 2002), Williams syndrome is not unlike dozens of other rare disorders. However, its discrete genetic etiology and distinctive phenotype—marrying moderate intellectual disability and a characteristic "elfin" facial structure with unusual sociability, verbal skills, and (arguably) musicality—has made it the subject of unusually intense biomedical and popular attention. Williams syndrome shows us how genetic mutations can be leveraged to explain not only disability and impairment, but also some of our most cherished human capacities. A survey of the scientific research and social action around Williams syndrome takes us on a dizzying tour. We encounter research programs on human capacities for language, sociability, and music; a 7q11.23 microdeletion and the *ELN* gene; mouse models; neuroscience labs; mass media; independent film; foundations; a global advocacy network; the elves and pixies of medieval lore; and, last but not least, Alan Alda. How then did Williams syndrome attract so much attention from such a motley crew of actors?

Within months of each other in 1961, a team of doctors in New Zealand and another in Germany independently reported a peculiar syndrome characterized by supravalvular aortic stenosis, mental retardation, and a distinct facial appearance (Beuren, Apitz, and Harmjanz 1962; Williams, Barratt-Boyes, and Lowe 1961). What has often been called Williams-Beuren syndrome soon entered into modern nosology, though Williams syndrome is now the favored term. More recently, beginning in the mid-1990s, Williams syndrome has been associated with a microdeletion at site 11.23 on the long arm of the seventh chromosome, and particularly the *ELN* gene, which codes for the protein elastin (see Nickerson et al. 1995; Osborne et al. 1996; Lowery et al. 1995; Donnai and Karmiloff-Smith 2000).

The landmark 1995 study that identified a deletion at 7q11.23 in around 90% of Williams syndrome cases (Nickerson et al. 1995) did more than establish etiology: it actually changed Williams syndrome. As the Williams Syndrome Association itself puts it, "It is important to stress that WS is a genetic diagnosis, and an individual who does not have the gene deletion does not have Williams syndrome (i.e., a person who was clinically diagnosed with WS but was later found not [to] have a deletion in fact, does NOT have WS)."[3] Williams syndrome is now strictly tied to the 7q11.23 microdeletion, excluding some who had been given the older clinical diagnosis and including others who would have been unlikely to receive it.

Since being affixed to the 7q11.23 microdeletion, Williams syndrome has attracted attention from both biomedical researchers and popular media. But why? A paper entitled "An Experiment of Nature" (Reiss et al. 2004:5009) began by pointing out that Williams syndrome's unusual cognitive phenotype and "well-defined genetic etiology . . . provides a rare opportunity for elucidating linkages among genetic, neurobiological, and neurocognitive levels of investigation." Similarly, at a symposium on Williams syndrome held at the annual meeting of the Cognitive Neuroscience Society in 1998, it was noted that Williams syndrome "is *the stuff geneticists' dreams are made of*":

the reason for the excitement over the map [of 7q11.2] is that if we could precisely define various aspects of the hypersociability and language abilities in WMS, we could differentiate the WMS markers and thus relate a small number of genes to complex phenotypes. . . . *If it is indeed the case that this region of chromosome seven is responsible for variability in traits such as hypersociability and language ability, we might in fact be looking at part of what makes us human.* To what extent are these genes variably expressed in each of us? Could these genes have something to do with the evolution of language? (St. George 1998:203; my emphasis)

A more recent paper by several leading Williams syndrome researchers proposed to "[use] WS as an example of an 'experiment of nature'" (Järvinen-Pasley et al. 2008:2–3). Thus "behavioral neurogenetics" research on Williams syndrome "holds wider relevance in illuminating the ways in which genetic and neurobiological pathways contribute to cognition and behavior in typically developing individuals" (3). There are many similar statements scattered throughout the biomedical literature on Williams syndrome (e.g., Meyer-Lindenberg, Mervis, and Berman, 2006:391).

This approach to the study of our core human faculties via Williams syndrome has also attracted significant attention from popular media. Take the 2001 episode of the PBS series *Scientific American Frontiers* (Chedd 2001). Host Alan Alda "enters the worlds of children who are 'Growing Up Different.'"[4] After a teaser, followed by an ad by Agilent Technologies that promises to turn the Cs, As, Gs, and Ts, of our genetic code into cures for disease, Alda looks into the camera to explain the show's rationale. Trying to understand the behavior of others, he avers against the backdrop of children playing at a picnic, is one of the most difficult parts of being a kid. Alda goes on to say that, for some kids, "the difference that they're born with is so profound, that the world is more baffling than usual." By showing the viewers at home some of these children and the researchers who are studying them, he explains, "We'll see how the insights that these researchers are achieving are not only helping the kids who are different make sense of the rest of us, but they're also helping the rest of us understand what it means to be human."

Alda's first stop is the Salk Institute for Biological Studies in San Diego and a gathering of people with Williams syndrome. Still at the same picnic, Alda explains, "At first glance the kids here are like most kids—certainly they're high-spirited enough. But they are all linked by possessing a rare genetic disorder called Williams Syndrome." He goes on to note that the "cause is literally visible under a microscope" before explaining the FISH test for the 7q11.23 microdeletion. "The missing chunk contains only about twenty-five genes," he explains, "so scientists are hoping to be able to trace not only the disabilities of people with Williams Syndrome but also some of their special strengths directly back to just a handful of genes." Then we cut to a conversation between Alda and Ursula Bellugi, perhaps the world's leading Williams syndrome researcher:

Alan Alda: I mean, are you going to find out there's a gene for compassion?
Ursula: Let's call it sociability and . . . goddamn it, we might.
Alan Alda: You what?
Ursula: We might. We might.
Alan Alda: You might? [. . .] That would be amazing.
Ursula: Yeah, it would be, wouldn't it? I think that's sort of the hunt we're on. And I think that's a possibility.

Alan Alda: So you're actually *by studying carefully what the roots of Williams Syndrome*
are, you're actually finding out what the roots of qualities that all of us have are,
huh? [. . .] I mean, *you're beginning to track down how we are who we are.*
Ursula: I think that's put very, very well . . .

While this might seem like the kind of utopian rhetoric that was popular in 2001 as the Human Genome Project was nearing completion,
Bellugi was the principal investigator on a $5.5 million grant awarded
by the NIH in 2010 "to link social behavior to its underlying neurobiological and molecular genetic basis using Williams syndrome as a
model" (Salk Institute 2011).

Williams syndrome continues to attract attention from biomedical
researchers and popular media, recently serving as the subject of a major documentary (Kent 2011) and a successful French film (Archambault 2013). Oliver Sacks devoted a chapter of his book *Musicophilia*
(2007) to this syndrome, entitled "Hypermusical Species." That same
year, David Dobbs explored Williams syndrome at length in a *New York
Times* magazine piece entitled "The Gregarious Brain" (2007) explaining why a neurogeneticist like Julie Korenberg would tell him that Williams syndrome "is the most compelling model available for studying
the genetic bases of human behavior." Dobbs recounts, "After being ignored for almost three decades, Williams has recently become one of
the most energetically researched neurodevelopmental disability [*sic*]
after autism, and it is producing more compelling insights." (Dobbs
somewhat overstates the scale of research on Williams syndrome.) The
reason, he went on to explain, is that it "arises from a known genetic
cause and produces a predictable set of traits and behaviors." This
makes Williams syndrome "perfect for studying not just how genes
create intelligence and sociability but also how our powers of thought
combine with our desire to bond to create complex social behavior—a
huge arena of interaction that largely determines our fates."

Remarkably, many even believe that Williams syndrome is a modern
way of categorizing and understanding the elfin "storytelling bands of
yore." This raises a fascinating question: Did the elves and pixies de-
picted in medieval European and other sources have a 7q11.23 microdeletion? According to Howard M. Lenhoff, a biologist with more than
140 publications to his name and also the father of a girl with Williams syndrome, the answer appears to be "very probably." Drawing
on "anthologies and secondary literature sources dealing with fairies"
(1999:154), Lenhoff explains, "I found a number of recurring physical
and behavioral characteristics remarkably similar to those of individu-

als with Williams syndrome." He listed the obvious facial features as well as "seven key characteristics: stature; kindness; sensitivity; love of music, song and dance; hyperacusis; fascination with circles and spinning objects; and orderliness and concern for the future." Lenhoff left readers in no doubt that he agreed with this hypothesis: "The similarities [are] too striking to be merely coincidental," he argued (154), and a "lack of understanding of genetics and human embryology led [the authors of these tales] to invent magical and mystical explanations [of their] encounters with individuals having Williams syndrome" (157–58). Making a similar argument in a *Scientific American* piece—complete with pictures (see fig. 3.1)—Lenhoff concludes, "In the past, storytellers created folktales about imaginary beings to help explain phenomena that they did not understand. . . . Today researchers turn to Williams people in a quest to understand the unknown, hoping to decipher some of the secrets of how the brain functions" (Lenhoff et al. 1997:73). This theory is widespread among advocates,[5] bloggers, and even experts. Still, there are some dissenting voices: Steven Pinker, for example, suggested (2007:52) that "they look more like Mick Jagger."

This hypothesis about the origins of mythic, elfin creatures was favorably reported in newspapers like the *Los Angeles Times* (Boucher 1994), and it crops up in the biomedical literature as well. A paper in *Neurology* commented on the striking similarities between "Williams subjects and folk such as pixies, elves, and leprechauns. . . . One wonders if people with Williams syndrome were not the inspiration for some of these folk tales." For this and other reasons, the authors note, *"Understanding the biochemical and genetic basis for this syndrome has a fascination that reaches far beyond the syndrome itself"* (Rossen and Sarnat 1998; my emphasis).

The Williams Syndrome Association (WSA) plays a central role in all of this. They are a registered charity dedicated to raising awareness and providing support for families affected by Williams syndrome. For our purposes, it is the fourth and final of their mission statements that is most pertinent. "We will uphold our mission by: Encouraging and supporting research into a wide range of issues related to Williams syndrome."[6] The WSA provides researchers with a self-organized community of potential subjects and their families motivated to participate in research. On the part of their site aimed at researchers, they note, "Williams syndrome is gaining wider popularity in the research field due to its unique characteristics and to the wealth of information it is providing to the Human Genome project." They also provide a link

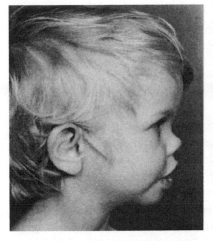
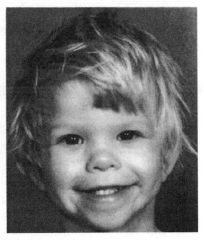
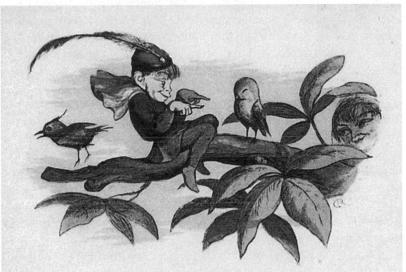

FIGURE 3.1. Williams syndrome images: (*top*) Williams syndrome facial phenotype from Kaplan et al. (2001); (*bottom*) *Poor little birdie teased*, illustrated by Richard Doyle, engraved and colored by Edmund Evans. The *Scientific American* article on Williams syndrome (Lenhoff et al. 1997:73) included an image from the Williams Syndrome Foundation UK and Doyle's "pixie" picture. (Phenotype photos copyright © 2001, SAGE Publications, reproduced by permission)

to a Williams Syndrome Registry that includes detailed clinical data on WSA members to "enable authorized researchers to find potential candidates for research programs that can offer new hope for our WS family member's [sic] well being."[7]

The WSA embraces efforts to leverage Williams syndrome and the 7q11.23 microdeletion to get at bigger questions in biomedicine and beyond: "By supporting the WSA, you will create life-changing opportunities for people with Williams syndrome and help accelerate research that could have far broader applications. . . . Because Williams syndrome is genetic, it's possible that findings from research will pinpoint genes affecting certain medical conditions (cardiovascular disease, diabetes); developmental challenges (visuo-spatial problems, ADHD); and even personality traits (affinity for music, anxiety)."[8] They also embrace the surge of attention from the media, the medical community, and biomedical researchers that comes with it. A report following a Williams syndrome feature on ABC's *20/20* program provides some insight into the role the foundation sees for media coverage. The WSA's executive director, Terry Monkaba explains (quoted in Lovett 2012),

"If we can say, 'As recently seen on *20/20*,' people tend to pay more attention. . . . Science editors have gotten more interested, so general media attention on WS went from slim to 25 touches." Monkaba reckoned WSA had received nearly as much media attention in the past year as in the previous 29. The most immediate impact has occurred in the medical community itself. "It's pieces like *20/20*'s that make all the difference," Monkaba said. "Doctors see it, they go to the website, get interested." Doctors' and the public's heightened awareness has caused more people to be diagnosed with Williams Syndrome, here and abroad, and at younger ages, she said.

As I argue in chapter 5, increasing awareness and the numbers of diagnosed patients is utterly essential for the movements built up around genomically designated conditions.

Yet it is not clear how the foundation and its registry can encourage work that truly provides hope for people with Williams syndrome and their families. They note that "Knowledge about the features, health problems, and genetic changes in people with WS has grown steadily over the past forty years. However, progress in developing new therapies has lagged behind." The WSA faces a conundrum: the condition and the population they advocate for are characterized by serious developmental and physical disabilities, but Williams syndrome is mostly used by biomedical researchers to study the genetics of its relative *strengths*. It is clear that the WSA welcomes research of all kinds. They also gladly welcome the all-important boon in awareness, membership, and resources that comes with it. Still, it remains to be seen whether the WSA-led movement will be able to leverage that research interest to help Williams syndrome patients themselves.

A Warrior Gene

In 1993 a pair of articles in the *American Journal of Human Genetics* and *Science* by Brunner and others (Brunner, Nelen, van Zandvoort, et al. 1993; Brunner, Nelen, Breakefield, et al. 1993) reported a multigenerational Dutch family with X-linked mental retardation. Brunner had been approached by a member of the family, in which a distinct condition affecting some of the males had been apparent for years (Brunner 1996). The severity of what we now call intellectual disability was mild, and the identification of X-linked mental retardation kindreds was certainly not an uncommon finding. However, Brunner et al. reported an unusual behavioral phenotype characterized by aggression and violence. Behaviors included arson, attempted rape, exhibitionism, and an attempted suicide. The urine of three of the affected males was found to have disrupted monoamine metabolism, and genetic linkage analysis indicated a disruption in the *MAOA* gene at Xp11 (Brunner, Nelen, van Zandvoort, et al. 1993:abstract). That same year, a point mutation that turned *MAOA* "off" in the probands was identified (Brunner, Nelen, Breakefield, et al. 1993). *MAOA* mutations that cause monoamine oxidase A deficiency resulting in mild intellectual disability and impulsive, aggressive behavior came to be known as Brunner syndrome.

There were fourteen affected cases in the family identified by Brunner and his colleagues, with ten of them actually exhibiting the phenotype of aggressive, impulsive, and/or violent behavior. To date, only two other families with deleterious *MAOA* mutations have been identified (Piton, Redin, and Mandel 2013:376). Unsurprisingly, then, there is very little biosocial mobilization around Brunner syndrome itself as an illness or identity category.

But the association between the *MAOA* gene and the human proclivity for aggression did not stop there. Brunner's findings led directly to further research on the *MAOA* gene and the discovery of a polymorphism in its promoter region that significantly reduces monoamine oxidase A expression (Sabol, Hu, and Hamer 1998)—a less severe variant than the fully deactivated gene found in Brunner syndrome.

Just under a decade after Brunner first reported the association between aggression and *MAOA* deactivation, a 2002 report appeared in *Science* that examined behavior in people with this less severe, but much more common *MAOA* variant (Caspi et al. 2002). That paper, entitled "Role of Genotype in the Cycle of Violence in Maltreated Children," would forever transform the history of *MAOA* research. The report examined rates of "antisocial behavior" (852) among the males in a sample of 1,037 children.[9] They compared composite antisocial behavior scores according to childhood maltreatment (none, probable, and severe) and, crucially, whether subjects carried the normal, high-functioning *MAOA* allele or the low-functioning variant that had been identified a few years earlier.

Caspi et al. found that maltreatment had a strong and statistically significant effect on the likelihood of engaging in antisocial behavior, while the low-functioning *MAOA* variant did not. However, when they examined the *interaction* between the *MAOA* variants and childhood maltreatment—"the gene-environment interaction"—a strong and significant finding emerged: if a person was maltreated as a boy, then low *MAOA* activity as measured by the variant in its promoter region becomes a strong predictor of antisocial behavior. Their provocative finding was that the *MAOA* polymorphism mediated the impact of childhood abuse on antisocial behavior. In other words, the *MAOA* findings suggested that traumatic experience combined with a genetic endowment confers the greatest risk of pathological behavior. By late-2018, the paper had been cited more than five thousand times. Despite mixed attempts to replicate Caspi et al.'s findings (e.g., Young et al. 2006), the field of research on the *MAOA* gene and aggression had come of age: from an extremely rare X-linked syndrome to an allele associated with antisocial behavior that is found in around *one-third* of the (European) male population, the *MAOA* gene was being turned toward broad questions about human aggression.

Ever since Caspi et al.'s 2002 study, the *MAOA* gene and its common, low-functioning variant have been used as a platform for discussing genetics and aggression in both biomedical journals and the popular media, not to mention the social sciences (e.g., Conley and Rauscher 2013). To take one of many examples, the United Kingdom's *Guardian* reported on Caspi et al.'s study as follows:

Scientists have identified a gene that plays a role in the cycle of violence in men abused in childhood. The discovery could explain why some survive unhappy childhoods, and go on to normal lives, while others turn to violence, crime or antisocial behaviour. . . . The discovery might help explain why violence tends to be male rather than female—the gene is found on the X chromosome. Men have only one copy of the X chromosome; women have two. The gene might also be a predictor for the ability to tolerate mental stress or trauma. The military, the police or firefighters might screen recruits to see if they have the more active form. But the discovery also raises the spectre of biology as destiny, and the argument that people with the less active form of the gene could be social risks, to be treated with drugs. (Radford 2002)

These reports almost invariably focused on the significance of the *MAOA* finding for our understanding of males' variable proclivities for aggression and violence. However, Caspi et al.'s focus on gene × environment interaction rather than genetic determinism was not lost in the coverage. As the *Los Angeles Times* put it (Singer 2002), Caspi et al.'s findings "underscore the interaction between genes and environment in influencing human behavior. 'People shouldn't think they have no choice of whether to be violent or not,' [one of the study's authors] said."

New fields quickly took up the low-functioning *MAOA* variant. A 2004 report in *Science* discussed work entitled "Tracking the Evolutionary History of the 'Warrior' Gene." The article opens with a disturbing but prescient observation: "For males, a bit of aggression and risk-taking can earn rewards—*just ask real-estate magnate Donald Trump*" (Gibbons 2004:818; my emphasis). However, the author continues, "inappropriate aggression can lead to violence, addiction, early death, and, the worst fate of all in evolutionary terms, no offspring." (Suffice it to say, at the time of writing, it is all too easy to imagine President Trump's behavior resulting in "violence, addiction, early death," and far worse evolutionary outcomes than his not having had any offspring.) We learn how research on the *MAOA* gene was being used to trace this evolutionary "balancing act" between aggression and its risks. After a German psychiatrist found a similar *MAOA* variant tied to aggression in macaques, a subsequent study took tissue samples from some six hundred apes and monkeys and found that *MAOA* variant in all apes and "Old World" monkeys, but not in "New World" ones. This was taken to indicate that the aggression-inclining gene variant has been around for at least the twenty-five million years since apes and monkeys split, but not as long as the split between New and Old World primates. Aggression and the low-expression *MAOA* variant are therefore advanced as a rare example of "balancing selection"—a genetic trait that can confer an adaptive advantage as long as it remains confined to a minority of the population. *MAOA* research now appeared to suggest that we have different biologically driven proclivities for aggression that evolved at a tandem repeat mutation at 11.3 on the short arm of the X chromosome. So where would this line of research go from here?

For several years, the *MAOA* gene's reduced-expression variant, unlike the extremely rare disrupted variant identified by Brunner et al., could only be associated with aggression and antisocial behavior in populations that had experienced some kind of environmental insult, usually some form of childhood abuse. However, a 2006 paper in *Proceedings of the National Academy of Sciences* by Meyer-Lindenberg et al. found differences in brain function between those with the high- and low-expression *MAOA* variants, independent of environmental factors. This finding, they argued, "point[s] toward potential targets for a biological approach toward violence" (6269).

Three years later, a study in the same journal by McDermott et al. (2009) catapulted *MAOA* variation to even greater levels of general significance and popular attention. Armed with seventy-eight male subjects who had been tested for *MAOA* high and low variants, a behavioral economics study design, and a plentiful supply of bottled "hot (spicy) sauce" (2118), McDermott et al. set out to examine behavioral differences in subjects' reactions to provocation. In each of four rounds, after earning money from a vocabulary task, subjects would have either 20% or 80% of their earnings taken from them by an anonymous (and in reality fictional) alter. In each round, they were given the opportunity to either punish the alter through the forcible administration of the unpleasantly spicy hot sauce or to trade the hot sauce in for money. Subjects with the "*MAOA-L*" variant had both higher rates of retaliation overall and a strong and statistically significantly higher rate of retaliation when 80% of their earnings were taken. In particular, those with the *MAOA-L* variant were more than twice as likely to administer the maximal punishment of three dollars' worth of hot sauce in response to a theft (2120). The *MAOA-L* variant's behavioral implications were no longer mediated by developmental trauma, as with Caspi et al., but simply "moderated by the environmental *stimulus*" (2120; my emphasis). This group of three political scientists and one "transdisciplinary scholar" with a background in molecular biology argued that the *MAOA-L* allele had important lessons for our understanding of genetics, evolution, and human behavior: "Although spite has been the 'neglected ugly sister of altruism,' there is good reason to expect it may have played a significant role in the evolution of human behavior. . . . Models of the evolution of cooperation might usefully be revisited with this in mind" (2122–23).

An even more recent finding by Beaver et al. (2010), using data from the National Longitudinal Study of Adolescent Health, found that males with a low-expression variant of *MAOA* were nearly twice as likely to join a gang. Furthermore, gang members with low *MAOA* expression were more than four times as likely to use a weapon in a fight, suggesting that "variation in violence among gang members may be partially circumscribed by genotype" (133). Beaver et al. situate their findings in the broader history of *MAOA* research: "An impressive amount of empirical research has demonstrated that the low *MAOA* activity alleles are associated with a range of antisocial phenotypes, including serious physical violence and criminal behavior." Their study, however, moves *MAOA* research into unfamiliar terrain for genetics research. "Although the study of gangs has largely proceeded as a sociological phenomenon," they argue that "this investigation shows that gang formation and activity, like most antisocial behaviors, involves gene-environment interplay" (133). With this latest foray into subjects that are usually the domain of disciplines far removed from genetics, *MAOA* research has clearly come a long way from its original purpose: the genomic designation of the exceedingly rare developmental disorder, Brunner syndrome.

Once again, media coverage quickly followed Beaver et al.'s paper. However, there does not appear to have been any considerable backlash. *Time* reported the finding enthusiastically (Kingsbury 2009). After gesturing toward the research "leading *MAO-A* to be referred to as the 'warrior' gene," the article explains that this latest set of findings "takes the association one step further." Beaver is quoted explaining, "For the first time, we were able to establish a direct connection between the MAO-A gene and the choosing of a violent lifestyle." Another *MAOA* researcher, Joshua Buckholtz, is quoted putting the findings in a broader context: "What all these risk gene studies show us is that genes do an important job in loading the gun. . . . But it's the environment that pulls the trigger." The piece concludes with Beaver noting that early intervention based on *MAOA* status, rather than gene-based drugs, would the best societal response to these findings. Even a critical article on the misuses of the "warrior gene" in *New Scientist* (Yong 2010) concludes, "Once we move beyond genetic determinism

. . . the discovery of genes related to mental or behavioural disorders can only improve our knowledge of ourselves. It will also help us make better decisions." For example, the author continued, "adoption agencies might want to place children with the *MAOA-L* gene with particularly stable families," and "perhaps we could tailor effective criminal rehabilitation programmes to the variant of *MAOA* and other crime related genes a prisoner has." Beaver captured the utopian, but perhaps terrifying tone of these discussions about *MAOA* variants very well: "It's a way to *harness this type of information and use it in a very progressive and humane fashion*" (37; my emphasis).

One particularly contentious area of research has been *MAOA* variants, race, and aggression. *MAOA* research ran into serious controversy in New Zealand when a 2005 conference paper (Lea et al. 2005) reported substantially higher rates of *MAOA-L* variants among Maori populations. The paper was quickly picked up by the popular press as an explanation for high Maori crime rates. Despite initially favorable coverage, a backlash ensued. Leaders from the Maori Party and leading New Zealand biologists roundly condemned the finding on both ethical and scientific grounds (e.g., *New Zealand Herald* 2009; Crampton and Parkin 2007; Stokes 2006). A detailed response (Lea and Chambers 2007) published in the *New Zealand Medical Journal* argued that "it is well recognised that historically Māori were fearless warriors," and that the "'warrior' gene hypothesis" provides "evidence of positive (natural) selection acting at the MAO-A gene. It suggests to us that Polynesian males who embark on long, dangerous canoe voyages and engaged in (and survived) war with other islander tribes carried the [*MAOA-L* variant] to Aotearoa (New Zealand), where they both increased in frequency due to rapid population growth" (7). Unsurprisingly, this response failed to placate the critics.

Subsequent studies have found that a majority of Asian/Chinese and African American males (more on this below) have *MAOA-L* variants as well. It may only be white and Hispanic populations for whom the "high-functioning" *MAOA* allele is the most common, yet we tend to treat it as "normal" and other alleles as "warrior gene" variants.

In just the last few years, *MAOA* research has taken an even more disquieting turn. It seems researchers had lumped two distinct alleles together under the moniker "*MAOA-L*." A high-functioning *MAOA* gene has four repeats (4R) of a thirty-base DNA sequence in its promoter region, while genes with three or two copies (3R or 2R) were considered low-expression (3R and 4R are by far the most common alleles).[10] A 2008 paper in the *European Journal of Human Genetics* found that most of the *MAOA-L* vs. *MAOA-H* differences in violent behavior among an Add Health sample of 2,524 participants were accounted for by the much rarer 2R allele (see esp. Guo et al. 2008). What makes this line of research so disturbing is a pair of recent papers by Beaver and his colleagues reporting a far higher rate of 2R allele carriers among African American males than Caucasian ones in the same Add Health sample. Beaver et al. (2013; Beaver, Barnes, and Boutwell 2014) found that only 0.1% of Caucasian males carried the 2R allele. In their 2013 paper, Beaver et al. reported that 5.2% out of "between N = 167 and N = 174" of the African American sample had the 2R allele. In 2014, it was 6% of 133. In both papers, Beaver and his colleagues therefore restricted their analyses to the African American males. In other words, their provocative finding that "the 2-repeat allele confers an increased risk of shooting and stabbing multiple victims over the entire life course" (Beaver, Barnes, and Boutwell 2014:262) was based on just *eight* African American males. Further confounding their results, all genotyped Add Health participants were part of sibling pairs. Other studies have reported broadly similar 2R allele rates of around 0.5% for white males and 5% for black males, though they reached more guarded conclusions (e.g., Reti et al. 2010; Roettger et al. 2016). Meanwhile, a 2014 paper in *Biological Psychiatry* (Haberstick et al. 2014) that examined the same data concluded the key associations were "probably false-positives . . . and should be interpreted with caution until replicated" (29).[11]

Despite its flimsy empirical basis, Beaver et al.'s focus on the *MAOA* 2R allele's implications for criminal behavior has already attracted the attention of several right-wing bloggers and far-right racist hate sites. For example, "WhiteRights" posted part of an article by Walter Ward on the notorious white supremacist forum Stormfront. After explaining Beaver et al.'s 2R findings, Ward writes, "If a single gene could offer some explanation as to why African-Americans commit roughly five times as many violent crimes per capita as whites, wouldn't studying it—and how to treat it—potentially save countless lives and deserve a Nobel Prize?"[12] It is all too easy to see how *MAOA*/"warrior gene" research could become a major vehicle for "scientific" racism.

In a few cases *MAOA* testing was invoked in criminal trials (Jorde 2012; Wolfson 2014), including a high-profile murder case. However, experts have pointed out that the information could be used to justify harsher sentences, leading defense attorneys to reconsider the strategy of invoking *MAOA* status in trials (Young et al. 2006). There have even been scattered calls for newborn screening that could inform early intervention for "children at risk of criminal behavior" on the grounds that "Brunner and Caspi's research can and should be used to prevent violent crime and to preserve the sense of peace and safety that is the foundation of free, civilized societies" (Brooks-Crozier 2011:531). Fortunately, prevailing norms about the use of genetic information, including the Genetic Information Nondiscrimination Act (Slaughter 2008), will severely prescribe the widespread use of *MAOA* testing by public institutions, even in the "progressive and humane" vein advocated by Young and Beaver.

The more straightforward answer to the "What is to be done?" question about *MAOA* variation and aggression seems to be—sell it. Since November 2010, Family Tree DNA has offered a "Warrior Gene" test for a mere $99 (2010). Their website, set to a backdrop of a football player, a medieval knight, and a cross-looking, middle-aged man in a dress shirt, proclaims:

WHETHER IN SPORTS, BUSINESS OR ANY OTHER ACTIVITY, SCIENTISTS FOUND THAT PEOPLE WITH THE WARRIOR GENE VARIANT WERE MORE COMBATIVE THAN THOSE WITHOUT THIS VARIANT . . . Order your DNA test now and find if you have the "Warrior Gene"![13]

Family Tree DNA had plenty of help from popular media in promoting direct-to-consumer *MAOA* variant testing. Around the same time, National Geographic's show *Explorer* aired an episode entitled "Born to Rage?" (Day 2010), in which the former Black Flag front man and famously angry Henry Rollins travels around the country meeting a coterie of easily aggravated people, as well as some Buddhist monks, exploring their anger and testing them for a low *MAOA* variant. The show opens with a montage of violent urban scenes set to a brooding soundtrack: "Are some people born to be violent?" the narrator asks. "An extraordinary discovery suggests they *are*. A single gene has been directly associated with violent behavior. This controversial science has ignited debate over genetic screening and eugenics. Now, for the first time, *Explorer* takes you inside the Warrior gene." The show features interviews with McDermott (of hot sauce fame) and discusses how "a new breed of genetic scientist is challenging" the consensus that nurture tends to trump nature in the production of human behavior, particularly with respect to violence. They are also said to be challenging the idea that "as a society, it's something we can try to put right. . . . The discovery of the warrior gene suggests that nature has a far bigger influence on our behavior than we'd ever imagined." The show reaches its denouement with the revealing of Rollins's "Warrior Gene" test result (it is negative) and concludes, "The link between our genes and our behavior makes it clear that the debate is no longer nature vs. nurture. It's nature *and* nurture that make us who we are. And whether we like it or not, the journey inside the warrior gene has only just begun." As the show's director, Philip Day, put it to *USA Today* (Della Cava 2010), "If you mix the experiences of a difficult childhood with this Warrior Gene, it can be incendiary."

On April 4, 2011, Dr. Phil aired an episode, also entitled "Born to Rage?" and again featuring Rose McDermott, with the tagline, "Scientists believe they may know why some people are quicker to anger than others. A new study suggests that inside a rageaholic's DNA, 'a warrior gene' may be pulling the strings. Could today's guests be genetically predisposed to fits of fury?" The show's web page recounts the highlights:

"We tested each of you for the warrior gene," Dr. Phil tells the three guests. "Do you think you have it?"

"I want to hope that I do," Scott says. "I think it would be a good thing," Bryan says. "You wouldn't have to look so hard to see what's troubling me." Lori says she doesn't think she has it. Even though the warrior gene is rarer in women, test results reveal that Lori does have the gene. "Well, it's an answer for me," Lori says. "It helps me understand why I get as angry as I do. It's a relief there's something linked to this anger, and it's not brought on because I want to do it." Bryan and Scott also carry the warrior gene.

"I wish it did explain everything," Dr. Phil says. "I want all three of you to know that when you have a gene, and you have the trigger from the environment, that means you're more likely, or more susceptible; it doesn't mean you have to. It doesn't mean you can't control it. . . . . This is not an excuse to go out and rage against people."

Then, at the bottom of the page we are given the link to the Family Tree DNA test, prominently featured in the show itself: "Think you could be a warrior? To get your own warrior gene testing kit, click here and enter promo code **Dr. Phil** to receive $30 off your order."[14]

In sum, Brunner syndrome and the *MAOA* mutation that causes it were leveraged toward more general issues about human aggression and violence. In all the major research papers, Brunner et al.'s findings are cited as the origin of *MAOA* research into this kind of behavior, even though Brunner himself has denounced much of that work (Brunner 1996). From *Science* and the *American Journal of Human Genetics* through to the *New York Times*, *National Geographic*, *Newsweek* (Wolfson 2014), and even Dr. Phil, gene × environment interaction is invoked to both ground statistically significant findings and create a firewall to charges of reductionism and eugenics. (Of course, one would struggle to find a genetic determinist crass enough to disagree.) The path from Brunner syndrome to the *MAOA-L* variant and then to the "warrior gene" shows how biomedical researchers can leverage rare genetic mutations in severely affected patients to create platforms for far-reaching questions and eventually even direct-to-consumer genetic tests. However, in the face of significant public criticism (see above and Horgan 2011), there is no clear path forward for serious *MAOA* research or social mobilization. We should probably hope it remains a fringe topic.

A Genetic Model for Autism

Fragile X syndrome's origins as a medical category bear a striking resemblance to those of Brunner syndrome: a woman came to a hospital in a major European city seeking support for a family member showing signs of "mental deficiency," which was understood by the family to be an inherited condition affecting only the sons. It was the early 1940s, and the setting was the National Hospital in London. Like Brunner et al. in Amsterdam half a century later, J. Purdon Martin and Julia Bell worked to establish a pedigree—the pattern of affected and non-affected members of a family that could be used to determine an inheritance mechanism. When Martin and Bell published their paper, "A Pedigree of Mental Defect Showing Sex-Linkage," on this particular family in 1943 they inaugurated a huge field of research about what came to be known as "X-linked mental retardation" or XLMR (Martin and Bell 1943). Subsequent studies identified additional cases of XLMR using family pedigrees (e.g., Allan et al. 1944; Losowsky 1961; Opitz et al. 1965), and over the last few decades, hundreds of XLMR conditions have been genomically designated according to specific mutations on the X chromosome (see Chiurazzi et al. 2008).

Unlike Brunner et al., Martin and Bell did not report a more detailed phenotype than mental deficiency, noting that "no peculiar features, either mental or physical, have been recognized which would serve to distinguish the disease which afflicts this family from other forms of dementia" (1943:154–55). Nor did they have at their disposal techniques that could identify particular genes or chromosomal abnormalities underlying these X-linked phenotypes. It was not until 1969 that a "fragile site" on the X chromosome was associated with XLMR (Lubs 1969). Even then, as historian Andrew Hogan (2016) has shown, it took years of cytogenetic and clinical refinement throughout the 1970s and 1980s to piece together a reasonably coherent syndrome—albeit one that went under a bewildering series of overlapping names. Yet, this 1943 study is now considered the foundational report on what came to be known as Martin-Bell syndrome and, nowadays, Fragile X syndrome.

Beginning in 1991, however, Fragile X came to be fixed to a distinct, newly observable mutation. From the early 1990s on, Fragile X syndrome has been diagnosed strictly according to an overabundance of trinucleotide CGG repeats (greater than two hundred rather than the normal complement of fewer than forty-five) on the *FMR1* gene at 27.3 on the long arm of the X chromosome. It is now characterized by variable degrees of intellectual disability, high rates of autism, a distinctive facial appearance, macroorchidism, and a host of other associated traits (Raspa et al. 2017; McLennan et al. 2011). This makes it quite different from the family with nonspecific XLMR described by Martin and Bell in 1943.[15]

Furthermore, what we now call the Fragile X mutation diverges considerably from the "fragile site" on the X chromosomes, which was rendered visible under a microscope beginning with Lubs's 1969 paper and with increasing reliability over the next twenty-plus years. Yet all the work done in the 1970s and 1980s to improve cytogenetic testing for the fragile site on the X chromosome and refine the differential signs for Fragile X syndrome quickly gave way to a new molecular test in the early 1990s. The new molecular test for Fragile X did not just make diagnosis clearer or easier: it remade the population and led to its being split up into at least two new, genomically designated conditions. While prevalence studies in the 1980s using cytogenetic tests for a "fragile site" put Fragile X prevalence as high as 1 in 1,000 (Webb et al. 1986), subsequent studies using molecular tests put rates at more like 1 in 4,000–6,000 (Morton et al. 1997; Turner et al. 1996).[16]

What are we to make of this? Once a molecular test for the CGG repeat expansion on *FMR1* was developed in 1991, Fragile X was *re*-designated according to a new genomic referent. "The" Fragile X mutation had changed. In fact, just a year later in 1992, the population with XLMR and the cytogenetically visible "fragile site" started being partitioned when another repeat expansion in the same chromosomal region was discovered and then associated with a "Fragile X mental retardation 2" or *FMR2* gene and a new genomically designated condition called FRAXE.[17] The genetic disorder that had been pieced together throughout the 1970s and 1980s was "split," à la the fourth pathway to genomic designation described in chapter 1, in order to correspond to more clear-cut mutations. Fragile X syndrome has been strictly tied to the CGG repeat expansion on the *FMR1* gene ever since.

However, even as it was found to be a much rarer condition than previously thought, the 1990s saw Fragile X syndrome grow in leaps and bounds as an object of biomedical research and social mobilization. Three related developments were primarily responsible. First, a reliable molecular test was developed that could identify the CGG repeat expansions at *FMR1* (Kremer et al. 1991; Rousseau et al. 1991; Verkerk et al. 1991). Furthermore, the tests developed for the CGG repeat expansion in the early 1990s allowed for the identification of "carriers." When a woman has the so-called Fragile X "premutation," her children are at high risk of having the full Fragile X mutation. (I take up the issue of Fragile X "carriers" in great detail in chapter 8.) Second, a patient advocacy group whose extraordinary success would make it a model for others to follow was starting to gain steam. Finally, Fragile X was increasingly associated with autism spectrum disorders (ASDs), which were beginning their steep rise in prevalence and salience during these years. Today, Fragile X is the most well understood and widely recognized of more than two hundred genetically specific forms of XLMR (Chiurazzi et al. 2008; Ropers and Hamel 2005). We have come a long way since Martin and Bell's work of the 1940s.

Beginning in the early 1980s, autism began to be noted in case reports on Fragile X syndrome (FXS) (Brown et al. 1982; Gillberg 1983; Hagerman and Jackson 1985; Watson et al. 1984). In 1986 a major study by Randi Hagerman and colleagues that examined fifty males with Fragile X for autism and autistic traits was published in the *American Journal of Medical Genetics* (Hagerman et al. 1986). They reported autism rates of up to ~30%, depending on the diagnostic criteria used (a wrinkle we delve into in the next chapter). Autistic traits were observed in almost all the children.

Around the same time, Hagerman founded the first major Fragile X advocacy organization along with some parents of affected children. From its humble beginnings around a kitchen table in 1984, that group would blossom into an extraordinarily successful foundation. Fast-forward twenty-five years from her first paper on Fragile X and autism, and Hagerman is able to report that "Targeted treatments to reverse these problems are currently being studied in patients with FXS. Many of these targeted treatments may also be helpful for ASD without FXS" (Hagerman, Hoem, and Hagerman 2010:9). How was so much progress made for a rare genetic disorder?

First of all, Hagerman was not reinventing the wheel. Another author on that 1986 paper was Bernard Rimland, a psychologist who played perhaps the key role in the development of autism advocacy and research as we know it (Eyal et al. 2010; Silverman 2011). Rimland's own *Autism Research Review International* reported these and future Fragile X–related findings enthusiastically (1987, 1989, 1991). Autism researchers and advocates saw in Fragile X the promise of a genetic model that could be leveraged to better understand their far more prevalent condition. Drawing on many of the repertoires pioneered by Rimland and the autism parents' movement, the new Fragile X community set off on the task of assembling an extensive network of biomedical researchers, parent activists, and political allies. As we will see in the next chapter, the rise of autism as a category of childhood abnormality, ideas about autism genetics, and Fragile X's emergence as a privileged site of biomedical research have been deeply intertwined for decades.

Crucially for us, the Fragile X community did not simply draw on the example of autism research and advocacy. They also *leveraged* the hope that their specific genetic disorder would help to unlock the biological mechanisms underlying autism more generally and welcomed the increased interest from biomedical researchers and funders that followed. As the autism "epidemic" loomed ever larger, Fragile X syndrome research grew accordingly. As a member of the US Interagency Autism Coordinating Committee put it, "There are these autism-associated disorders which are monogenic and can give really interesting insights into how the brain doesn't develop normally and actually causes symptoms that are very similar to autism" (Koroshetz 2007: 103–4). Koroshetz explained, "These genes give scientists tools. They now have animal models, mouse models that they can really work with. Sometimes having the tool is what really attracts the really good scientists. . . . So we are hoping that this research will help these kids with these really bad things, but it may also pay off in the general autism research." This rationale plays a key role in justifying Fragile X's status as a priority area for the NIH, not to mention considerable pharmaceutical investment.

At the same meeting, a leading neurobiologist representing the Simons Foundation described the situation like this (Fischbach 2007:226–28): "The great majority of autisms we just don't understand. We call them idiopathic." In the face of genetic complexity, he explained, "One [strategy] is to look at the single-gene disorders, these syndromic autisms of Fragile X, Rett syndrome, and others, and say what is it about those diseases that may teach us something about autism. . . . We are funding several groups doing that." In other words, when you know a genetic mutation often leads to autism, as is the case for Fragile X and several other genomically designated conditions, a range of experimental strategies come into view. For geneticists, and especially neurogeneticists, the preferred point of entry is an animal model. By inducing a mutation like the CGG repeat expansion in *FMR1* in mice (it is almost always mice), you can try to infer autistic behaviors, dissect and examine brain structure and function, and, eventually, begin to experiment with the compounds that can lead to pharmaceutical treatments. You can also conduct all kinds of IRB-approvable studies on people with genomically designated conditions, making small populations like the one diagnosed with Fragile X syndrome objects of intense biomedical interest.

The Fragile X community has worked hard to promote and facilitate biomedical research. The National Fragile X Foundation blossomed from a meeting at a kitchen table in 1984 to a registered charity whose 2017 revenues came in at more than $1.75 million (see National Fragile X Foundation [2018]). Their core missions are to fund and facilitate research, provide information and support to affected families, raise awareness, lobby, and establish a network of specialist clinics. They have set up a biobank and a patient registry for researchers, and they also help to recruit Fragile X patients to take part in studies. While they provide their own postdocs and research fellowships, it is their lobbying that has helped to make Fragile X syndrome a major topic of biomedical research with diverse funding streams. Taking the NIH alone, Fragile X is now priority topic with some $117 million allocated to relevant projects that were active in 2018—part of a steady upward trajectory over recent years and far more than the other two cases discussed in this chapter (see table 3.1 below). Fragile X advocates have even successfully lobbied for millions in research funding from the US Department of Defense as well as the CDC and raised their own funds from corporate donors, foundations and individual donations.

And yet, as effective as their activism has been, the potential for leveraging from Fragile X to speak to autism more generally remains something of an obligatory passage point (Callon 1986)—the sine qua non of justifying the allocation of so many resources to a rare disorder. The most recent NIH research plan for Fragile X (The Trans-NIH Fragile X Research Coordinating Group and Scientific Working Groups 2008) noted that

as many as 30 to 50 percent of individuals with FXS meet the diagnostic criteria for autism or autism spectrum disorders (ASDs). FXS is considered a portal for understanding a variety of neurobehavioral disorders, including autism, ADHD, and anxiety disorders. . . . There are currently multiple research efforts aimed at developing treatments and novel interventions. One such effort is related to clinical trials of pharmaceuticals for FXS [and] includes an ongoing cooperative agreement led by the NIMH in partnership with the NICHD, NINDS, FRAXA, and Autism Speaks to develop therapeutics related to metabotropic glutamate receptor (mGluR) antagonists to treat FXS and autism. . . . The NIH's focus on efforts to understand the relationships between FXS and autism continues through the Program Announcement (PA) soliciting research to study the *Shared Neurobiology of FXS and Autism*. (4, 8)

Later in the report, this goal was spelled out even more clearly (twice, no less): "Objective 4.5. *Leverage* knowledge about biological pathways in FXS to design treatment studies for individuals with other developmental disabilities that share common pathophysiological mechanisms" (18, 33; my emphasis). This confluence of concerted activism by Fragile X advocates and the hope that research on a rare syndrome can provide novel insights about neurodevelopmental disorders like autism has made the National Fragile X Foundation perhaps the single greatest success story among foundations for rare genetic disorders. It also made NFXF a model for others to follow.

As the NFXF's longtime and widely hailed executive director, Robert Miller, put it to me in a 2015 interview in Pleasant Hill, California, the association with autism was something of a "double-edged sword" (see chapter 5):

I'd say the best side of that sword is the side that it brings attention to Fragile X. We used that, as an organization. We utilized that relationship frequently, to help bring awareness to Fragile X, and help improve the diagnosis. . . . The mantra was always, "Hey, this is a single-gene disorder. It is relatively easier to study." I don't know if any of it's easy to study, and I'm not a scientist. If we understand this single-gene disorder, it's going to help us understand lots of other things—not just autism, but lots of other genetic disorders. That argument was used a lot, also with the NIH.

It was a very effective argument, and one that led to great success in garnering funds and attention for Fragile X.

Their work may soon bear fruit. At an autism research meeting in 2005, MIT geneticist Mark Bear and colleagues presented evidence that autistic symptoms could be reversed in "Fragile X mice." As Bear put it in a paper entitled "Toward Fulfilling the Promise of Molecular Medicine in Fragile X Syndrome" (Krueger and Bear 2011:411), "FXS is therefore poised to be the first neurobehavioral disorder in which corrective treatments have been developed from the bottom up: from gene identification to pathophysiology in animals to novel therapeutics in humans."

But, Bear explained in the very next sentence, this was not just about Fragile X: "The insights gained from FXS and other autism-related, single-gene disorders may also assist in identifying molecular mechanisms and potential treatment approaches for idiopathic autism" (Krueger and Bear 2011:411). Today, several pharmaceutical companies have brought Fragile X products to late-stage trials (e.g., Beck 2012; Javitt et al. 2011; but see Pollack 2013 on a recent setback). The company Bear founded, Seaside Therapeutics, actually had two.

Alas, trials of Fragile X compounds for the general autism population were tried and failed at Seaside, pushing them to the brink of bankruptcy. Meanwhile, despite some parents reporting enormous improvements in their children, the initial Stage 3 trials for Fragile X patients failed as well. Those improvements did not reach statistical significance for the aspect of the Fragile X phenotype that was designated as the primary target prior to the trial.

Still, advocates and researchers are undeterred. New trials are underway, with Novartis and other pharmaceutical companies joining the fray and the NIH recently funding an $11.5 million drug trial aimed at improving language skills in children with Fragile X.[18] The National Fragile X Foundation is helping recruit and refer patients for the trials. In fact, they are now lobbying the Food and Drug Administration (FDA) to modify the trials process and the very idea of outcome measurement for neuropsychiatric pharmaceutical compounds. Meanwhile, we will see how other mutations and the genomically designated conditions they index are being used to investigate autism and other neurodevelopmental disorders as well. A recent review in *Science* sums this approach up quite succinctly. The authors acknowledge that the results of "clinical trials have been mixed so far," but insist, "Only when we are able to *leverage* the heterogeneity of neurodevelopmental disorders into precision medicine, will the mechanism-based therapeutics for these disorders start to unlock success" (Sahin and Sur 2015; my emphasis).

In sum, Fragile X syndrome is leveraged by biomedical researchers to get at prevalent conditions—primarily autism but also conditions like ADHD and intellectual disability—that have proven recalcitrant to the molecular gaze. The Fragile X community has used this form of leveraging to attract the sort of research and pharmaceutical investment that can only be rationalized on the basis of Fragile X's capacity to speak to much larger populations of patients. Where this biosocial juggernaut will go next will be fascinating for the social studies of science and medicine. In any event, if Fragile X represents an important landmark in the surprisingly intractable project of "fulfilling the promise of genetic medicine" (Krueger and Bear 2011), it was accomplished via a complex admixture of social mobilization and biomedical research spanning rare disease and common forms of childhood developmental difference.

Understanding Leveraging Today

In each of our three cases, a genomically designated condition was leveraged to pry open new and far-reaching lines of research. The process of affixing a population to a specific genetic mutation can take years. However, once they were tied to genetic mutations, all the disorders discussed in this chapter were leveraged as what Star and Griesemer called "boundary objects"—"plastic" enough to allow for multiple interpretations and usages but also sufficiently "robust" to be treated as a single object of knowledge across sites (Star and Griesemer 1989; see also Star 2010). We saw how multiple scientific disciplines and a range of actors from far-flung fields converged on genetic mutations as objects of knowledge production and mobilization, leveraging them toward different ends.

Not only are the goals of the various groups divergent—so are their frameworks for understanding genomic abnormality. A genetic mutation means very different things to a molecular biologist, a neuroscientist, a pharmaceutical researcher, a doctor, a psychologist, the parent of an affected child, or a person who is grappling with its effects. Nevertheless, in each of our cases a genomically designated syndrome served as a boundary object around which a wide range of actors was able to coordinate action and pursue overlapping projects.

Simply noting that genetic mutations can serve as boundary objects that enable various projects of leveraging, however, raises the question, Boundary objects for whom? The different contours of these networks shape the research conducted on a mutation, not to mention its myriad ramifications. Leveraging always takes place in particular circuits of knowledge production and social mobilization—circuits that invariably change the very meaning of a mutation itself.

Table 3.1 summarizes some of the findings from our three cases. *MAOA-L* and Williams syndrome received far more popular attention, at least until recently, due to their roles as platforms for investigating general human traits and capacities. The Williams Syndrome Foundation and Family Tree DNA have worked to facilitate media coverage and reaped the attendant rewards. We see that Fragile X is alone in *not* being leveraged to speak to general traits. However, Fragile X researchers and advocates moved early to forge alliances with their counterparts concerned with autism. Today, it is Fragile X that has become by far the largest object of research and investment: among current NIH grants, a total of $117.3 million has been allocated for current projects that list Fragile X in their title or abstracts, compared to around $19.1 million for Williams syndrome and $9.1 million for projects related to *MAOA*.[19]

Table 3.1 only tells part of the story. In order to really grasp the contrasting ways in which these disorders have been used and transformed by leveraging projects, we need to consider the way they became boundary objects in the first place. The potential for leveraging with respect to general traits, albeit ones with very different valences, drove media interest in *MAOA* and the Williams syndrome mutation from early on. In Fragile X syndrome, by contrast, the potential for leveraging toward medical conditions, and an early alliance with autism researchers and advocates, fueled the success of groups like the National Fragile X Foundation. It was only much later that pharmaceutical concerns and the mass media took serious interest. The CGG repeat expansion on the *FMR1* gene became a major object of "biocapital" investment, not because of "overdetermined" circuits of speculation and

Table 3.1 Leveraging, alliances, and resources in *MAOA*, Williams syndrome, and Fragile X

	MAOA	Williams syndrome	Fragile X
Leveraging for general traits	✓	✓	X
Leveraging for medical issues	X	Minimal	✓
Advocacy for the disorder	X	✓	✓
Alliances with other advocates	X	Minimal	✓
Commercial uptake	DTC testing	Minimal: independent films and clinical genetic testing	Pharmaceutical industry, clinical and carrier genetic testing
Mass media interest	✓	✓	✓ (recent)
NIH current funding	$9,124,372	$19,144,233	$117,305,441

accumulation (see Sunder Rajan 2006:6), but because of a complex network that spans fields, marries rare and common disorders, and blurs distinctions between biomedical research, advocacy, and enterprise.

The differences in NIH funding reflect Fragile X syndrome's current status amid a more general *medicalization* of biological research.[20] While Canguilhem and Jacob discussed leveraging toward basic questions about the nature and organization of life, medical concerns have now become paramount in human genetics. As McKusick, often dubbed its "founding father," put it (1993:2351), "Medical genetics must be almost unique among clinical specialties; it arose out of a basic science [human genetics] rather than beginning as a craft that later sought out a scientific base." McKusick notes that human genetics has gone from a discipline dominated by PhDs to one where MDs are firmly in the majority, and the premium placed on research with medical relevance is unrivaled. In his review of early research on human chromosomes, Harper (2006:55) is even more blunt, noting that the early cytogenetics research was almost all done in basic research labs, for which "the human species had previously had no special significance and indeed was unpromising material by comparison with insect and other species with larger and fewer chromosomes." Furthermore, the field "had no incentive to pursue human cytogenetics [and] no medical links" (55). Few had even considered that cytogenetics might one day serve as a valuable clinical tool. As we saw in chapter 2, change in this regard was slow and halting.

Leveraging mutations today, by contrast, works within the context of the thorough medicalization of human genetics and biology more generally. The focus on "translation"—work that can bridge the surprisingly intractable gap between information about our genomes and the practice of medicine—is partly a result of patient advocacy, but it is also a way of justifying biomedical research expenditures. The potential to speak to common medical conditions now attracts the most powerful allies and abundant resources in the world of genetics research. None of our cases are as sociologically straightforward as the "monsters" discussed by Canguilhem and Jacob. In each instance, alliances had to be forged. Esoteric questions about human morphology and development have been sidelined in favor of topics that can attract the interest of activists, commercial enterprises, consumers, and/or mass media.

Brunner syndrome gave rise to a research program on *MAOA* variants and aggression that has probably garnered the most publicity and (for now) commercial profit of our three cases. In some ways, the scope of the biological knowledge produced by leveraging from the Brunner syndrome mutation—from social psychology and criminology to evolutionary theory and people's direct-to-consumer genetic test results—far outstrips that of our other two cases. However, there is no clear path forward for the *MAOA* network. Despite interest from media and commercial concerns, the only significant political agitation in this case has been directed *against* the use of *MAOA* gene variants as a means to understand human difference. It is certainly tempting to simply write the "warrior gene" off as "bad science" with disconcerting eugenicist undertones (Horgan 2011). That said, many *MAOA-L* studies were well-grounded in existing research paradigms and published in leading peer-reviewed journals. If it is an example of "bad science," then, like XYY research decades earlier, it is because *MAOA* researchers lacked robust alliances, stoked fears about eugenics, and came into conflict with prevailing norms and concerned activists. That said, we should certainly not fool ourselves into thinking that *MAOA-L* research on race, gender, and violence/deviance could never catch on and inform practice.

Williams syndrome has also been the topic of considerable popular media coverage for its remarkable phenotypic profile and capacity to speak to quintessentially human abilities. The Williams Syndrome Association seems primed to reap significant gains from this surge in attention and awareness. However, it has been less successful in leveraging that attention and interest toward its own goals. The challenges faced by people with Williams syndrome and their families are simply not the phenotypic features that have attracted biomedical and popular interest.

Fragile X syndrome may not receive the kind of enthralled media coverage as the "warrior gene" and Williams syndrome. Nevertheless, a robust network of researchers and advocates has been assembled around it that operates in a close, sustained alliance with the field of autism research and advocacy. Through this dual process of leveraging, the interests of Fragile X activists and researchers and their counterparts concerned with autism are coupled and advanced in unison. In this way, they have garnered hundreds of millions of dollars in funding, a huge increase in caseloads, an extensive network of clinics, and advanced-stage pharmaceutical trials. Cases like Fragile X show how leveraging is now likely to be at its most powerful when the researchers and advocates dedicated to a genomically designated condition are able to align their interests with major categories of biomedical research and social mobilization.

Conclusion

We have seen three very different paths from rare genomically designated conditions to broader understandings of the relationship between genes and human difference. Brunner syndrome and the *MAOA-L* gene variant received considerable popular attention for their supposed association with aggression, violence, and antisocial behavior, culminating in a highly publicized direct-to-consumer genetic test for a "warrior gene." Williams syndrome and the 7q11.23 microdeletion that causes it served as a platform for genetics research and popular speculation about the relationship between the genome and human capacities for language, sociability, and even musicality, bringing unprecedented attention to the condition and its foundation. Finally, Fragile X syndrome was carved out of the broader category of X-linked mental retardation before going on to become a model for autism research. In short, we have seen how rare genetic mutations are leveraged to get at enormous topics in the study of human difference. This sort of leveraging comes up again and again throughout the rest of this book. Indeed, it probably makes certain groups with genomically designated conditions among the most intensively studied people in the world.

And yet nowadays, it is leveraging projects directed toward questions of health and illness that are likely to attract the most funding and allies. As the Fragile X case illustrated, genetic mutations and the patient populations who have them can become major objects of interest not only for biomedical experts, but also for a panoply of actors and organizations ranging from patient advocates, genetic counselors, and health care providers to state agencies, charitable foundations, and highly capitalized pharmaceutical and biotechnology concerns. In fact, many other genomically designated conditions have been taken up as models for common medical issues. The next chapter shows how several have directly followed Fragile X's path as genetic models for autism, while chapter 5 explores the links between 22q11.2DS and psychiatric issues like anxiety, ADHD, and schizophrenia.

Still, it is important to keep in mind that this is not *only* an issue for neurodevelopmental and psychiatric disorders. Take Prader-Willi syndrome, which has long been fixed to 15q11–13 deletions or the total silencing of genes in those regions. A pair of recent *New York Times* articles explored the relationship between Prader-Willi syndrome and obesity (Pollack 2014; Tingley 2015). "Once an obscure and neglected disease," Pollack explains, "Prader-Willi is starting to attract more attention from scientists and pharmaceutical companies for a simple reason: It may shed some light on the much broader public health problems of overeating and obesity." The story notes that a drug targeting obesity in this population is already being developed, and goes on to quote both leading researchers and Prader-Willi patient advocates:

"These are remarkable human models of severe obesity," said Dr. Steven B. Heymsfield, a professor and former executive director of the Pennington Biomedical Research Center in Baton Rouge, La. "When we discover the underlying mechanism of these very rare disorders, they will shed light on garden-variety obesity." . . . Prader-Willi patient advocates are actively encouraging the association in hopes that linking the syndrome to the broader problem will attract more academic and pharmaceutical industry research on their disease. "The more interest and research there is on it, the more it helps our kids," said Janalee Heinemann, director of research and medical affairs at the Prader-Willi Syndrome Association.

In other words, researchers and advocates alike are doing everything they can to make the most of the connection between the mutation that causes haploinsufficiency in Prader-Willi kids and the vast public health problem represented by obesity. The second *Times* article goes into less detail, but still offers this sweeping assessment: "Prader-Willi's specific genetic roots, while not expected to explain all forms of obesity, could offer universal truths about the biology of hunger and fullness."

These leveraging projects can produce strikingly divergent forms of knowledge, with radically different implications for the people whose genetic mutation has become an object of biomedical fascination. Some of this undoubtedly has to do with the mutations themselves, but it also very much a question of the contrasting networks mobilized around them. "Biosocial" group formation may be initiated by knowledge about our genomes, as Rabinow ([1992] 1996) famously suggested. However, activism is not just one possible outcome of genetics research: it also shapes the way that knowledge about a mutation develops. Indeed, the more closely you look, the harder it is to tell where knowledge production ends and social mobilization begins. By studying these networks of research, capital accumulation, and activism, we can better understand not only how knowledge about the many is leveraged out of rare genetic mutations, but also how knowledge about those mutations is produced and used.

The model pioneered by the Fragile X network has proven to be particularly powerful, and we will soon see how many other groups dedicated to genomically designated conditions are now emulating it. In terms of reiterated fact-making, this kind of network building and collective action has emerged as the leading way to turn rare genetic mutations into truly powerful facts. Even if a mutation cannot be rendered *the* gene for an established disorder, leveraging can turn it into *a* gene for even the most common conditions. The attendant rewards can be nothing short of game-changing for a rare disease advocacy movement. Nevertheless, as the larger project of finding meaning in the human genome continues its inexorable, if unexpectedly halting march forward, we should look to the many varied ways in which rare genetic mutations can be leveraged to speak to far-reaching questions about human difference.

FOUR

The Loops That Tie: Mutations in the Trading Zone of Autism Genetics

It's our turn to leverage these mutations to get at bigger issues. Genomically designated conditions like Fragile X and XYY allow us to see how looping can change the genetic makeup of a population. As the categories through which we diagnose disease shift over time, sometimes as a result of genetics research, so too do findings about what we take genetic mutations to be etiological *for*.

To recap, rare genetic disorders can become prized models for biomedical research. A known mutation can serve as a privileged biological vista—a way into the molecular processes underlying human endowments like language, traits like aggression and sociability, or complex forms of illness like heart defects or schizophrenia. This strategy has proven especially fecund for research on autism, the *FMR1* gene, and Fragile X syndrome. It has helped turn the Fragile X movement into a beacon for other groups organized around genetic disorders.

But how do these intersections between rare mutations and common forms of illness come to pass in the first place? To answer that question, we have to delve into the social processes that made the autism–Fragile X nexus possible at a population level. For many years, autism was not something that experts saw when they examined children with Fragile X. They were not disorders that meaningfully overlapped at a symptomatological or population level, and so there was obviously very little scope for mobilizing the Fragile X mutation as a biological model for autism. The autism–Fragile X association depended upon a host of major developments in psychiatry, genetics, and patient advocacy—trends that have likewise brought dozens of rare, highly penetrant genetic mutations into autism's powerful orbit.

Yet that is just the end of the beginning for these intersections between mutations and psychiatric disorders. Toward the end of this chapter, I show how researchers and advocates for conditions like Fragile X and 22q13DS on the one hand, and their counterparts dedicated to autism on the other, had to overcome a series of obstacles in order to work so productively together. They had to create a "trading zone" where divergent goals and understandings about the very nature of disease, cause, and symptom are set aside in favor of cooperation and mutual exchange.

As Hacking convincingly argued, looping renders kinds of people like autism "moving targets." But as those kinds of people loop, they can drag their underlying biology along with them on their travels—transforming what it means to have a genetic mutation in the process. Looping remakes the relationships between mutations and kinds of people. Tracing mutations like the microdeletion at 22q13.3 or an extra Y chromosome across years and decades allows us to get at this process empirically for the first time, unveiling the rich social history underlying autism's much-discussed genetic heterogeneity.

Human Kinds and the Human Genome

Telling people that they have a genetic mutation can set a complex series of processes into motion. They suddenly have a new label, complete with its own expectations and presumed commonalities with other people who have the same mutation. However, once a group with that mutation gets together, along with their families and the biomedical experts who want to study and treat them, new forms of looping emerge. Those new groups may confound experts' expectations. New and surprising forms of difference may be discovered among its members. The population with the mutation will probably turn out to be more phenotypically varied than expected. In turn, the reported phenotype of the condition will be updated, creating new indications for a medical geneticist to work with when trying to provide a diagnosis, as well as new expectations for patients, families, and caregivers. Then, the whole process of looping begins anew. Genomic fixity may alter looping dynamics, but it certainly does not bring them to a halt.

Making matters even more complicated, clinical diagnostic categories change all the time and for all sorts of reasons (see, e.g., Fleck 1981; Aronowitz 1999; Rosenberg and Golden 1992). The very terms we use to interpret a mutation's phenotype shift along with these ever-changing practices of clinical, psychiatric, and developmental classification. Saying that a mutation causes intellectual disability in 80% of its bearers depends on the cutoff point for intellectual disability, just as labeling someone with "ADHD" depends on shifting diagnostic protocols, or diagnosing them with hypocalcemia or failure to thrive depends on the thresholds established for biochemical tests and growth chart percentiles. In other words, what it means to have a genetic mutation cannot help but depend on the way we classify human difference at a phenotypic level. If a mutation causes its bearer to have an IQ of 72, for example, then the collective decision to set the cutoff for intellectual disability at 70 rather than 75 has enormous implications for them. If we were to raise that cutoff to 80 or 85, then significant proportions of people with conditions like 22q11.2DS or even XYY syndrome would suddenly fall under a new surveillance umbrella. (This is no empty hypothetical: prior to 1973 children with IQs as high as 85 could be classified as mentally retarded [MacMillan, Semmel, and Gerber 1994:467–68].) In other words, genomically designated conditions do indeed loop, but they do so in a broader ecology of looping kinds (Hacking 1998a, 1998b). The very phenotype of a genetic mutation depends on spirals of looping that shape medical and psychiatric classification.

In order to get at the loops that tie mutations to common conditions, I explore the case of autism and its changing relationship to genetics. Autism is a human kind, as Hacking himself argued (1995:374–79), that is "doubtless biological, . . . [yet] nevertheless has been wandering." I want to show how that "wandering" had huge implications for autism's biological etiology: as autism became a more inclusive diagnosis, it began to absorb previously unrelated genetic mutations into its population.

At the same time, the way we understand and classify difference can itself be shaped by biological evidence. Since the late 1970s and the release of *DSM-III* (1980), for example, American psychiatry has been committed to the "neo-Kraepelin" idea that the classification of mental disorders should be valid—that is, reliable—and that validity would one day give way to soundness—that is, a biologically grounded system of psychiatric classification (Horwitz 2002). We are nowhere near a neat alignment between psychiatric illnesses and biology, but that is the agreed-upon goal. In practice, this means that evidence from fields like genetics has sometimes played an important role in the classification and reclassification of psychiatric disorders. This was very much the case for autism.

Hacking was well aware of the fact that biological explanations could have powerful looping effects. In one of his first pieces on looping, he gave the example of how "the scientific (biological) knowledge about alcoholics *produces a different kind of person*" (1995:373; my emphasis). But Hacking did not pursue this line of thought. In this chapter, I continue where Hacking left off and show how ascribing a genetic etiology to a condition can indeed "produce a different kind of person." However, I also show how this new kind of person can defy expectations and then loop back to change the findings of genetic research.

In order to unpack the relationship between looping and biology, we need to do two things. First, we must take stock of the way findings from genetics research can change how people understand themselves and are understood by others. This can happen, for example, because, as Hacking (1995:373) put it, "By and large, biology is exculpating"; the discovery of genetic etiology can remove stigma or the attribution of blame. This destigmatization-through-biologization is intuitively easy to grasp, and it is central to the story about autism told in this chapter. Yet destigmatization is only one way that the imputation of genetic etiology can reshape a kind of person. "Geneticization" can actually increase stigma (Phelan 2005; see Shostak, Conrad, and Horwitz 2008 for a more nuanced account). It can also have effects that go far beyond stigmatization. In the case of autism, ideas and evidence about genetic origins played a direct role in recasting it as a broad continuum of impairment and difference. Evidence from genetics research, in short, can play a direct role in the looping processes that make and remake kinds of people over time.

Second, we need to consider how changes in diagnostic practice can shift the distribution of genetic mutations found in a population. Every time diagnostic criteria are changed—whether to better capture phenotypic variability, to better conform to genetic evidence, or for any other reason—the genetic makeup of the population picked out by the classification may change as well. This new population then shifts the material conditions for understanding the genetic etiology of the classification, which in turn creates new spirals of looping. A genetic explanation for a human kind—be it a "gene for" or the invocation of heritability—will not pin it in place: it may actually initiate new loops. In the case of autism, "geneticization" had unintended consequences: it helped autism loop into a broad spectrum that is now associated with hundreds of genetic mutations.

None of this is meant to imply that diagnostic categories are in any way "false" or "fake." Hacking deployed the term "dynamic nominalism" in large part to reject the staid opposition between what is real (and therefore supposedly immutable) and what is merely a name or a social "construction" (and therefore ephemeral) (see esp. Hacking 1995, 2007). A genetic mutation may indeed be a more rigid scientific object than a psychiatric illness like depression or multiple personality disorder, but it does not follow that the of people with that mutation are stable and unchanging. Genomic designation is not a clean and timeless way of carving up human difference at its joints. There is no knowledge about human difference that is independent of its conditions of possibility or immune to looping effects. Through spirals of looping, rare genetic disorders, broad surveillance categories, and everything in between reverberate and transform one another over time.

Autism, Genetics, and Looping

At first glance, autism genetics presents us with an intractable riddle. Consider four seemingly contradictory statements about autism: (1) The estimated prevalence of autism has increased dramatically over the last four decades, from around 2–5 per 10,000 in the 1960s through 1980s to perhaps 1 in 59 American eight-year-olds today (Kogan et al. 2009:1396; Baio 2018). (2) Autism is highly heritable. Indeed, "Autism has the highest estimated heritability (>90%) among behaviorally defined neuropsychiatric disorders" (Brkanac, Raskind, and King 2008:599). (3) Autism spectrum disorders (ASDs) are highly genetically heterogeneous, having already been associated with hundreds of rare mutations in the human genome (see Betancur 2011; and below). (4) *All* of the mutations associated with autism can also cause intellectual disability and other developmental disorders (Pinto et al. 2014).

How is this possible? If autism is, at least in large part, a genetic disorder, and almost all the mutations that are known to cause it are also associated with intellectual disability, how can autism have become so much more common without a corresponding explosion in intellectual disability rates? (The rate of intellectual disability has actually declined.) What possible mechanism could make a strongly genetic disorder like autism spread so quickly and so widely?

As with any good riddle, the answer is surprisingly simple: autism itself changed.

Social scientists have already showed how diagnostic expansion accounts for much of the meteoric rise in ASD prevalence (Eyal et al. 2010; King and Bearman 2009; Silverman 2011). This helps us untangle the loops that tie autism to genetic mutations. As looping led autism to be a more inclusive category, it brought previously unassociated mutations into the autism population in the process. Our four facts about autism now fit together quite seamlessly: intellectual disability and autism only came to be associated with the same genetic mutations *after* autism looped into a far broader kind of person and absorbed a host of previously unrelated mutations into its population. The fourfold riddle is dissolved when we recognize that looping transformed the genetic makeup of the autism population.

This all had sweeping implications for conditions like 22q13DS and XYY syndrome. Autism can now be used to understand their respective phenotypes, suggest treatment strategies, and provide a rationale for the sort of leveraging projects that are so key to the Fragile X model of mobilization. In this way, looping processes radically changed the way we understand both autism and the genetic mutations that are now understood to cause it.

Geneticization, Genetic Evidence, and the Four Loops of Autism Genetics

There is ample evidence that autism's dramatic rise in prevalence can largely be attributed to diagnostic expansion (Eyal et al. 2010; Grinker 2008; King and Bearman 2009)—this is what people mean when they say things like, "We are just better at recognizing autism nowadays." Another surprisingly strong driver of autism diagnoses, it turns out, is social influence in the form of friends, schools, and neighborhood effects (Liu, King, and Bearman 2010). A powerful parents' movement has changed the image of autism, secured vast resources for treatment and educational support, and therefore made autism a more desirable diagnosis for a family seeking the best for a developmentally challenged child (Silverman 2011; Singh 2010). Finally, even the long-term demographic trend toward higher average parental age, leading to more de novo mutations, may have played a small but significant role (Liu, King, and Bearman 2010).

So where is autism genetics in all of this? Clearly, population-level changes in our chromosomes or DNA cannot account for such a dramatic change in ASD rates.[1] The human gene pool simply could not have changed enough in just a few decades to explain how a phenotype could become orders of magnitude more common throughout the United States and many other countries as well. Nevertheless, I show how genetics did help usher in autism's transformation from a rare and narrowly defined psychiatric condition to a highly common spectrum disorder. As other scholars have pointed out, the idea that autism was a genetic condition played a key role in the development of the powerful autism advocacy movement—an important driver of the increase in ASD caseloads and prevalence. In addition, I show how genetics research on autism—especially in the form of heritability studies—provided important evidence in support of diagnostic expansion. There may not have been significant changes to a whole population's gene pool, but these changes in diagnostic practice did transform the genetic makeup of the *autism population*. This transformation, in turn, made it possible to diagnose ASDs in many people with the genetic mutations discussed in this book.

This story is best told as a tale of four loops.

Loop 1—The Origins of Autism and a Parent-Blaming Etiology

Let's start at the beginning. Our first loop centers around the initial delineation of autism. Leo Kanner's foundational paper reported eleven children characterized by "profound aloneness," insistence on sameness, and "islets of ability" (Frith 2003; Kanner 1943). Kanner wrote that they "have come into the world with innate inability to form the usual, biologically provided affective contact with people" (42–43). Yet a few years later, he also noted how "the children have been brought up in emotional refrigerators, . . . [lacking] the warmth of genuine parental affection," and spoke of the children as having "removed themselves" from the world in response to this atmosphere (Kanner 1949:27). It seems as though Kanner could not decide between a psychogenic or biogenic theory of causation. As a clinician, etiology was probably not foremost in his mind. What he was sure of, however, was that the parents of autistic children, though psychiatrically normal, resembled their children in telltale ways. They were highly intelligent, but also obsessive and cold: "The parents, grandparents, and collaterals are persons strongly preoccupied with abstractions and limited in genuine interest in people" (Kanner 1943:42). This observation became received wisdom about autism and remains so to this day (despite long-standing evidence to the contrary; see Allen et al. 1971). The new human kind therefore applied to a *dyad*—the autistic person and the "autism parent," bound together through both kinship and deep similarity.

In the decades after Kanner's seminal report, the prevailing psychodynamic interpretation held that autism was caused by cold parenting, especially on the part of "refrigerator mothers" (Bettelheim 1967; Silverman 2011). This was obviously a highly stigmatizing account of autism's etiology, but it did ensure that "autism parent" became a powerful identity. This identity was the point of departure for geneticization.

Loop 2—Parent-Led Geneticization

The second loop witnessed the initial geneticization of autism. Geneticization did not originate in a bona fide biomedical research program. It was the father of an autistic boy, Bernard Rimland, who in 1964 published the first notable work arguing that autism was a genetic disorder. Rimland wanted to dispatch the psychogenic explanation of autism and the stigmatizing trope of the "refrigerator mother." To this end, he mobilized a great deal of evidence in support of a genetic explanation, though it would be years before the biomedical community followed suit in a sustained way. By exculpating parents, the project of geneticization that Rimland inaugurated had far-reaching implications. Above all, it made autism a far more desirable diagnosis and enabled the surge of autism advocacy that followed (King 2008; Silverman 2011). The very next year, Rimland founded the National Society for Autistic Children (NSAC)—the forebear of today's powerful autism advocacy organizations. The NSAC became increasingly assertive, formed ties to therapists and researchers, and saw its parent membership grow (Eyal et al. 2010:167–93). From the very start then, the geneticization of autism was animated by parents interested in destigmatization and advocacy (Bumiller 2009; Nadesan 2005).

Geneticization also allowed Rimland to argue that autistic children were not retarded. "Autistic children," he said, "were to have been endowed with unusually high intelligence" (1964, 124)—a potential inherited from their parents that had somehow gone awry (127). No wonder that the NSAC was dominated by middle-class parents or that autism was considered for many years to be a disorder characteristic of upper-middle-class families (Wing 1980). The dyad, for Rimland and those who followed in his footsteps, went from a matter of parents' cold behavior causing their child's autism to one of shared genetic inheritance (albeit differentially expressed).[2] Furthermore, the notion that the parents are similar to their children because of a common genetic endowment also bolstered the parents' claims to be unrivaled "experts on their own children" (Silverman 2011:142–43). The genetic reinterpretation of the dyad connecting autistic children and their parents therefore played a singular role in autism's early looping processes.

However, this move toward geneticization initiated a spiral of looping with unforeseen consequences. Rimland (1964:52, 59–60) insisted that autism was *rare*, because he thought rarity was evidence of genetic causation. If cold parenting caused autism, he reasoned, the diagnosis ought to be much more widespread, and it should come in gradations, as in a spectrum. But autism *was* rare, Rimland argued, and "there is an absence of gradations of infantile autism which would create 'blends' from normal to severely afflicted" (52) With hindsight, we can appreciate the irony that Rimland's foray into genetics helped to inaugurate the very looping processes that made autism both widespread and gradated.

Loop 3—Genetics Points toward Diagnostic Expansion

While geneticization began with autism parents, it was solidified as a fact through biomedical research. When genetics researchers did join the fray, however, their findings were interpreted as evidence in favor of expanding what we mean by *autism*.

In 1977, Susan Folstein and Michael Rutter published the results of a study comparing monozygotic (MZ) and dizygotic (DZ) twin concordance for autism, demonstrating that it was highly heritable (Folstein and Rutter 1977b). Their study was hailed as a breakthrough, and a summary version appeared in *Nature* (Folstein and Rutter 1977a). It is still remembered as "one of the most significant studies in the history of autism" (Feinstein 2010:147–48).

Yet there is cavernous wrinkle in this story. What Folstein and Rutter actually found was an autism heritability estimate of 36%—significant evidence of a genetic contribution, but much lower than subsequent estimates of 80–90% based on similar methods. It was a secondary finding that put the MZ concordance of a "broader linguistic or cognitive impairment" or simply "cognitive disorder (including autism)" at 82% (1977b:302, 310, 1977a:727). "What is inherited," they said, "is a form of cognitive abnormality which includes but is not restricted to autism" (1977b:310). To be more specific, four out of eleven MZ twin pairs were concordant for autism (none of the DZ pairs were). Crucially, five of the seven MZ twin pairs who were not concordant for autism per se shared some form of "cognitive impairment" (303). One could interpret what Folstein and Rutter found in 1977 as indicating that autism was only partly heritable, or that the distinction between autism, mental retardation (as it was called), and other "cognitive abnormalities" was problematic. However, this is not how the finding was cast.

As Rutter (2000) put it years later, "The replicated evidence from both twin and family studies undertaken in the 1970s and 1980s indicated both strong genetic influences and the likelihood that they applied to a phenotype that *was much broader than the traditional diagnostic category of autism. . . .* This implied that *genetic liability extended beyond 'autism proper.'* It also raised questions about the diagnostic boundaries of autism and led to an appreciation of the need to consider the likelihood of a *broader phenotype of autism*" (3–4; my emphasis). Clearly then, Folstein and Rutter interpreted their results as evidence that autism's diagnostic criteria should be considerably expanded (see also Folstein 1996). This is all the more remarkable given that only *one* of the twins with this broader "cognitive or social impairment" actually "had social or behavioral problems *at all reminiscent of autism*" (1977b:303; my emphasis). While three sets of twins presented with "social or emotional disability" (they counted shyness, dog phobia, and a "psychiatric disorder of uncertain nature"), Folstein and Rutter's findings remained ambiguous at best (1977b:303–4; Bailey et al. 1995:63).

Over the years that followed, a concerted effort was made to change autism's diagnostic criteria to capture just such a "broader phenotype." In quick succession, NSAC (Ritvo and Freeman 1977), Wing and Gould (1979), Schopler et al. (1980) and Rutter himself (1978) all published spectrum-type diagnostic criteria emphasizing a trio of communicative, social, and behavioral impairments. Significantly, all four versions were formulated in close coordination with either the British or the American parents' associations, and the main researchers sat on the *DSM-III-R* committee that radically revised autism's formal diagnostic criteria (Waterhouse et al. 1992). The finding that a broader phenotype was far more heritable therefore served as key evidence in support of diagnostic expansion.

In the years since, the observed heritability of autism increased as its diagnostic criteria were loosened. A 1995 study by Bailey et al., for which Rutter was the senior author, sought to replicate Folstein and

Rutter's 1977 findings by combining nineteen twin pairs from the original study with twenty-eight new ones. Bailey et al. found a 60% MZ concordance rate for autism proper (69% in the new sample) vs. 0% DZ concordance. Crucially, they found 92% MZ vs. 10% DZ concordance for a "broader spectrum of related cognitive or social abnormalities." They defined autism using the *ICD-10* criteria (Bailey et al. 1995:66), which were similar to the broader criteria introduced in *DSM-III-R* (1987). Because they were using a sample that significantly overlapped with the older study, this strongly suggests that the observed heritability of autism changed because its diagnostic criteria had been revised in accordance with the more heritable, "broader autism phenotype" (see also LeCouteur et al. 1996; Piven et al. 1997). More recent twin studies using even more inclusive diagnostic criteria yield ASD heritability estimates as high as at ~95% (Nordenbæk et al. 2013).[3] A broader conception of autism and increasing evidence of heritability went hand in hand.

In this way, the movement that began with Rimland's focus on genetics, rarity, and severity looped to render autism a broad, highly heritable spectrum. Genetic evidence did more than just change how we understand ASD etiology: it helped remake the category of autism itself.

Loop 4—Autism's Genetic Heterogeneity

The unintended consequences of geneticization did not end with diagnostic expansion. Rutter and Folstein's findings also served as the opening salvo in a rapid expansion of autism genetics research. Figure 4.1 shows us that there were only a handful of papers making reference to both autism and general genetics terms in their titles before the 1990s; by contrast, there are now more than two hundred such papers published annually. The precipitous increase follows the 1995 publication by Rutter and his team that replicated the seminal 1977 study and found considerably higher autism heritability (Bailey et al. 1995; above). It is the most cited paper in the history of autism genetics, while Folstein and Rutter's original 1977 papers are the only pre-1990s autism genetics studies still widely cited today.

The goal of finding a gene for autism, or perhaps a few genes for autism, animated the field for years (Singh 2015). Folstein and Rutter knew that autism was not a clear-cut case of Mendelian inheritance (1977b:309). However, they still hoped to show that autism is caused by mutations in a very small number of genes (Bailey et al. 1995:73).

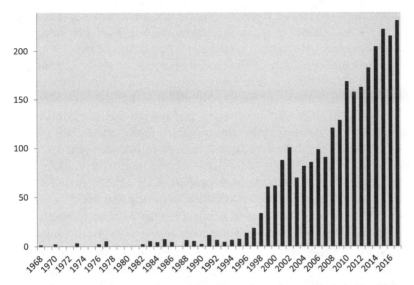

FIGURE 4.1. Papers published per year with autism and genetics terms in their titles, 1968–2017. Web of Science search string: "TI=(autis* AND (gene OR genes OR genetic* OR DNA OR GENOM* OR CHROMOSOM* OR heritab* OR mutation*))." Restricting the analysis to titles undoubtedly misses a huge swath of the field, but given the change in Web of Science capture for topic terms from 1991 onward, it is the only valid metric over this time period.

Yet, as the evidence piled up, it became clear that autism, like most common conditions, is extremely genetically heterogeneous. A review of the genetic abnormalities associated with autism noted that no less than 124 gene mutations and 55 "chromosomal loci," or CNVs, have been strongly associated with autism spectrum disorders (Pinto et al. 2014; see also Abrahams and Geschwind 2008:352–53). Meanwhile, a recent paper in *Nature Genetics* helped matters a little by reporting that only around 70% of the nearly *six thousand* de novo genomic variants identified in large samples of ASD patients and their families were likely pathogenic for autism (Kosmicki et al. 2017).

There were two sources of increased heterogeneity, both traceable to these same looping processes. First, there was undoubtedly an increase in *observed* heterogeneity. Rapid technological innovation in genetic testing and ever-increasing scrutiny of the autism population meant that more and more mutations would inevitably be found in people with ASDs. NIH funding for autism research began to increase rapidly, from $22 million in 1997 to $108 million in 2006, when the Combating

Autism Act mandated a further increase of NIH funding to $210 million by 2011.[4] Of all the fields funded by the NIH's autism budget, genetics has grown the fastest (Singh et al. 2009). In addition, 1997 also witnessed the formation of the Autism Genetic Resource Exchange—the most widely used autism repository pooling together biosamples from more than twelve thousand families—and the Autism Genetics Cooperative (AGC), a framework for pooling samples among the top researchers in the field (Silverman 2011:155–60; Singh 2010; Tabor and Lappé 2011). These developments were all initiated and driven by parent-led activist groups like Autism Speaks and Cure Autism Now. Working with organizations like the NIH, CDC, the Simons Foundation, and other major players, autism organizations have organized huge biobanks, raised their own funds for genetic research (Singh et al. 2009), and used their status as the gatekeepers of research subjects to speed up research and encourage data-sharing (Silverman 2011:155–59).[5] All considered, it is hardly surprising that researchers have found a bevy of new mutations in autism patients over the last few decades.

The second explanation of autism's increased genetic heterogeneity is more contentious. It goes like this: shifts in diagnostic practice brought previously unrelated mutations into the autism population and, in so doing, transformed its *actual* genetic heterogeneity.

Looping and the Human Genome

But how could I possibly show that a looping process transformed the actual genetic makeup of the autism population? Studying findings from autism cohorts will not do the trick: genetic testing techniques have changed too much for longitudinal comparisons, and most of the mutations in question are so rare that we would need studies of many thousands of people, going back decades, to gain statistical power on their incidence among autism patients.

Instead, we will go in the other direction, from research cohorts selected for specific genetic mutations—that is, people with genomically designated conditions—to rates of autism diagnoses. That way, we can effectively control for genetic mutations and see changes in whether or not they can be understood as genetic etiologies for autism. In this way, we will see how genetic mutations that were not associated with autism twenty, thirty, or forty years ago have nevertheless become powerfully linked to it. As ASD rates in genomically designated populations rose at a vastly higher rate than for the population as a whole, autism absorbed new genetic mutations into its ranks. This proves that looping helped create autism's staggering genetic heterogeneity.

Consider a highly telling counterfactual. If autism had remained the thing that Kanner diagnosed—a disorder that was mutually exclusive with mental retardation and defined by "cardinal symptoms"—this growth in autism's genetic heterogeneity would have been impossible. As I demonstrate below, few to none of the kids with genomically designated conditions, even the ones most strongly associated with autism, could have been diagnosed with the disorder delineated by Kanner in 1943. *All* of the mutations that are associated with autism are also linked to mental retardation. If a concurrent diagnosis of autism with mental retardation was not meaningful—as Kanner argued— diagnosing most of the people bearing these mutations with autism would simply be a nonstarter. Moreover, even as *DSM-III* (1980) permitted a concurrent diagnosis of autism with mental retardation, it still required a "pervasive lack of responsiveness to other people (autism)." It would have been impossible to identify 179 genetic mutations and chromosomal loci associated with *both* intellectual disability and ASDs (Pinto 2014; above), let alone accommodate them all within a single framework, if one was still working with Kanner's or even *DSM-III*'s conception of autism. The expanded diagnostic criteria introduced by *DSM-III-R* and *DSM-IV* (1994), as well as the creation of intermediary categories like "pervasive developmental disorder (not otherwise specified)" (PDD-NOS) and "atypical autism," formed the bridge that linked so many genetic disorders to autism.

The Pioneering Case of Fragile X

Even Fragile X—perhaps the leading biological model for autism research—could never have been strongly tied to the disorder delineated by Kanner. The first scattered reports of single individuals with Fragile X and autism were published in the early 1980s (e.g., Brown et al. 1982; Gillberg 1983; Watson et al. 1984), but they had little effect. That all began to change when a group of authors, including leading figures in autism and Fragile X research and advocacy, started to see that association as both strong and important. Take the very first study to claim that there were high rates of autism in patients with Fragile X. As we saw in the last chapter, its authors included Randi Hagerman, the leading Fragile X expert and cofounder of the main Fragile X advocacy organization, and the aforementioned autism parent/pioneer, Bernard Rimland. In 1986, Hagerman, Rimland, and coauthors reported that among the fifty males with Fragile X they were studying, "Sixteen percent of patients fulfilled all of the DSM III criteria for Infantile Autism and an additional 30% fulfilled criteria for Infantile Autism Residual State. Thirty-one percent of patients had autism using the ABC checklist. . . . Some autistic traits were seen in *almost all* of the 50 fra(X) patients." The newer and more encompassing the autism diagnostic, the more Fragile X kids could be seen as autistic. Perhaps most striking of all, they found that *"none of the patients fit the classical Kanner syndrome* as described by the E2 questionnaire" (Hagerman et al. 1986:359; my emphasis). Clearly, a meaningful link between Leo Kanner's autism and Fragile X would have been unthinkable.

For one thing, autism and mental retardation had to become valid comorbid diagnoses with the publication of *DSM-III* in 1980.[6] With widespread deinstitutionalization and the rise of early intervention, eminent autism expert/parent/activists, such as Rimland and Lorna Wing,[7] could accept the idea that autistic children would score poorly on an IQ test, but insist that these findings masked underlying abilities and forms of intelligence.[8] But that was just the first step. Rimland and Hagerman found that only 16% of Fragile X males met the *DSM-III* criteria for autism. It was the ABC checklist, which broke down Kanner's "cardinal symptoms" and "profound alones" into separate scales of variable impairments in language, communication, and repetitive behaviors, that produced the startling finding that *all* Fragile X males exhibited autistic traits, and 31% of them had full-blown autism. As this approach gained steam, more and more Fragile X probands could be given ASD diagnoses.[9]

But diagnostic expansion is just one part of the story, albeit an essential one. It would be some time before Hagerman and Rimland's findings were widely accepted in the genetics or autism communities. For years, many experts rejected the very idea of an association between Fragile X and autism. Fragile X researchers and advocates did not simply wake up one day to find that the label *autism* suddenly fit their kids. Instead, they had to actively work within the broader currents sweeping over genetics and psychiatry in order to forge an interface between autism and Fragile X.

It took years for the main autism parent organizations to embrace the link with rare genetic disorders like Fragile X. For them, as Hagerman explained in our 2015 interview in Sacramento, California, a strong association implied that autism was irreversible. As Robert Miller, the longtime executive director of the National Fragile X Foundation, told me in a 2015 interview in Pleasant Hill, California, "When I first started at the foundation . . . autism organizations really did not want to hear [about Fragile X]. They were not interested. It muddied their message."

Meanwhile, skepticism among autism researchers was just as pronounced. Hagerman explained that most psychologists just "don't order blood tests." She also recalled how "a lot of people in the autism field felt that Fragile X autism wasn't true autism." Many psychologists thought that whatever autistic features one found in Fragile X were simply artifacts of their low IQ scores, while others simply saw them as wholly distinct behavioral phenotypes (e.g., Einfeld, Molony, and Hall 1989; see Cohen et al. 1991 for a review of this debate). The idea that Fragile X might provide a window on the biology of autism would have never crossed their minds. As late as 1994, leading figures in autism genetics like Rutter dismissed the likelihood of an association between autism and Fragile X as "quite low." Rutter argued, citing Hagerman herself, "that *some* autistic features were indeed quite common but the overall clinical picture was rather different" (Rutter et al. 1994:316; emphasis in original).[10] We will see how a similar obstacle had to be overcome around twenty years later when it came to autism and 22q13.3 Deletion Syndrome.

Most rare genetic disease researchers rejected the autism–Fragile X association out of hand as well. Hagerman told me that she "talked about the high rate of autism in Fragile X," to a group of leading genetics experts at a conference in around 1986 and showed them how "it varied depending on what autism measure you utilized, and what questionnaire to diagnose autism." One senior colleague told her "it must be the air in Denver [where Hagerman was based], or the high altitude, because they didn't see any behavioral problems, and they didn't see any autism in Fragile X." In short, she explained, "they didn't believe [us] about the association with autism." Hagerman recounted a similar instance a couple of years later when a video of a child with Fragile X was shown at a conference in Sicily. In our 2015 interview, Hagerman recalled two towering figures in human genetics, Gillian Turner and John Opitz, discussing the behavioral phenotype:

Gillian said to John, "John, I don't see any autism here." John Opitz said, "You're right, Gillian, there's no autism in this patient." I thought, oh my God. I mean this patient had classical autism: hand flapping, poor eye contact, mannerisms, no social interaction, hand biting, was going like this. I thought, hmm, I wonder what these geneticists think autism is? . . . As a young researcher, it was devastating to me because I felt shot down by these great geneticists. I mean, I am great friends with all these people, but it depends on what background you come from. The thing about Fragile X is it pulls together all kinds of backgrounds.

When it came to the field of medical genetics, the idea that there were high rates of autism in the Fragile X population was quite simply a very hard sell. In sum, Hagerman and her allies faced a kind of pincer resistance from the geneticists who had pioneered the early Fragile X research *and* the psychologists who still held sway in autism research and treatment.

Eventually, things began to change. The hype surrounding the Human Genome Project gained steam throughout the 1990s. Autism advocates, confronted with the failure of much-lauded behavioral therapies for many patients, started to come around to the idea that genetics research might be their best way forward. Meanwhile, Hagerman told me that her husband, the leading Fragile X geneticist, Paul Hagerman, introduced the idea of Fragile X as a biological "portal." The National Fragile X Foundation took the idea that Fragile X could hold the genetic key to autism and ran with it. Miller told me that cultivating that link was "often discussed" by the NFXF. Hagerman said the movement "uses the idea of Fragile X as a portal" for autism and other conditions "all the time" in their outreach and lobbying. That is how Fragile X became the most studied "autism gene" and one of the most well-funded and widely recognized genetic disorders in the world.

At the same time, we should keep in mind that the Hagermans probably construed the FXS-autism findings quite differently from their colleagues focused on autism itself. Like many Fragile X researchers and advocates today, Hagerman thinks of the *FMR1* mutation as the fundamental diagnosis and autistic behaviors, mental retardation/intellectual disability, and so on, as part of the Fragile X phenotype (Brown et al. 1986:344–45; Hagerman and Jackson 1985; Reiss and Freund 1990, 1992). At NFXF conferences to this day, parents and researchers alike discuss how many children with Fragile X display autistic traits, even as they exhibit strong social proclivities that stand in sharp contrast to classic autism. As Hagerman herself put it in a Q&A session at a National Fragile X Foundation meeting in 2014, people with Fragile X do exhibit classic autistic traits like repetitive behaviors and an aversion to eye contact. However, in Fragile X an aversion to parties or meeting another person's gaze is caused by anxiety resulting from an *acute awareness* of others, not the detachment or absence of a "theory of mind" seen in classic autism.[11] Robert Miller told me how "kids with

Fragile X [generally] seek social interaction out. They may not be real good at it, but they seek it out, or at least seem to find some pleasure in it." Again, it is not Kanner's "profound aloneness," but difficulties in social interaction that tend to put children with Fragile X in range for an autism diagnosis.

Miller also stressed the importance of seeing Fragile X as the fundamental diagnosis. When I asked him during our 2015 interview how he would explain things to a parent whose child had been diagnosed with both Fragile X and autism, he replied, "Well, we'd say they have both because Fragile X Syndrome is a *medical condition*. There's a blood test. You have it or you don't. Autism is a behavioral condition. . . . It's *a description of part of what the Fragile X Syndrome is causing in your child.* Usually, people get there." NFXF and its allies work to leverage the connection to autism even as they situate autistic behavior as a symptom of the real medical condition, Fragile X.

The rise of ASD rates in FXS patients over the last thirty years from 0% to ~40% and beyond 80% in some studies did not happen automatically or straightforwardly. Like the early heritability studies on autism before it, the initial evidence linking Fragile X and autism produced ambiguous, contested results. Only now, in hindsight, can we say that Hagerman et al. established an important biomedical fact. Fragile X thrives precisely because it is at once a distinct disorder and a genetic model for autism. That is why we turn, toward the end of this chapter, to a discussion of the "trading zone" of autism genetics.

Long-Standing Mutations Pulled into Autism's Orbit

The autism–Fragile X connection, however, is just the beginning of the story. Fragile X totally dominated the early literature on autism and genomically designated conditions, but it also paved the way for a series of important new associations between ASDs and many of the mutations discussed in this book. This section traces those associations over time (for a far more detailed version of this analysis, see Navon and Eyal 2016:1444–51). By turning to these long-standing cases of genomic designation, we see how the very same rare, highly penetrant mutations that were not associated with autism prior to the fourth loop discussed above have, in recent years, become strongly tied to it. Indeed, some of these genomically designated conditions are now, like Fragile X, being leveraged as biological models for autism.

There are thirteen genomically designated conditions that have been in the literature for at least twenty years and have also been associated with autism in more than just scattered case reports. We have already encountered most of them—Fragile X, 22q13DS, 22q11.2DS, 5p–, Williams syndrome, 2q37DS, and the sex chromosome aneuploidies: XYY, XXYY, Klinefelter (XXY), and Turner (monosomy X) syndromes. The others—WAGR/11p13 Deletion Syndrome, and the Smith-Magenis and Potocki-Lupski syndromes (17p11.2 deletion and duplication)— were first reported between 1978 and 1991.

When we look at the changing ASD rates in people with those mutations over time in table 4.1, clear patterns emerge. First, almost all these mutations were associated with a "cognitive phenotype"—most often mental retardation or developmental delay—well before they were associated with autism. This association often came in the same paper that reported the mutation (nine of thirteen cases), or very shortly thereafter (four cases), with a mean "lag" time of 0.4 years. Put differently, most of these mutations were first observed in children who came to medical attention because of developmental delay, sometimes alongside various congenital abnormalities.

Second, in contrast to the very short or nonexistent gap between discovering the mutation and associating it with a cognitive phenotype, there is generally a long lag before autism is reported in probands. The mean lag is 16.6 years. In 2q37 Deletion Syndrome it only took three years, and Smith-Magenis syndrome only four, but those were among the most recently discovered mutations (1989 and 1982 respectively). For XYY, it took ten years (1961–1971), but it was another thirteen years before a report of autism in an XYY proband was ascribed anything more than incidental significance (see below). In most cases it took well over a decade, and for the 5p–, Klinefelter/XXY and Turner syndromes (monosomy X), it took more than thirty years. Yet the literature makes it clear that research subjects with genomically designated conditions *were* being evaluated for psychiatric issues, and therefore that autism would likely have been reported when "it" was encountered. Indeed, when an association with autism was first noted, usually in a case study, it was often published in a leading journal, demonstrating that finding autism in probands was considered a significant finding that was not likely to have been simply missed or ignored.

The third and most striking pattern is the marked increase over time in reported autism rates, mostly taking place after 2000, as seen in table 4.1. With the exception of Fragile X syndrome, there were no reports of autism rates in research cohorts with these conditions prior to 1990, even though most of the mutations (eleven of thirteen) were

Table 4.1 Histories of autism association in thirteen genomically designated conditions

Syndrome/locus	Mutation reported	First cognitive phenotype	First autism report	Mean ASD rate, pre-1990 (n studies)	Mean ASD rate, 1991–2000 (n)	Mean ASD rate, 2001–2012 (n)
Fragile X syndrome/ FMR1 CGG, Xq27.3	1969	1969	1980	22.2% (13)	21.5% (6)	41.7% (28)
WAGR/11p13 Deletion Syndrome	1978	1978	1995	NA (0)	NA (0)	29.9% (3)
22q13 Deletion Syndrome	1988	1988	2000	NA (0)	NA (0)	38.7% (6)
22q11.2 Deletion Syndrome	1981	1982	1998	NA (0)	NA (0)	30.4% (10)
Cri du Chat/5p– syndrome	1963	1963	1994	NA (0)	NA (0)	39.6% (2)
Williams syndrome/ 7q11.2 deletion	1993	1993	2006	NA (0)	NA (0)	26.0% (3)
Smith-Magenis/ 17p.11.2 deletion	1982	1984	1986	NA (0)	NA (0)	76% (2)
Potocki-Lupski/ 17p.11.2 duplication	1991	1992	2000	NA (0)	14.3% (1)	51.7% (2)
2q37 Deletion Syndrome	1989	1989	1992	NA (0)	12.5% (1)	52.7% (2)
XYY syndrome	1961	1962	1971	NA (0)	NA (0)	37.4% (7)
XXYY syndrome	1961	1961	1977	NA (0)	NA (0)	41.4% (4)
Klinefelter/XXY syndrome	1959	1959	1999	NA (0)	NA (0)	17.2% (9)
Turner/Monosomy X syndrome	1959	1959	1997	NA (0)	3.5% (2)	0% (1)
Summary		Mean lag	Mean lag	Total studies	Total studies	Total studies
		0.4 years	16.6 years	13	10	79

discovered earlier. During the 1991–2000 period, there was still just a trickle of case reports and only four studies reporting autism rates in syndromes other than Fragile X. From 2001, however, autism diagnoses have been reported in significant proportions of people with twelve out of thirteen of these genomically designated conditions. Fragile X saw its mean ASD rate roughly double to 41.7% across twenty-eight studies. In nine syndromes with no reports of ASD rates prior to 2001, average rates of 17.2%–76% across forty-six studies were reported over the next twelve years. In two of the three other cases, average ASD rates increased roughly four times to around 50% as well.

This trend, which is also reflected in the review literature on autism genetics,[12] provides strong evidence that the actual genetic heterogeneity of autism increased over time. It is likely just the tip of the iceberg. These thirteen long-standing disorders do not, by themselves, account for very much of autism's increased prevalence, heritability, or genetic heterogeneity. But that is not my claim. Instead, they represent strong evidence for the fourth loop described above: as autism's diagnostic criteria were broadened, the ASD population expanded to include not only greater phenotypic range, but also new mutations hitherto unassociated with autism. Human geneticists have known about these thirteen mutations for decades. They have always been understood as highly penetrant causes of developmental disorders. And yet, prior to 2001 there were very few reports of people with these mutations who were diagnosable with autism. From 2001 onward, however, many individuals carrying these mutations were being diagnosed with ASDs, thereby increasing autism's genetic heterogeneity. They go from little or no association with autism to rates that could not possibly be found in common genetic variants. The same is probably true for the hundreds of rare mutations only discovered after autism had already looped to into a broader, more heritable condition.

Three Case Studies

A few case studies will help us get a better sense of the way looping brought new mutations into the autism population. Each of the three cases outlined below revisits a genomically designated condition already encountered in chapters 1–3 and shows how they came to be tied to autism. Each one speaks to a particular looping trajectory that bound genetic mutations to autism, changing how both are understood in the process.

Williams Syndrome

In chapter 3, we saw how Williams syndrome and the 7q11.23 micro-deletion that it is tied to are being leveraged as a biological model for human language and sociality. It may come as quite a surprise then to see it listed as a disorder that overlaps with autism. It probably should come as a surprise. Williams syndrome represents a strikingly decisive confirmation of the looping argument: it is associated not only with moderate intellectual disability, cardiac problems, and a distinctive facial phenotype, but also with a distinctive trait of "hypersociality" and strong relative strengths in language and musicality.

Williams syndrome's remarkable sociability and strong language skills even led some to describe it as the "anti-autism." As the leading Williams syndrome researcher, Ursula Bellugi, and her colleagues put it (Jones et al. 2000:41), the "social behavioral contrasts between WMS and autism are striking." Indeed, they are *polar opposite groups when it comes to social behavior. . . .* WMS seek out social interaction and eye contact and, generally, do it in a polite and friendly manner." Like others in the field, they hoped that "future studies examining the neuro-anatomical differences between WMS and Autism may reveal clues to aspects of the neural and genetic bases of social behavior" (44; see also Einfeld, Tonge, and Rees 2001). Williams syndrome was seen as a biological model because it provided such a striking *contrast* to autism.

But while early discussions emphasized the differences between autism and Williams syndrome, today the two are increasingly reported as comorbid diagnoses. How did it become possible for these "polar opposite" diagnoses to overlap to such an extent? The answer is that the "overfriendliness" of individuals with Williams syndrome—their easygoing manner in approaching others and holding a conversation—is now interpreted as merely *apparent* evidence of social skills and empathy. On closer scrutiny, while they may indeed be quite well attuned to social cues, their behavior also indicates an impairment in the capacity to reason about the mental states of others. As one study put it, "social perception was spared in comparison with other neurodevelopmental disorders, but social cognition was not."

In this way, researchers were able to point to behavioral characteristics that *do* resemble autism: "problems with establishing friendships," "disinhibition and social isolation," as well as "pragmatic language impairment (PLI), including excessive chatter, the propensity for socially inappropriate statements and questions, and for talking to themselves," and generally not being well attuned to the conversational partner. In this rendering, individuals with Williams syndrome suffer from "social difficulties" that can place them on the autism spectrum. Thus: "Far from representing the polar opposite of autism, as suggested by some researchers, Williams syndrome would seem to share many of the characteristics of autistic disorder" (Laws and Bishop 2004:45; see also Tager-Flusberg and Sullivan 2000). People with Williams syndrome may be friendly and social, but they struggle to establish and maintain a group of friends; they may initiate lots of conversations, but in the wrong sort of way.

Kanner's "autistic aloneness" could never have been mistaken for Williams syndrome's "problems with establishing friendships." And yet, we have gone from Williams syndrome and autism as "polar opposite groups" (Jones 2000) to a mean ASD rate of 26% in three studies of molecularly confirmed Williams syndrome patients. One of those studies found full autism in three of thirty children with "genetically-confirmed Williams syndrome" and ASDs in 50% of those thirty cases (Klein-Tasman et al. 2009:3). Thus, an influential review of mutations associated with autism noted (Betancur 2011:55) that "50% of patients with Williams syndrome meet the diagnostic criteria for ASD." That is why the Williams Syndrome Association's executive director, Terry Monkaba, could exclaim on ABC News: "Our 15,000 kids may hold the key to helping millions with autism. . . . What a great legacy!" (cited in Lovett 2012).

XYY Syndrome

Autism's diagnostic expansion at the "high-functioning" end of the spectrum has also increased the scope for associating genomically designated conditions and ASDs. Take the case of XYY syndrome (i.e., males with an extra Y chromosome). Let's quickly recap what we learned in chapter 2. XYY had infamous beginnings in the 1960s and 1970s as a common genetic disorder that was intensively associated with aggression and antisocial behavior in the guise of a "Super Male" syndrome. Today, by contrast, XYY syndrome is primarily associated with moderately increased stature, acne, mild behavioral problems and around ten fewer IQ points than unaffected siblings (e.g., Leggett et al. 2010; Ross et al. 2012).

XYY is not as rare as Williams syndrome or the 22q13.3 microdeletion. It is found in around one in one thousand male births, so it is hardly surprising that there were a couple of case reports of autism in people with an XYY karyotype in the 1970s (Abrams and Pergament 1971; Nielsen et al. 1973; Gillberg, Winnergard, and Wahlström 1984). Researchers, however, were unanimous that the association was "most probably coincidental" (Nielsen et al. 1973:22). For the first few decades of XYY's existence as a biomedical fact, that is as far as it went.

Yet when we fast-forward to the period since 2001, we find an important association between XYY and autism. Unsurprisingly, this link was forged by the same group of blacksmiths: the argument that XYY might be a genetic cause of autism was first advanced by Christopher Gillberg (Gillberg, Winnergard, and Wahlström 1984), who was also among the first to link autism to both Williams and Fragile X syndromes. Just like the 1970s researchers, he was reporting on a single case study where an XYY proband also qualified for the diagnosis of infantile autism. However, Gillberg did not think the association was merely incidental. He connected XYY to autism in two ways. First, drawing on Lorna Wing's and Simon Baron-Cohen's speculations that autism is somehow linked to maleness, he implicated the existence of an extra Y (i.e., "male") chromosome. Second, he accounted for the fact that so few cases of XYY were found to be diagnosable with autism by resorting to the idea of a spectrum of autistic-like behaviors, ranging from severe to mild: "The XYY karyotype may predispose the child to speech-language delay, difficulties in establishing social relationships, and overall immaturity of brain development. All these features . . . are typical of autism, *but in autism there is another dimension to the problems, regarding severity and quality.* The XYY constitution per se does not cause autism, but rather might predispose the boy to milder disturbances of the kind seen in 'the triad of language and social impairment' described by Wing and Gould (1979)" (358; my emphasis). For XYY syndrome, as with Fragile X, a broader spectrum made it easier to associate autism with a genetic mutation. Still, in the mid-1980s Gillberg's speculation probably seemed far-fetched, and nobody bothered to follow up on it for almost twenty years.

Beginning in 2003, however, a series of XYY cohort studies began to report autism rates. We find no less than seven studies reporting a mean ASD rate of 37.4% in XYY cohorts between 2003 and 2012. A paper by Tartaglia et al. (2007) (leading Fragile X expert Randi Hagerman, discussed above, was a coauthor), found 36% (8/22) were diagnosable with an ASD—one with autism and seven with PDD-NOS. A 2011 study found that eleven of fifty-eight cases of XYY syndrome had an ASD, while "communicative profiles indicative of mild autistic features were common" among the remainder (Bishop et al. 2011:954). Finally, in 2012 a pair of studies found that half of a sample of forty *already* had an ASD diagnosis, while nine of the remaining twenty were in the mild-to-moderate range (Cordeiro et al. 2012; Ross et al. 2012). We have come a long way from the "coincidental" association reported in the 1970s: a 2010 *Neurology* paper by Roeltgen and Ross was entitled, "XYY Syndrome: A Possible Model for Autism Spectrum Disorder (ASD)."

Phelan-McDermid Syndrome

As we saw in chapter 1, a person who has a 22q13.3 microdeletion is diagnosed with 22q13 Deletion Syndrome, now known as Phelan-McDermid syndrome (PMS). While there are no clinical diagnostic criteria, most people with PMS have moderate-to-severe intellectual disability and severe language delays. They are also likely to suffer from a subset of many other associated symptoms. As with Fragile X, autistic behaviors are common. However, even though mental retardation was considered a core feature of the 22q13 deletion from its discovery in the late 1980s (see Phelan, Rogers, and Stevenson 1988; Phelan et al. 1992; Wong et al. 1997), it was another twelve years before an association with autism was even noted in the literature (Goizet et al. 2000).

Even then, in 2001, the medical geneticist most associated with Phelan-McDermid syndrome, Katy Phelan, specifically ruled out a comorbid autism diagnosis. She agreed that most 22q13DS patients display significant "autistic features," but also explained how "it is somewhat difficult to make an additional diagnosis of autism for children with severe to profound mental retardation," because "to be diagnosed with autism there must be qualitative differences in language and socialization when compared to non-autistic children with retardation of similar degree." This makes it very hard to see autism in people with 22q13DS. Phelan explains why: "With a cognitive age equivalent of 9.3 months, these children are expected to show some autistic-like features. All children in this sample appear to have language and socialization skills consistent with their general mental ability" (Phelan et al. 2001:95). Phelan made a nearly identical assertion two years later (Phelan 2003:2). Essentially, she agreed with the critics of Hagerman and Rimland's studies from the mid-1980s, who argued that the rates of autism in Fragile X were no different than in IQ ("cognitive age")-matched controls. A diagnosis of autism was superfluous for understanding a genetic disorder already associated with severe developmental and linguistic delays.

And yet by 2008, Phelan had abandoned her reluctance to countenance ASD diagnoses in 22q13DS patients, as long as it was cordoned off as a distinct form of "syndromic autism" (Phelan 2008:14; my emphasis): "Behavioral features of Phelan-McDermid syndrome include poor eye contact, stereotypic movements, decreased socialization, and language impairment consistent with autism spectrum disorders. . . . *Deletion 22q13 has been shown to be one of the common chromosome defects associated with autism.*" Toward the end of this chapter, we will see how Phelan came to embrace the link between autism and 22q13DS.

Reported rates of autism in PMS are now consistently in the 40%–80% range (see Sarasua et al. 2011). Meanwhile, 22q13.3 deletions are estimated to account for around 1% of ASD caseloads, and mutations in the key 22q13.3 gene, *SHANK3*, may account for another 1% (Abrahams and Geschwind 2008:344). As we will see below, the association with autism has been utterly transformative for 22q13.3/*SHANK3* research and the fortunes of the PMS Foundation.

So here we have three trajectories of diagnostic expansion that brought genomically designated conditions, which is to say rare genetic mutations, into the autism population: from hypersociality and relative strengths in language to autistic difficulties in social communication in the case of Williams syndrome; from mild behavioral challenges and slightly depressed IQ scores to high ASD rates in XYY syndrome; from mental retardation to a comorbid diagnosis of autism in the case of Fragile X. In each case, there can be little doubt that the high ASD rates now seen in these disorders would have been unthinkable twenty years ago, never mind to Kanner. Even Fragile X—*the* leading genetic cause of ASDs—could only be strongly tied to autism after a series of important changes in psychiatry and medical genetics. All these mutations have displayed fairly constant associations with mental retardation/intellectual disability at the same time as they witnessed a dramatic spike in ASD rates across disparate geographical and institutional contexts. There are no plausible environmental or biological mechanisms that could account for these shifts. The only reasonable explanation is that they were the result of a series looping processes that allowed actors to forge powerful ties between autism and these genetic mutations. In this way, tracing genomically designated conditions over time provides decisive evidence that looping transformed the genetic makeup of the autism population.

The Trading Zone of Autism Genetics

The alliances between the autism community and the much smaller networks dedicated to rare genetic disorders are not devoid of challenges. First of all, they often have to navigate divergent "disease ontologies," or conceptions of the real condition to be understood and treated. One side sees a biologically grounded genetic disorder and a series of behavioral/cognitive *symptoms* that can include autism; the other side sees a psychiatric condition that can be *caused* by mutations like Fragile X or the 22q13.3 microdeletion.

Second, even though changes in diagnostic practice have made it possible to find ASDs in kids with genetic disorders like Fragile X or XYY, there are still important phenotypic discordances. In various ways, many kids with genomically designated conditions simply do not look like classic cases of autism. Experts, advocates, and parents are well aware of these discordances. Yet they find a way to work with an autism label even as they question and qualify its meaning.

Finally, even when these two kinds of groups come together, their goals are not quite the same. Advocates for people with genetic disorders want to advance research that may lead to treatments for the rare condition that they care about. Without a doubt, they would be delighted if that research also led to a major breakthrough in autism treatment more generally. Still, that is not their primary goal. Conversely, autism experts and parents undoubtedly care about children with genetic disorders—after all, the constituencies directly overlap. However, their objective is to use a rare genetic condition's biological specificity to unpack the underlying pathophysiology of autism and treat it *tout court*.

In order to maintain these alliances, experts and advocates have created what Peter Galison would call a "trading zone" (1997)—a site for cooperation despite contrasting frameworks and goals. As Galison explains (1997:783), "Two groups can agree on rules of exchange even if they ascribe utterly different significance to the objects being exchanged; they may even disagree on the meaning of the exchange process itself. Nonetheless, the trading partners can hammer out a local coordination, despite vast global differences." Using Galison's trading zone metaphor highlights the way that autism genetics brings together a host of actors with very different goals and ways of understanding the terms *autism* and *genetics*: there are researchers from many different fields of biomedical research, clinicians with varying backgrounds in genetics, pharmaceutical companies seeking targeted compounds, politicians, and government agencies directing research funds. Last but certainly not least, we find the patients and parents, advocacy groups, and foundations dedicated to rare genetic disorders, and their counterparts dedicated to autism.[13]

In this trading zone, autism researchers and activists get human subjects bearing mutations and actual segments of DNA that they interpret as autism-susceptibility genes. Fragile X and PMS advocates, on the other hand, get ASD diagnoses and the recognition and funding that comes from being associated with autism. These two groups have been able to develop what Galison calls a "contact language" (1997:783) based around the idea of a "final common pathway." It allows them to productively talk past one another without confronting their different perspectives and goals.

Coming Together along a Common Pathway

You cannot seamlessly transition from the chimerical quest for a gene for autism to a genes-for model. In some ways, the goal remains the same. The leading autism advocacy organization is unequivocal: "Autism Speaks funds genetic and genomic research to advance understanding of autism in ways that can lead to improved diagnosis and treatment." That much is hardly surprising. At the same time, even they embrace syndromal forms of autism as important diagnoses in their own right: "Genetic testing is particularly important for detecting a number of syndromes associated with autism. These include fragile X syndrome, Angelman syndrome, tuberous sclerosis complex, chromosome 15q duplication syndrome, Pheland [sic]-McDermid syndrome and DiGeorge syndrome [i.e., 22q11.2DS]."[14]

So how can research on rare mutations helps us understand and treat autism? Some argue that autism should be split up into a handful of more biologically specific conditions. As Christopher Walsh, a professor of pediatrics at Harvard, head of genetics at Children's Hospital Boston and chair of the Scientific Advisory Board for the Autism Consortium, put it, "I would like every kid on the spectrum to have not 'autism,' but a more specific disorder" based on specific genetic mutations (cited in Pettus 2008:29). From this point of view, the genetic mutations constitute the "real" disorders, while autism is merely a symptomatic diagnosis. Indeed, the Betancur piece cited above describes itself (2011:43; my emphasis) as a "review [of] the different *genetic and genomic disorders* in which *ASDs have been described as one of the possible manifestations."* More broadly, a growing number of researchers, not to mention important institutions like the NIMH (Insel 2013), would have genomic designation play a much larger role in psychiatry.

For the most part, however, autism genetics has not fully embraced this "splitting" strategy. It is not hard to see why: autism advocacy organizations wield too much power to have their raison d'être chopped up into a series of rare genetic disorders. They control a great deal of funding and many of the DNA samples and databases that make autism genetics research possible. Take the heir to the Autism Genetic Resource Exchange (above)—the Autism Speaks–Google collaboration, MSSNG, that aims to sequence the genomes of more than ten thousand autism patients and make the data available to researchers. Here is how the Autism Speaks main page on "Genetics and Genomics" puts it: "MSSNG will identify many *subtypes of autism,* which may lead to more personalized and more accurate treatments."[15] Rutter himself was clear about the promise autism researchers see in rare genetic disorders: "There is the potential of molecular genetic findings for leads on effective drug treatments," although "the research route is likely to prove long and arduous" (2000:11).

The splitting vs. subtypes perspectives are bridged by the idea that hundreds of mutations converge on a "final common pathway" (or a small number of pathways) that can *explain* autism (see Reiss, Feinstein, and Rosenbaum 1986:725–29 for an early articulation; and Sahin and Sur 2015 for a recent review in *Science*). This burgeoning line of thought was part of a much broader turn in human genetics toward the biological *pathways* that lead from genetic mutations and wind their way through a complex set of molecular and physiological processes to common conditions (Jacob 1993:265–66; Müller-Wille and Rheinberger 2012; Rheinberger 2010:159–69). One sees this style of reasoning quite clearly in the FXS literature very soon after its molecular basis was discovered in 1991 (see Baumgardner, Green, and Reiss 1994 for a key example).

With the turn to common pathways, the potential clash embedded in the FXS-autism association—"What is it *really,* autism or FXS?"—is dissolved. Hence in a 2008 paper in *Nature Reviews Genetics*—probably the most widely cited review of autism genetics ever published—Abrahams and Geschwind described the focus on "molecularly defined syndromes" and autism *tout court* as "two contrasting but valid and *potentially compatible paradigms*" (2008:344, 352–53; my emphasis). As they explain (344; my emphasis): "Although these ASD-associated syndromes involve genes with multiple molecular functions, it seems increasingly plausible that they *converge on common biological pathways or brain circuits to give rise to ASDs.*" The turn to common pathways therefore "provides hope that common treatments could be developed for those with etiologically distinct genetic forms of ASD" (Bill and Geschwind 2009:5). The senior author of both these papers, Daniel Geschwind, has long been a leading figure in autism research and an active collaborator with the key advocacy organizations like Cure Autism Now and Autism Speaks.[16] Yet in a 2008 paper in the leading life sciences journal *Cell*, he argued that our "molecular knowledge" about autism etiology means that *"our concepts of disease boundaries are likely to change"* (Geschwind 2008:395; my emphasis).[17]

One even sees both approaches at play simultaneously. In a recent *Annual Review of Medicine* piece, Brandler and Sebat provide a detailed, emphatic endorsement of genomic reclassification (2015:491; my emphasis): "The spectrum of *autism is breaking up into quanta of related genetic disorders* . . . whose definition is based entirely on genotype." And yet, they also endorse mutation-specific research into treatments for autism itself. "[R]ecent discoveries implicating de novo mutations," they argue, are being "coupled with downstream functional work" to understand autism biology and develop targeted treatments. "The large number of ASD drugs currently in the pipeline leaves us with cautious optimism for the future" (501). In this one review piece, intended for doctors and medical researchers of all sorts, we see these two approaches to the genetics of autism functioning side by side. They argue for "breaking up" autism according to underlying genetic mutations *and* research on treatments for ASDs that target shared biological pathways.[18] In this way, Fragile X and many other genetic disorders can thrive as models for autism research.

Autism, 22q13, and the Trading Zone in Action

Over the last few years, there has been a huge surge of interest in the 22q13.3 microdeletion, its key deleted gene, *SHANK3*, and people with Phelan-McDermid syndrome/22q13DS. *SHANK3* is now considered perhaps the most highly penetrant autism gene (Vorstman et al. 2017:365), and interest from autism researchers and organizations has exploded as a result.

The Phelan-McDermid Syndrome Foundation has wholeheartedly welcomed and encouraged this interest. Geraldine Bliss, a 22q13DS parent and longtime chair of the PMSF Research Support Committee, explained the situation in an Autism Speaks Official Blog post:

There has been growing scientific interest in *SHANK3*. . . . While only about 1% of people with autism spectrum disorders (ASD) have *SHANK3* mutations, *SHANK3* research has broad implications for many people with ASD. It plays an important and central role in synaptic structure, learning, and memory in autism. It interacts with many other proteins critical to neurological functioning, and some of these proteins are already implicated in other genetic forms of autism. . . . *Unlocking the mystery of SHANK3 will open the door to understanding its partner proteins, providing a research path towards effective drug treatments for many ASDs.* (Bliss 2011; my emphasis)

Once again, the notion of a "path" helps explain why autism researchers should devote so much attention to a rare mutation. Meanwhile, *SHANK3*'s status as a genetic model for autism attracts increased awareness for PMS and opportunities for the PMSF, not to mention biomedical research and funding on a scale that would be otherwise unimaginable for such a rare disorder. The PMSF is consciously trying to emulate the autism–Fragile X alliance discussed above—it even tried to hire the longtime NFXF leader, Robert Miller, as its first paid executive director.[19]

I was fortunate enough to see this trading zone in action at a 2011 meeting at the New York Academy of Medicine. The occasion was the International Phelan-McDermid Syndrome Symposium, co-organized by the PMS Foundation and Joseph Buxbaum, a leading expert on autism genetics from the Seaver Autism Center at the Mt. Sinai School of Medicine. Geraldine Bliss—the leading organizer from the PMSF side—succinctly stated the purpose of the symposium: "to bring together our stakeholders to develop a plan to maximize scientific resources through coordinated efforts and to find the fastest pathways from bench to bedside." The sixty-odd researchers participating in the symposium came from a range of fields: neuroscience, psychiatry, pediatric medicine, biology, medical genetics, genetic counseling, basic genetics, stem cell research, physiopathology, and pharmacological development. A small cadre of long-standing 22q13DS experts and PMSF advocates were joined by dozens of autism researchers and leading advocates from organizations from Autism Speaks and the Simons Foundation Autism Research Initiative, as well as researchers from pharmaceutical companies. The president of the PMSF at the time, Sue Lomas, captured the moment in a speech at the symposium. Even though "neither [group] expected to be brought together by the worldwide efforts to understand and treat autism," she marveled at how "our paths cross today and tomorrow as we the stakeholders—families, basic scientists, clinicians and clinical researchers, trainees and representatives from the autism community—come together with a common goal: to share, learn and plot a course to treatment."

Katy Phelan herself, we saw, was for many years skeptical of the idea that kids with PMS also had autism. In an interview during the conference in New York (2011), I asked Phelan about new findings that put the rate of ASDs in PMS patients at 78%. She exclaimed, "That's amazing," especially with "so much interest and money available—I shouldn't say money—but autism is so hot right now." For autism researchers, she explained, the PMSF means you "have a community" and "you have an identified genetic cause of autism and you have a group—a defined group of individuals that are eager to participate in a study to learn more about their condition." And that, Phelan explained, is "an autism researcher's dream come true. So it is definitely beneficial to the researchers and it's beneficial to the families." In short, researchers turning to PMS as a genetic model for autism found a highly organized community ready and waiting for them—a "dream come true" indeed.

This joint endeavor did not involve an agreement about the basic relationship between condition, cause, and symptom. Catalina Betancur presented tables of the dozens upon dozens of genetic mutations associated with ASDs and explained, "Autism, like intellectual disability or epilepsy, is not a single disorder but a behavioral manifestation of tens and probably hundreds of genetic and genomic disorders" (my emphasis). For John E. Spiro of the Simons Foundation Autism Research Initiative, by contrast, genetic mutations like the 22q13.3 microdeletion or a SHANK3 mutation were "causes of Autism Spectrum Disorder." Throughout the symposium, some spoke of PMS as the real condition and autism a symptom, while others discussed ways to understand and treat autism by looking at SHANK3 disruption as one of its many causes.

Yet this deep gulf in thinking did not dampen the sense of excitement among PMSF activists. As one of the main PMSF leaders told me in an interview following the 2011 symposium in New York, "You know, this autism connection has just changed our lives . . . totally changed our lives." She also told me that, while she was certain her son was diagnosable with an ASD, she had never sought such a diagnosis because, to her, autism was merely a "subjective" classification. PMS, by contrast, is the "real, scientific" condition, grounded in causal biological mechanisms and offering the better basis for community organization, research, and treatment strategies. For her, the "deletion in chromosome 22 . . . is his diagnosis," so when "people ask me, 'Does he have autism or does he have Phelan-McDermid first? What does he have first?' And I say, 'He has Phelan-McDermid, because that is his scientific *answer, right? And possibly he has autism as a symptomatic thing.'"* The 22q13/PMS movement can clearly leverage their rare, "more specific" and "scientific" forms of illness without somehow being subsumed by the massive field of autism research and advocacy.

Even though it is only estimated to account for at most 2% of autism diagnoses (Abrahams and Geschwind 2008:344), *SHANK3* had become what Autism Speaks called "the new 'it' gene for autism" (Kouser 2011). A multi-lab discussion about building mice models of autism where the *SHANK3* gene would be turned off generated a huge rush of enthusiasm. A constant refrain in talks about mouse models goes something like, "Of course a mouse can't have autism, *but* . . ."[20] Autism is a human disorder that centrally involves language and social responsiveness. Nevertheless, a mouse's squeals, responses to the scent of other mice, and tendency to choose between isolation or proximity to other mice in experimental settings are used to infer something that resembles autism. A mouse with a genetic mutation may not have an ASD per se, but it can display behaviors that are said to resemble autism. So, when researchers show that a mouse with *SHANK3* haploinsufficiency displays autistic-like behaviors, they can claim to have developed an animal model for both PMS and autism. A paper marking a major step forward was presented at the symposium, and it was published just days later in *Nature* (Peca et al. 2011). (There are now several lines of mouse models for PMS, as well as at least one viable rat model and a primate [marmoset] model in development.) The autism and PMS devotees were all ecstatic about a possible glimpse into the pathophysiology of the condition they care so much about, not to mention the potential for developing a targeted pharmaceutical treatment. They just happened to have different conditions in mind.

No less than three speakers invoked Krueger and Bear's (2011) influential paper on Fragile X research as the first true realization of the "promise of molecular medicine" (411). Indeed, the enormous influence of the Fragile X model was evidenced with exquisite clarity by a talk subtitled "Lessons from Fragile X." Mark Bear himself, probably the leading figure in Fragile X pharmaceutical research, explained how we could go from groups with specific genetic mutations to the development of animal models and on to pharmaceutical development. He then provided a succinct, suitably future-oriented formulation of the "final common pathway" logic: "ASD is one common consequence of altered synaptic regulation of protein synthesis. . . . Do many genetic lesions converge onto a few pathophysiological mechanisms? Will treatments developed for one cause of ASD be effective for others?"

With the Fragile X model to draw upon and *SHANK3*'s status as the new "it" gene for autism, pharmaceutical studies soon took off. A phase 1 clinical trial was conducted on PMS patients at the Mount Sinai School of Medicine's Seaver Autism Center for a pharmaceutical compound, insulin-like growth factor-1 (IGF-1), that has been shown to reverse abnormalities in *SHANK3*-deleted mice (Bozdagi, Tavassoli, and Buxbaum 2013; Kolevzon 2012). In addition to physical and neurological exams and medical and psychiatric histories, PMS subjects were assessed using no less than *six* protocols that pertain to ASD diagnoses. Only children with a score of twelve or higher on the ABC Social Withdrawal subscale were included. In 2014, the trial results were published, showing that IGF-1 had significantly reduced autistic symptomatology in PMS patients and providing "proof of concept to advance knowledge about developing targeted treatments for additional causes of ASD associated with impaired synaptic development and function" (Kolevzon et al. 2014; see also Costales and Kolevzon 2015). Another such trial is underway at Harvard and Children's Hospital Boston, just as pharmaceutical products for Fragile X syndrome are still winding their way through the trials process.

Meanwhile, the PMSF has established a patient registry for research modeled on the Autism Genetic Resource Exchange and has started directly funding PMS studies. It has also worked to cultivate a small field of dedicated researchers for whom PMS is more than just a biomedical lens on ASDs.[21] As a PMSF newsletter put it, "The Foundation feels strongly that by facilitating research into autism scientists will be able to discover new things about PMS and help all PMS families, even those that don't have a member with an autism diagnosis" (Assendelft 2012). The rare genetic condition thrives on its strong relationship with a common psychiatric disorder.

The chair of the PMSF Research Committee also discussed the importance of directing biomedical research: "We can help *shape the direction* that researchers are going. We can use our 'moral authority' to get researchers to share information and resources (like animal models) that they would otherwise not be willing to share with competing researchers, and we can use our influence to bring attention to issues that need further research" (Bliss 2012). PMSF advocates know that they possess a very valuable biomedical commodity—people with a 22q13.3 microdeletion—and that they cannot let PMS become *solely* a model for autism research.

Things are moving quickly for PMS and its foundation. Their February 2013 Research Update marveled, "when we began executing our ambitious strategic plan for science just two years ago, I had no idea how quickly we would progress. With limited funds . . . *we've leveraged existing resources* to minimize capital investments by PMSF." The very next line provides insight into exactly how they "leveraged" their situation:

Did you know that 80% of individuals with Phelan-McDermid Syndrome have autism? Scientific discoveries related to the gene, *SHANK3*, implicated in Phelan-McDermid Syndrome, have been among the most promising in the field of autism research. *Not only are these discoveries hastening translational efforts related to Phelan-McDermid Syndrome, but they are yielding new insights into the causes of autism and possible treatments.* (Phelan-McDermid Syndrome Foundation 2013:2; my emphasis)

This one community update is testament to the way the PMSF has pursued its "singular purpose [t]o improve the quality of life of individuals with Phelan-McDermid syndrome" (2) by focusing on the idea that their rare genetic disorder actually holds great promise for autism research.

For better or worse, people with Phelan-McDermid syndrome may soon be receiving pharmaceutical products from researchers and companies who hope that what works for one genetically specific form of autism will work for the ASD population more generally. We will have to wait and see whether these projects, conducted in the trading zone of autism genetics, will help people with mutations like the ones discussed in this book.

Conclusion

This chapter added a new layer to the question, What does it mean to have a genetic mutation? We saw how the answer depends on prevailing forms of phenotypic classification—the way we draw distinctions between people on the basis of what they are like—and therefore on broader currents that are constantly reshaping classification in medicine, psychiatry, and many other fields. How else could we even begin to describe a mutation's phenotype? When a condition like autism changes, so too does the scope for associating it with this or that mutation. In other words, tracing the relationship between autism and genomically designated conditions over time allowed us to see how looping processes can rework mutations' phenotypes and transform the genetic makeup of populations.

The kinds of people the wider world cares about—whether it is the media, a senator, the NIH, or large business concerns—are always in flux. In the early 1970s, our fixation on issues of crime and social disorder laid the stage for an extra Y to become the "criminal chromosome" and turned XYY syndrome into a biomedical lightning rod for some of the most charged social issues of the day. In recent years, the very same mutation—and many others besides—has been swept up in the project of understanding and treating conditions like autism and ADHD. In a sense, this is hardly surprising: researchers will look to genetic mutations to get at the most common, salient, and therefore resource-rich forms of difference of the day. This sort of story is playing out in other fields as well, as we will see with ADHD,[22] schizophrenia, and 22q11.2DS in chapter 5.

Yet it is not just a question of which categories of difference receive the most attention and from whom: the kinds of people themselves may have to change before they can be tied to known mutations. When clinical classification changes, as it constantly does, so too does the very language for describing a mutation's phenotype. Yes, we care more about autism now than we did in the late 1960s and 1970s when XYY attracted so much attention as a gene for deviance and crime. But even if autism, despite its rarity, had somehow become a cause célèbre and a top NIH priority back then—if Richard Nixon had made it a campaign centerpiece and Elvis had headlined autism fund-raisers—it would not have mattered to people with the XYY, Fragile X, 5p–, or XXYY syndromes. The "autism" of the early 1970s was just not part of those syndromes' symptomatology. It was not meaningfully associated with any of those mutations.

In other words, the ties that bind mutations and psychiatric disorders depend on dual looping processes. Psychiatric categories are born, discarded, and shifted over time, changing the scope of associating them with genetic mutations. Once an association between a mutation and a psychiatric condition has been established, however, parents and expert specialists then know to look for that phenotype or symptom in kids with the relevant genomically designated condition. The association is then likely to become stronger over time. When an alliance like the autism–Fragile X one is formed, a whole host of actors become even more invested, sometimes quite literally, in the association between a mutation and a phenotype. Complicating things further still, we have seen how evidence from genetics—including knowledge about various forms of "syndromic autism"—has changed our understanding of autism itself. In short, genomically designated conditions loop, but they do so within a broader ecology composed of other kinds of people that are also looping, albeit in very different ways. As researchers aim to uncover the genomic basis of different categories of human difference, we should therefore keep in mind that they are aiming at "moving targets" (Hacking 2007)—ones that can in fact be moved by the very attempt to ascribe and uncover a genetic etiology.

The trading zone of autism genetics helps us grasp the dizzyingly complex task of conducting "translational" genetics research on psychiatric illness. A growing chorus is calling for a wholesale reclassification of disease according to genetic mutations and other kinds of biomarkers (Insel 2013). However, when we turn our attention to places where genomic designation is *already* in play, it becomes clear how naive this self-proclaimed "revolution" really is. "Fulfilling the promise of genetic medicine" at the intersection of mutation-specific disease and autism (Krueger and Bear 2011; above), it turns out, took complex processes of looping and intricate cooperation in the face of divergent goals and frameworks of understanding. Most genetic conditions are simply too rare to attract the levels of attention and resources that they need on their own. Even initiatives like the Orphan Drug Act are not strong enough to truly shift the political-economic dial of contemporary biomedicine. Meanwhile, existing psychiatric disorders like autism, schizophrenia, and ADHD will not be cast aside any time soon. As the next few chapters show, advocates and specialist experts therefore have to work within existing systems of medical classification, even if they are really thinking and dreaming in terms of a mutation and what it means for a child's future. Cooperation and interfacing, not wholesale replacement, are the name of the game in the world of genomic designation. To paraphrase Marx, the new system can only develop in the womb of the old.

FIVE

Assembling a New Kind of Person

Disney World might seem like an odd venue for a conference about a genetic mutation. For the myriad actors united by an interest in the 22q11.2 microdeletion, however, it was just the place. When you take a step back, it is easy to see why the International 22q11.2 Foundation chose Disney World for their eighth biennial meeting in 2012. For one thing, it has ample hotel space and all the requisite facilities for a small scientific conference. For another, it was a very appealing destination for families, with its nearly endless sources of entertainment for kids—those with 22q11.2 Deletion Syndrome, their siblings, and experts' children alike.

To top it all off, Disney World provided a novel twist on the usual role of mutant mice at a genetics conference. Take the main reception. After dinner, I found myself chatting to a cognitive psychologist about therapeutic approaches for children affected by rare genetic disorders. Mid-sentence, he burst out laughing and pointed to the other side of the room. A little confused, I looked over and saw a geneticist and his daughter having their picture taken with Mickey and Minnie Mouse. "That's an incredible photo," the psychologist exclaimed, "he basically slaughters mice for a living!" By then, a long line had formed as an array of biomedical researchers, clinicians, activists, parents, and children waited for their turn with the murine guests of honor.

The next day, the same room was host to a session entitled "Of Mice and Men" about 22q11.2DS research on a very different sort of mutant mice: ones with carefully induced mutations that "knock out" genes homologous to the human genes affected by the 22q11.2 microdeletion. The parents and researchers in the room were united by the hope that research on these genetically modified mice might shed light on the condition of many of the same children who had been waiting in line for Mickey and Minnie Mouse the night before. Perhaps, they hoped, the mutant lab mice would play an instrumental role in developing pharmaceutical compounds for 22q11.2DS, and maybe even a cure.

By then, we had turned to the Family Program portion of the conference and talk of increased awareness, the work of the International 22q11.2 Foundation, treatment options, and the challenges patients and their loved ones might face over the coming years. A packed, two-day program dedicated to biomedical research on 22q11.2DS, which also included an "Of Mice and Men" panel, had ended the previous evening. But even as the meeting program was split in two, the attendees, despite their very different backgrounds and stakes in 22q, were not. One of the most striking things about this meeting, focused on both biomedicine and families, was how many of the parents arrived early to hear about the latest 22q11.2DS research and how many of the researchers stayed to talk about the 22q movement and spend time with 22q families.

In the halls between sessions and during the evenings, they all exchanged stories, knowledge, and advice with one another. Kids with 22q11.2DS played together and talked to the doctors and caregivers they had come to know over the years. Almost everyone shared their hope for a future where 22q11.2DS was widely recognized, where it was diagnosed earlier and more frequently, where it had the research funding and care resources that patients needed, and where groundbreaking treatments had become available. A presentation about soon-to-be-published research on prenatal testing for 22q11.2 mutations appeared to show that 22q11.2DS prevalence is much higher than previously estimated, setting everyone abuzz. These findings seemed to vindicate the long-standing belief of many of the experts in attendance that 22q11.2DS is actually *not* a rare condition.

At the same time, there was widespread frustration. Families and experts alike discussed the daunting obstacles they faced in pursuit of the goals inscribed in the longtime motto of the International 22q11.2 Foundation: "Detection, Care, Cure." They lamented the lack of funding and attention dedicated to 22q11.2DS. They recounted the "diagnostic odyssey" many families go through before finally discovering the microdeletion at the source of all their problems, and the uphill struggles they then face trying to implement the expert 22q guidelines in local clinics and schools. In short, they wrestled with the many challenges of mobilizing a mutation.

During the five-day conference, we heard from patients, parents, activists, genetic counselors, psychologists, and representatives from numerous fields in genetics, medicine, psychiatry, and special education, as well as a celebrity photographer and a commercial pharmaceutical researcher. Outside in the parking lot sat the "22q Mystery Tour Bus." It represented the Dempster Family Foundation, which had entered the field a few years earlier when the daughter of Ryan Dempster—the longtime Chicago Cubs and, most recently, Boston Red Sox starting pitcher—was neonatally diagnosed with 22q11.2DS. This motley crew, gathered together in Orlando, Florida, hailed from all over North America, Europe, and beyond—twenty-one countries were represented in all.[1]

We learned about the DNA breakpoints that demarcate the key protein-producing regions of 22q11.2, the haploinsufficiency that causes heart defects in mice with homologous mutations, and the spectrum of physical and developmental challenges faced by people with 22q11.2DS. We also heard about the latest research on treatment, counseling, and education for people with 22q11.2DS. We heard about the pressure that had to be brought to bear in Washington to get 22q11.2DS added to the US newborn screening regime, the past and future for the foundation, a 22q summer camp, and the networks of support and mutual aid developed between families. We listened to detailed discussions of when parents should tell a child about their 22q11.2DS diagnosis and how to explain what the microdeletion means for them and their future. Finally, we heard story after story that culminated with someone being diagnosed with 22q11.2DS and their family discovering the 22q community.

In order to get at the new model for mobilizing mutations that has become so powerful in recent years, I spend most of this chapter unpacking the network organized around the 22q11.2 microdeletion. I show how that network has made great strides in building up knowledge about 22q11.2DS and then using that knowledge to inform patient evaluation, treatment, and education. However, I show how they have also run up against a range of deep-seated obstacles. Throughout, I draw on interviews with experts, clinicians, advocates, and parents as well as fieldwork visits to several 22q11.2DS-themed conferences; Elwyn Services in Pennsylvania; Children's Hospital of Philadelphia; a

US Department of Health and Human Services committee meeting on newborn screening conditions; Geisinger's Genomic Medicine Institute and Autism and Developmental Medicine Institute in Lewisburg, Pennsylvania; and a 22Q at the Zoo awareness-raising event. In addition, I draw extensively on a range of publicly available materials ranging from newsletters and websites to treatment guidelines and close readings of the pertinent biomedical literature. In this way, I use 22q11.2DS to examine the cutting edge of genomic designation today even as I try to remain true to 22q's specificity as a disease, illness, and cause.

The Rise of Genomic Designation

Studying 22q11.2DS helps us understand how some mutations have far outstripped their onetime status as esoteric objects of human genetics research. Geneticists can still simply report new mutations in the literature, and that alone is enough to constitute them as thin biomedical facts. But in order to develop a detailed understanding of a mutation's phenotype or turn it into a diagnosis that can reshape clinical practice and the lived experience of patients and their families, a mutation must be made to travel far beyond the labs and journals of contemporary genetics research. Advocates dedicated to conditions like 22q11.2DS have therefore developed innovative strategies for mobilizing mutations. By tracing mutations as facts across different times, places, and fields, we make sense of the growing but still vastly uneven power of genomic designation today.

Assembling a New Kind of Person

Turning a mutation into a robust medical condition is no easy task. The challenge for actors working in the name of conditions like 22q11.2DS is far more complex than simply garnering resources for an established disorder, even a rare one. They need to mobilize the mutation they care so much about in institutions and fields that are geared toward other systems of classification and sometimes even hostile to genetics. The seed is almost invariably planted in the biomedical literature, but it also needs to take root in alien environments like Facebook pages, support groups, pharmaceutical companies, the local doctor's office, or a special education team. To return to Fleck's example (1981:113), discussed in the introduction, we need to unpack the way an esoteric finding about a biomarker can metamorphose into a diagnosis that a doctor can relay to a patient or parent. We need to understand how a genetic mutation can become a life-changing piece of clinical information and self-knowledge, turning something like 22q11.2DS into what Hacking would call a kind of person. So how do the networks built up around mutations like the 22q11.2 microdeletion accumulate the sorts of knowledge, resources, and alliances it takes to change patients' lives?

In order to really matter, these kinds of networks must take the form of what Foucault called an "apparatus" or "*dispositif*" (Foucault 1977, 2010:19–20). When a genomically designated condition truly gains traction, it takes the form of "a thoroughly heterogenous ensemble" that brings together scientific statements, discourses, institutions, laws, and many other things besides—"in short, the said as much as the unsaid" (1977:194). For Foucault, the apparatus is a "system of relations" between these many different elements that "has as its major function at a given historical moment that of responding to an urgent need" (194–95).

As we will see, genomic designation can lead to a radically different relationship between observation, classification, and intuitional practice. It involves the philosophical commitment to make the genome a privileged site of classification—natural enough for human geneticists, perhaps, but less obvious for parents who want to understand their child's developmental difference. It responds to the need for personalized medicine and care, the need to understand difference according to biological lesions, and the need to find common cause, mutual aid, and support for people whose difference does not fit neatly into established categories. Of course, Foucault tended to deal with matters much broader in scope and scale than genomic designation.[2] Still, we can think of genomic designation as an embryonic dispositif, albeit one that is unlikely to supplant or even fully break free of its gestational environment: modern allopathic medicine.

Geneticists can isolate a mutation and delineate a new "syndrome" very quickly. Still, what it means to have that syndrome—as well as the meaning of the mutation itself—is contingent on the shifting apparatus of knowledge and practice that has been assembled around it. Complicating matters further still, those networks often grow quite unevenly across fields, locales, and institutions. In short, mutations must be made to work as categories of human difference in each and every site. The status of a genomically designated condition in the biomedical literature certainly helps. Still, mutations have to be *translated* in every new domain and locale in which actors seek to mobilize them.[3] That is how a mutation can morph from an uncertain biomedical finding into a full-fledged kind of person.

In order to make this happen, activists have developed what scholars as diverse as Tilly (e.g., 1993, 2003) and Swidler (1986, 2001) have termed "repertoires" of collective action. We will see how they have learned how to establish foundations and create specialist clinics, biobanks, and research consortia for genomically designated conditions. They have seen how invaluable it can be to forge alliances with experts and advocates interested in common, overlapping conditions like autism and ADHD. In short, they have adopted the kind of awareness-raising and outreach strategies that are most effective for genetically specific disorders. These different strategies of action were developed the hard way by pioneering advocates, creating a toolkit that can be creatively adapted by others.

The reiterated fact-making framework outlined in the introduction helps us understand how this can happen: it allows us to historically situate and then unpack the kinds of research and mobilization that can turn a mutation like the 22q11.2 microdeletion into a real kind of person. In other words, we can see how the meaning of a genetic mutation depends on the work of a dedicated network, even as it is caught up in the vast currents sweeping over science, medicine, and society.

New Opportunities and Enduring Challenges

A series of broader trends helped to pave the way for genomic designation. From deinstitutionalization and the disability rights movements to the cultural ascendancy of the genome and innovation in communications and genetic testing technologies, recent decades have transformed the terrain for mobilizing mutations.

Perhaps most important of all, 22q11.2DS, like other genomically designated conditions, is part of a growing field of disease research and advocacy that has been extensively reviewed in other social scientific work (Best 2012; Bishop 2010; Epstein 2007b, 2016; Heath, Rapp, and Taussig 2004; Novas 2006; Panofsky 2011; Rabeharisoa and Callon 2002; Terry et al. 2007). There have been support groups for conditions like Tay-Sachs and cystic fibrosis since the 1950s; various philanthropic projects devoted to conditions like polio, tuberculosis, cancer, and alcoholism throughout the twentieth century; and organizations devoted to causes like women's health that can be traced back even further. Partly inspired by the success of HIV/AIDS and breast cancer activism, disease-related advocacy has reached new heights in the last few decades (Best 2012:781; Epstein 2007b:501–2; Terry et al. 2007). Not only are there now far *more* advocacy organizations devoted to conditions both rare and common, but they have also taken on increasingly important roles in organizing and even collaborating on biomedical research itself.[4] When it comes to genetic disorders, advocacy groups can now redirect research toward translational projects that might actually help patients (Terry et al. 2007)—a key task when so many researchers enter the field hoping to leverage mutations to get at much broader questions.

In many ways, this is by now a familiar story in the world of disease advocacy. To be sure, the networks formed around genomically designated conditions are indelibly embedded in this new world of disease advocacy. They lobby, raise funds, and work with biomedical experts to organize programs of research. Indeed, they see themselves as part of that broader shift, draw upon the examples of others, and cooperate under the remit of umbrella groups like the Genetic Alliance.[5]

However, we have to home in on a very particular corner of contemporary patient advocacy. As useful as the social scientific literature on these new health movements is, more work needs to be done in order to understand the rise of genomic designation. Being tied to a mutation surely provides some advantages for a disease advocacy movement. At the same time, genetic specificity also raises enormous obstacles. For one thing, we have seen how genomic specificity often begets phenotypic complexity (a point that I develop even further in the next two chapters). For another, when you start with the seemingly simple fact of a pathogenic mutation, building up the knowledge, numbers, and resources that it takes to turn it into a powerful category of illness is actually even more complex than working with long-standing clinical diagnoses. In many cases and in most places, people simply do not know what you are talking about when you mention 22q, Fragile X, *MECP2* Duplication Syndrome, or some other weird-sounding condition named after a gene or chromosomal locus. It certainly is not easy to explain it either. It is a challenge just to get people referred for the right sort of genetic testing, never mind convincing nonspecialist experts to reorient their practice based on the fact that someone has a mutation.

For these and other reasons, actors dedicated to a genomically designated condition cannot blindly adopt the strategies developed by more long-standing disease advocacy movements, even ones for genetic disorders like Huntington's or cystic fibrosis. They undoubtedly benefit from the broader "social movement spillover" (Meyer and Whittier 1994) created by HIV/AIDS and autism advocates, among others. But 22q advocates cannot simply wait for the world to come to them. They must also creatively adapt existing repertoires for raising awareness, increasing rates of diagnosis, developing care strategies, and convincing experts that a mutation can really be the key to understanding the medical and developmental challenges that a person faces. They have to forge points of interface with groups and institutions geared toward fundamentally different modes of classification, be it in special education, clinical medicine, or insurance bureaucracies. In other words, conditions like 22q11.2DS must be mobilized to work through but also *transform and realign* prevailing epistemic and institutional frameworks for understanding and acting on human difference.

But before we turn to the network organized around the 22q11.2 microdeletion, let's trace the development of the Fragile X network. It is, after all, the great pioneer and model for mobilizing mutations that advocates for 22q and many other genetic disorders are so determined to emulate.

Fragile X, Genetic Counselors, and the Development of a New Model

At the end of chapter 2 we saw Patricia Jacobs hail the emergence of a new test for "X-linked mental retardation associated with a marker at Xq28" as the dawn of a new era in human genetics. She was more right than she could have imagined. We saw how that condition, now known as Fragile X syndrome, gave rise to a pathbreaking model of expert-advocate collaboration, alliance formation, and activism for genetic disorders. It took another decade for a reliable test to enter into circulation. By then, in the early 1990s, Fragile X was increasingly associated with autism as well as mental retardation, rates of institutionalization had long since plummeted, and parents were usually the primary caregivers for their children.

This was the context in which Fragile X families and researchers, who began working together at a "kitchen table" in 1984, were able to go from strength to strength. When the foundation was first formed, however, it had surprisingly mundane goals. A group of Fragile X experts that included both Randi and Paul Hagerman had published a book about Fragile X in 1983 as well as a series of articles throughout the early 1980s. Unsurprisingly, they wanted to disseminate their findings to colleagues and Fragile X parents. Randi Hagerman told me that the initial impetus for the foundation came from the need to pay for xeroxing, of all things. She explained it like this in our 2015 interview in Sacramento, California: "Then we started the foundation, the

National Fragile X Foundation, with several interested parents and other colleagues. We really started the foundation because the hospital, Children's Hospital in Denver, was really mad at us for xeroxing. We had written a couple of papers, and we were xeroxing chapters from our book. They said, 'These xeroxing costs are breaking the hospital. You can't xerox anymore.' We thought, oh gosh, we have to be able to disseminate information separate from the hospital. That's why we started the National Fragile X Foundation." Hagerman immediately explained that the foundation's early goals were "to also educate families and professionals, and also to carry out biannual conferences, every other year conferences, and eventually to support research."

Back then, there were no ready-made models for an advocacy organization dedicated to a genetic disorder like Fragile X. The fledgling foundation had to take a trial-and-error approach as it sought to broaden its remit from xeroxing and undertake a series of ambitious initiatives. Over time, that group developed into today's expansive National Fragile X Foundation, which campaigns, raises funds, and lobbies in Washington, DC. As we saw, they have made their relatively rare condition a priority for the NIH. Fragile X is now a well-recognized disorder and a major subject of biomedical research and pharmaceutical investment. It all began with a relatively simple innovation in genetic disease advocacy. As Hagerman put it to me in the interview mentioned above, "The good thing about the National Fragile X Foundation meetings is we thought it was really important to combine researchers with families. I think we were the leading edge in doing this."

When Robert Miller was hired as the executive director of the fledgling National Fragile X Foundation in 1999, the organization was run out of his dining room in Pleasant Hill, California. By the time I interviewed Miller in that same dining room in 2015, his tenure as NFXF director had just recently come to an end. I asked him to cast his mind back to those early days. The first thing he said was, "Well, the joke back then was, 'Fragile what syndrome?' . . . Awareness was obviously one of the biggest challenges." But awareness among whom? Miller recounted, "In the early days, we did, somewhat naively, focus on national awareness. We had license plate frames, and we had all these different schemes." Later on, however, their focus turned to "getting the awareness out to the people who matter. . . . We really started zeroing in on the medical world and the therapy world. . . . [M]y instinct is that it was very effective." Since then, Miller has always pushed for a much more targeted goal when it comes to "awareness" for genetic disorders. As he explained in the interview,

One of the challenges that I have to deal with, both back then as an executive director and now as a consultant, is trying to help *define what the awareness goal ought
to be.* . . . I often encourage organizations to focus, at least initially, on the people
who matter. That would be the doctors and the scientists, the people who are likely
to encounter someone with Fragile X or any other rare disorder, and therefore diagnose it or refer the family for testing. Because our parent support organizations,
or advocacy organizations, or whatever you wanna call them, often have limited
resources, limited funds. They can't be all things to all people. That's often hard for
some boards, who are usually comprised of parents, to understand. (my emphasis)

Parent advocates understandably want the whole world to know about
their child's condition. But what really matters for care—as well as for
building up numbers, knowledge, and resources—is targeted awareness-
raising toward the constituencies who can truly make a difference.

It is hard to underestimate the importance of this line of thought for
rare-disorder advocacy. With limited money and manpower, it may just
not be realistic to push for awareness throughout society. Instead, what
matters most is getting a disorder onto the relevant experts' radar. That
is how you get the genetic tests for a condition ordered, how you get
more people diagnosed with a particular genetic disorder, and therefore how you recruit new patients and families to the movement. That
is how you get researchers interested, obtain prevalence estimates, spur
the creation of a medical literature, and create the kinds of resources
that turn a genetic diagnosis into a rubric for organizing treatment and
care. It is only now, after years of this kind of concerted, targeted work,
that the National Fragile X Foundation has the membership, knowledge base, and resources to turn back to the goal of general awareness.
It took a stepwise process to mobilize the Fragile X mutation, and that
process cannot be easily circumvented or reversed.

The work of these early Fragile X syndrome experts and patient advocates represented a major breakthrough for genomic designation.
Time and again during my fieldwork, the National Fragile X Foundation was cited as a beacon for others to follow. Take Brenda Finucane,
a genetic counselor who has dedicated much of her career to genomically designated syndromes. Finucane, like Jacobs, was excited by the
molecular test for Fragile X syndrome and carrier status. However,
Finucane was equally enamored with the work of Fragile X advocates.
In our 2011 interview in Indianapolis, Finucane outlined some of the
National Fragile X Foundation's achievements, like having lobbyists in
Washington and priority status at the NIH, and explained, "It is the
model that support groups want to be like. . . . They are unbelievable, they

are fantastic." Fragile X experts and advocates took the ability to test for *FMR1* CGG repeat expansions and turned that mutation from an undifferentiated form of X-linked mental retardation into a leading object of genetics research, the raison d'être of a powerful social movement, and the essential referent of a richly detailed kind of person. They also created a network of specialist clinics that is coordinated and regulated by the National Fragile X Foundation.[6] There are now almost thirty such Fragile X clinics in the United States alone.

This new model for mobilizing mutations rests, in no small part, on a new breed of genetic counselor. Following Brenda Finucane's career makes this very clear. In her decades of work as a genetic counselor, Finucane has had a considerable impact on the literature, but also a huge impact on the ground. Finucane has not only counseled thousands of people with genetic disorders, but she has also been at the forefront of a complex invisible college (Crane 1969) that works to make genomically designated syndromes matter in schools, hospitals, advocacy networks, and homes. Since helping to found the pathbreaking Fragile X group, she has sat at a number of other "kitchen tables" and helped to start new organizations, such as Parents and Researchers Interested in Smith-Magenis Syndrome (PRISMS) and IsoDicentric 15 Exchange Advocacy & Support (IDEAS) committed to advancing the cause of genomically designated syndromes. Finucane has also served on the boards of several others, including the International 22q11.2 Foundation. She is a regular speaker at conferences and workshops for rare genetic disorders, helping parents and experts alike learn how to turn a mutation into a powerful category of difference. In 2012, she was aggressively poached from Elwyn by Geisinger Health System, a large health care provider and widely recognized leader in the rollout of precision medicine. The status this kind of work has attained in the field is perhaps best captured by Finucane's election as the 2012 president of the National Society of Genetic Counselors.

The new breed of genetic counselor seeks to advance the cause of genetic disorders as objects of research, care, and community formation. This stands in stark contrast with decades past. When medical sociologist Charles Bosk conducted fieldwork at a pediatric hospital in the late 1970s and 1980s, he found that "genetic counseling as a service is generally a matter of transferring information to individuals who request it, and then leaving those individuals alone to make the tragic choices based on that information" (1992:xix). Bosk's book, *All God's Mistakes*, is a nuanced and closely observed account of genetic counseling in a particular time and place. But for us, it provides a striking comparison with the kinds of advocacy and community organizing work that genetic counselors are engaged in today. Genetic counselors may not always receive the same accolades as their colleagues in genetics and biomedical research, but they are indispensable when it comes to setting up support groups, facilitating research, and helping to establish specialist clinics. Their profession, after all, is geared precisely toward translating genetics research for patients and families, leaving them ideally placed to help raise awareness among doctors, and especially among broader lay audiences.

Genetic counselors have become the key mediators—the glue that holds everything together and allows a movement to grow. I saw this time and again during my fieldwork. Far from imparting information and then leaving, genetic counselors are often found hard at work deploying the Fragile X model for mobilizing mutations.

Assembling 22q

Back in chapter 1, we saw how knowledge about the microdeletion at 22q11 unified the biomedical literatures on several rare clinical syndromes and led to the delineation of a qualitatively new condition called 22q11.2 Deletion Syndrome. But 22q11.2DS is far more than just an object of knowledge in the biomedical literature. Beginning in this chapter and into the next, I grapple with the way 22q11.2DS functions as an object of clinical practice and social action. Yet 22q11.2DS remains in a sometimes uneasy interface with the "clinical gaze." I therefore use 22q as a case to analyze not only the power of genetics to realign illness, but also the manifold challenges that actors face when they seek to turn mutations into truly powerful categories of illness. First, we briefly see how 22q advocates have sought to emulate the model for mobilization pioneered by Fragile X and how that effort came to be spearheaded by the International 22q11.2 Foundation.

Emulating the Fragile X Model of Mobilization

The 22q11.2DS network has made great strides in recent years, but 22q advocates still have a long way to go before they realize anything close to their full potential. Nothing makes this clearer than the comparison with Fragile X. At a 22q conference that she organized in 2011, Finucane told me that she thought the International 22q11.2 Foundation was where the Fragile X group was perhaps fifteen years prior, despite the fact that its population prevalence is probably much higher and reliable tests for their respective mutations were developed around the same time. It is plain to see that Fragile X advocates have simply had far more success building a social movement, forging alliances, and mobilizing their mutation in many different fields.

Advocates for 22q are well aware of this gap in mobilization. Rather than being disheartened by it, however, they see Fragile X as a proven model that they can draw upon. As Donna McDonald-McGinn—one of the leading 22q11.2DS experts/activists in the United States—told me in a 2011 interview, the International 22q11.2 Foundation leaders talk about emulating the Fragile X group at every planning meeting. At the aforementioned International 22q11.2 Foundation conference at Disney World, there was even a talk entitled "Lessons from Fragile X." Advocates for 22q are working hard to develop the sorts of alliances and strategically targeted outreach initiatives that lifted the Fragile X movement to new heights.

More recently, the 22q Foundation went even further in its quest to emulate Fragile X advocacy. When the longtime executive director of the National Fragile X Foundation and one of the key architects of the Fragile X movement's success, Robert Miller, became available, the International 22q11.2 Foundation pounced and hired him as acting director. The International 22q11.2 Foundation outlined its rationale very clearly in a January 2015 press release announcing the appointment: "During his time at the NFXF, Robert was able to guide the organization from being a one-person office representing an unknown condition to a robust and internationally recognized organization that substantially improved awareness, diagnosis and treatment of Fragile X." Thinking ahead, they explained, "We are looking forward to Robert bringing that experience to the 22q community and helping us with the many, similar challenges."[7]

Advocates for 22q are far from alone in their explicit and assiduous work to follow in the Fragile X's movement's footsteps. In fact, they are not even alone when it comes to hiring Robert Miller. PRISMS hired him to consult on a range of issues related to what used to be called 17p11.2 Deletion Syndrome. The Association for X and Y Chromosome Variations (AXYS), which we encountered toward the end of chapter 2, also hired Miller as an interim director.[8] AXYS, which represents people with sex chromosome aneuploidies like the XYY, XXX, and XXYY syndromes, faces many of the same challenges as 22q advocates: widespread underdiagnosis, considerable uncertainty regarding their mutations' clinical range and developmental trajectory, a lack of awareness on the part of nonspecialist medical professionals, and insufficient resources for the treatment and care of affected persons. More than any other network built around a genetic mutation, the Fragile X movement has made enormous progress on all of these fronts, and many others besides. It is no wonder then that they are the envy and guiding light when it comes to advocacy for genomically designated conditions.

Miller left no doubt that he sees the International 22q11.2 Foundation as having an enormous amount of work to do in its quest to catch up to NFXF. Advocates for 22q have the numbers, the potential severity of their phenotype, and the opportunity to leverage their overlap with conditions like schizophrenia, autism, heart defects, and many others. They also have the Fragile X model to draw upon, the help of veterans like Miller and Finucane, and the support of at least a couple of celebrities whose kids have 22q11.2DS. So, if 22q advocates can directly emulate their Fragile X counterparts, one might think it would be quite easy for the 22q11.2DS movement to catch up to and perhaps even leapfrog the trailblazing Fragile X Foundation. The same could be said for the common sex chromosome disorders represented by AXYS. Even though rarer disorders like Smith-Magenis or 5p– syndrome may face more of an uphill struggle, Fragile X advocacy has shown how much a small but dedicated group of experts and parents can accomplish when they mobilize a mutation in just the right way. And yet, surveying the landscape for 22q11.2DS reveals a picture of important progress alongside continuing frustration.

Experts, Advocates, and the International 22q11.2 Foundation

Today, the International 22q11.2 Foundation is the leading advocacy organization for 22q11.2DS in the United States. It is also the organization that most effectively coordinates between different national 22q groups. Thanks in large part to their efforts, as well as allied organizations in at least sixteen countries and smaller support groups scattered throughout the United States,[9] more and more people are being diagnosed with 22q11.2DS and having their care rerouted accordingly. Physicians are increasingly likely to be familiar with 22q11.2DS, at least in certain subfields, and families are more and more likely to have a specialist 22q clinic within a reasonable distance.

Like other disease advocacy organizations, the International 22q11.2

Foundation has fostered deep ties with biomedical experts. In fact, those ties can substantially erode the distinction between expert and activist altogether. On the one hand, we see the sort of impressive lay/activist expertise discussed elsewhere (see esp. Epstein 1995). On the other, leading biomedical experts have also become bona fide devotees of the cause. That is why, for Peter Scambler, the medical geneticist most responsible for establishing the link between Velocardiofacial syndrome (VCFS) and 22q11 deletions, what began as a straightforward finding has become a life's work. He openly acknowledged in our 2011 interview in London that 22q has become a cause for him. He also hazarded that, were it not for the personal relationships built with families and colleagues over the years, he would have moved on to topics that were "sexier, like stem cells or something." Instead he keeps working on 22q, runs marathons to raise money for the foundation, and gives support to their activism when he can.

The 22q movement counted biomedical experts among its most dedicated activists from the very beginning. Donna McDonald-McGinn has been working with parents and activists since at least the mid-1990s, when the name "22q11.2DS" first appeared in the literature. In 2003, she teamed up with a handful of parents in the Philadelphia area to establish a dedicated group for people and families dealing with 22q11.2DS. Soon after, they established the registered charity that eventually became the International 22q11.2 Foundation. Just like the National Fragile X Foundation, it all began with a group of parents and biomedical experts gathered around a kitchen table. Like Randi Hagerman before her with Fragile X, McDonald-McGinn pioneered research on the 22q11.2DS phenotype and how best to manage it, even as she worked doggedly alongside the parent activists who drive the 22q movement. Still, it was McDonald-McGinn's work that drew her to the cause, not the other way around. "I never went in wanting to do this," she told me when I interviewed her in Philadelphia in 2011. Rather, the original idea was simply "what is the diagnosis, keep moving." Ever since she found herself with a group of parents around that kitchen table in Philadelphia in the mid-1990s, however, she has dedicated her career to 22q11.2 Deletion Syndrome, working closely with that group through its metamorphosis into an international foundation. She organizes both research programs and foundation events, and she agrees that 22q is now a deeply held cause for her.

Researchers and advocates encounter a series of unusual opportunities and challenges with regard to 22q11.2DS. Take McDonald-McGinn's insistence that she "can't stop until every clinician is familiar

with 22q11.2 Deletion syndrome." Why has 22q11.2DS, which is actually *not* so rare at all, been so slow to achieve recognition in the medical community in general and the pertinent specialties in particular?
Why do rates of diagnosis remain so low? How does one communicate
such a diagnosis, with its highly variable clinical profile, to the relevant
professions and broader publics? Finally, how does one work to improve
care for people with 22q11.2DS in health care and education systems
that were not developed with this kind of genetic disorder in mind?

These questions help us begin to see how the International 22q11.2
Foundation's longtime motto, "Detection, Care, Cure," with all its
seeming straightforwardness for a disease advocacy organization, actually belies a profound set of challenges that any genomically designated condition must confront in one form or another. In the next two
chapters, we explore the various ways in which conditions like Fragile
X, 22q11.2DS, and 16p11.2DS can reshape clinical judgment and practice. The rest of this chapter focuses on the 22q movement, beginning
with the foundation's fascinating move to expand its constituency to
include 22q11.2 duplications. Then, we follow 22q experts and advocates down the long and arduous path of improving *detection* and
awareness of the 22q11.2 microdeletion, developing strategies and resources to *care* for people with 22q11.2DS, and the largely promissory
goal of developing a *cure*.

Absorbing a New Mutation: The 22q11.2 Duplication

The word *deletion* was not dropped from the International 22q11.2
Foundation's name simply for the sake of concision: it is part of a bold
strategy to absorb people with the 22q11.2 micro*duplication*, as well as
some other rare mutations involving 22q11.2, into their constituency.
The 22q11.2 duplication phenotype includes most of the clinical problems seen in 22q11.2 Deletion Syndrome, but it is also more likely to be
very mild. Unlike 22q11.2DS, it appears that most 22q11.2 duplications
are inherited from a parent who had no idea that they had been dealing with a genetic disorder their whole life. Chances are, therefore, that
most people 22q11.2 microduplications do not suffer from *any* of the
kinds of maladies that usually lead to a referral for genetic testing. No
one knows how many mostly normal people with 22q11.2 microduplications will be unearthed as genetic testing becomes more commonplace, but it will probably be a lot.

The first 22q11.2 microduplication was reported in 1999 in a four-
year-old female. This young girl presented with developmental delay,

failure to thrive, hypotonia, sleep apnea, "seizure-like episodes," velo-pharyngeal insufficiency, language and motor-skill delays, and dys-morphic facial features. In other words, she had features that had led to testing for a 22q11.2 micro*deletion*. In addition, familial testing re-vealed that her mother and grandmother also had the 22q11.2 micro-duplication. However, they appeared normal except for "a history of pre-auricular ear pits" (a dent or dimple on the external ear) (Edelmann et al. 1999:1159–60). Although only a couple of additional very short case reports appeared over the next few years, it would not be long be-fore the 22q11.2 duplication was designated as a new genetic condition.

By 2003, a paper in the *American Journal of Human Genetics* appeared with the title, "Microduplication 22q11.2, an Emerging Syndrome: Clinical, Cytogenetic, and Molecular Analysis of Thirteen Patients" (Ensenauer et al. 2003). A series of papers on the new 22q11.2 duplica-tion syndrome quickly followed (e.g., Carolina et al. 2005; Hassed et al. 2004; Portnoï et al. 2005). Research on this new 22q11.2 syndrome be-gan to gain steam during the late 2000s, though it remains far less de-veloped than 22q11.2DS (e.g., Courtens, Schramme, and Laridon 2008; Portnoï 2009; Wentzel et al. 2008). More recent work by a team that in-cludes leading 22q11.2DS experts like Beverly Emanuel, Elaine Zackai, and Donna McDonald-McGinn found high rates of ASDs among peo-ple with the 22q11.2 duplication, along with increased risk for a range of medical problems. However, many patients had very mild pheno-types (Wenger, Miller, et al. 2016). The duplication also exhibits wide variability even within the same family.[10] The NIH's *GeneReviews* sum-mary put it as follows: "The 22q11.2 duplication phenotype appears to be generally mild and highly variable; findings range from apparently normal to intellectual disability/learning disability, delayed psycho-motor development, growth retardation, and/or hypotonia. The high frequency with which the 22q11.2 duplication is found in an appar-ently normal parent of a proband suggests that many individuals can harbor a duplication of 22q11.2 with no discernible phenotypic effect" (Firth 2013). As the foundation explains on its website, "Many people with the duplication have no apparent physical or intellectual disabili-ties. Often times, parents of children with the duplication find out that they also have it only after their child is diagnosed." The page then goes on to list many of the same clinical associations as the deletion.[11] This is fairly typical for many of the microduplication syndromes that have been discovered through the course of research into their more serious, "reciprocal" microdeletion syndromes.[12]

What is *not* typical, however, is the way the 22q network is moving to absorb the 22q11.2 microduplication and therefore the people and families affected by it. In particular, the International 22q11.2 Foundation is making the duplication part of its raison d'être. At the meetings and conferences I have attended, it is discussed more and more. The foundation's website now includes it in its informational FAQ and member stories sections.[13] The fact that they even went so far as to drop "Deletion Syndrome" from the foundation's name shows just how seriously they are pursuing this goal. This has two important implications. First, it dramatically increases the potential constituency of the International 22q11.2 Foundation and the 22q network more generally. Second, it means that the 22q11.2 duplication is being parachuted into an existing network geared toward mobilizing its sister mutation. The 22q11.2 duplication therefore finds itself with an established group of interested researchers. Meanwhile, patients and families affected by the duplication have a foundation and network of resources ready and waiting for them. In recent years, database entries and management guidelines on 22q11.2 Duplication Syndrome have started to appear (e.g., Firth 2013; Hughes et al. 2016:201). There is a multigenerational family with a series of YouTube videos on 22q11.2 Duplication Syndrome, and growing interest from researchers and advocates interested in autism, ADHD, and schizophrenia.[14] The 22q11.2 duplication may have never achieved this kind of interest and investment if it had not been able to piggyback on the network established around its reciprocal deletion syndrome.

Detection (and Awareness)

The problem of ascertainment looms large for a condition like 22q11.2DS. Nothing matters more for the 22q movement than increasing the detection of 22q11.2 microdeletions and then bringing the people who bear them into the fold. Indeed, it is the key to achieving many of the 22q movement's other goals.

The more we learn about 22q11.2DS, the more we realize that it might not be very rare at all. With a relatively low profile and such a broad spectrum of clinical indicators (i.e., a phenotype), there is reason to believe that there are many, many people with 22q11.2 microdeletions (and duplications) who have not been diagnosed, in part because they do not conform to the long-standing but biased profile of 22q11.2DS in the medical field. Indeed, a recent study of more than 9,500 pregnant women found a far higher prevalence of 22q11.2 deletions and duplications than previous prevalence studies that were based on (biased) clinical ascertainment (Grati et al. 2015). They found 22q11.2 microdeletions in 6 out of 5,953 (~1 in 922) low-risk pregnancies and 25 of 2,311 (~1 in 92) high-risk pregnancies. Meanwhile, 7 of 5,953 (~1 in 850) low-risk and 7 of 2,311 (~1 in 330) high-risk pregnancies tested positive for a 22q11.2 duplication (806–8). Even at the low end of their confidence intervals, this study suggests that 22q11.2 deletions and duplications are staggeringly common when ascertainment is not biased by 22q11.2DS's clinical profile (primarily the presence of an infant cardiac malformation).

The International 22q11.2 Foundation (and other 22q groups) enthusiastically reported these findings to their members. They now state that 22q11.2DS's prevalence is probably around 1 in 1,000.[15] For the 22q social movement, after all, 22q11.2DS detection is also a question of *recruitment*. Each newly diagnosed person represents not only a tiny increase in total numbers, but also a client for treatment, care, and services; a potential research subject; and a new family that might join the International 22q11.2 Foundation or another support group. Indeed, the move to absorb the 22q11.2 *duplication* into their constituency can be seen as a new front in this endeavor. Sheer numbers of affected patients are key for disease advocates when they advance claims for resources (see, e.g., Best 2012; Bishop 2010), and social movement scholars have noted that it is also a central basis for claims-making more generally (e.g., Tilly 2004). Increased detection would therefore help unlock many of the precious resources that the 22q movement and its constituents so desperately seek. And yet, even as detection is essential for mobilizing mutations, it brings with it a host of challenges for a movement trying to establish itself in a health care system built up around clinical categories and evaluations.

Barriers to Detection

Although the detection of people with 22q11.2DS may seem like a straightforward goal, the reality is anything but. Advocates for 22q face a series of obstacles when it comes to identifying people with 22q11.2 microdeletions, never mind convincing them, their families, teachers, and caregivers that 22q11.2 Deletion Syndrome is the most salient category for understanding what makes them ill or different.

If a general practitioner, a specialist, or a genetic counselor orders a test for 22q, or a parent successfully demands one, a definitive result will most likely come back: either they have a 22q11.2 deletion, or they do not. The rub, however, is this: How do you get the tests ordered in the first place? On the basis of which clinical signs? How do you get 22q higher up on clinicians' differential diagnostics for children with heart and palate malformations, developmental delays, and certain cranio-facial features without exasperating ascertainment bias and missing mild or atypical cases? It is not just a question of having people referred to the correct clinical specialist. After all, there are no clinical diagnostic criteria for 22q as such, just differential indicators. A clinician may simply treat each presenting problem individually, without thinking to order a test for 22q11.2DS. Even those familiar with the typical symptoms are likely to miss all but the most classic cases of 22q11.2DS—that is, those who would have been eligible to receive a clinical DiGeorge syndrome (DGS) or VCFS diagnosis. But again, 22q11.2DS is characterized by more than two hundred associated symptoms ranging from serious congenital heart defects, cleft palate, and schizophrenia to small ears, tapered digits, and ADHD, with some patients affected by dozens of serious ailments and others by only a few or even none. So how do you get clinicians to think about the value of a genetic diagnosis, especially among patients who do not match the classic dysmorphic profiles?

There are also deep-seated racial, ethnic, socioeconomic, geographic, and sometimes gender barriers to the detection of genomically designated conditions. It is plain to see that patients are far more likely to receive careful genetic testing and analysis if their parents have the right kind of health care, the resources to pay out of pocket where necessary, and the social and cultural capital to push for better answers from biomedical experts. Parents often have to fight to get the kind of testing that can bring a diagnostic odyssey to an end, and they can only wield the resources they have access to in their battle.

People from racial and ethnic minority backgrounds face even greater barriers to detection, even net of socioeconomic disparities. Why? It turns out that facial appearance is often the only feature that is thought to indicate a particular genetic disorder and, even when not specific, it is often the basis for referral for a genetics evaluation (Hammond 2007; Morelle 2007; Shaw et al. 2003).[16] Yet as several 22q11.2DS experts told me at various points in my fieldwork, the craniofacial features in nonwhite 22q kids are "less distinct," especially in black patients (see Kruszka et al. 2017). What this means, of course, is that most biomedical experts are not used to dealing with nonwhite 22q kids, and that they are less used to dealing with nonwhite children altogether. Put simply, they are not as good at picking out unusual black and brown faces as they are white ones. When it comes to 22q11.2DS, and probably other genomically designated conditions as well, the "craniofacial abnormality" pathway to genetic testing leads to decreased ascertainment of nonwhite patients.

Ultimately, only population-level screening will remove all the barriers and biases that limit detection of genomically designated conditions like 22q11.2DS. This is anything but lost on 22q experts and advocates.

The Move toward Newborn Screening

In 2012, American 22q advocates made an audacious attempt to circumvent these manifold obstacles to increased ascertainment in one fell swoop: they appealed to have 22q11.2DS added to the universal newborn screening panel. If they were successful, virtually every newborn in the United States would be screened for 22q11.2DS. Not only would patient numbers likely explode, but researchers would finally be able to grapple with the true scope and range of the 22q11.2DS phenotype. To top it all off, these new 22q11.2DS patients would have the cherished opportunity for early intervention. Advocates for 22q even hoped that newborn screening for 22q11.2DS would be replicated abroad. As the leader of the main 22q group in the United Kingdom put it, the members of the International 22q11.2 Foundation "are like vanguards who drive things forward, and I can only hope that when we will get Washington to agree, the North Atlantic Drift will bring it over to Britain."

How did they make their case? Take this excerpt of a speech by Sheila Kambin—who subsequently became the lead chairperson of the International 22q11.2 Foundation—submitted as testimony in support of this bold bid. "My son Aiden's diagnostic odyssey incorporated 27 specialists over a 5-year period at major medical centers. Despite having 18 findings associated with 22q, Aiden remained undiagnosed. The cost was over $500,000, but what cannot be measured in dollars is Aiden's lost chance for early interventions, interventions which I believe could have substantially improved his prognosis. What would Aiden's IQ and speech be like today if he had come to attention in infancy? We will never know." Kambin is presenting her audience with a poignant "what if?" story. She regularly recounts her family's story at 22q meetings in order to hit home the promise of increased awareness and early diagnosis for 22q11.2DS. We will encounter one of those speeches, delivered to an International 22q11.2 Foundation conference, in the next chapter. But this time, Kambin was speaking along with a group of leading 22q11.2DS advocates, clinicians, and researchers at a meeting of the US Department of Health and Human Services' Secretary's Advisory Committee on Heritable Disorders in Newborns and Children that I attended in January 2012. They were making the formal case for adding 22q11.2DS to the US universal newborn screening panel.

Kambin closed her short speech by emphasizing that only screening could ensure that a majority of young children with 22q11.2 deletions received the all-important genetic diagnosis: "I am a parent. I am also an obstetrician/physician who has coped with her son's medical diagnosis by medicalizing every aspect of it. I can recite every anomaly associated with the syndrome. I also work on a special delivery unit which was built to deliver babies with congenital anomalies, specifically babies with congenital heart disease. And I came here to tell you today that I could not reliably make this diagnosis in a delivery room. *Newborn screening is the only solution to this complex problem. Please do right by these wonderful children and recognize having newborn screening for 22q.*" Kambin's son was never tested for 22q11.2DS per se—he was only diagnosed after a chromosomal microarray test was ordered—despite exhibiting many of the relevant signs. More surprising still, Aiden was treated at probably the leading center for 22q research and treatment in the world, Children's Hospital of Philadelphia (CHOP), and his parents were clinical specialists in pertinent subfields. If he did not receive an early 22q11.2DS diagnosis, Kambin asked, what chance do most kids with a 22q11.2 microdeletion have?

In the end, despite a series of well-received statements from Kambin, Donna McDonald-McGinn, and other 22q experts and activists, their bid to have 22q11.2DS added to the newborn screen failed due to insufficient evidence about the viability of the 22q11.2 screening technique, the specificity of the phenotype, and the efficacy of early intervention. Still, the 22q team were not discouraged: first attempts to add a condition to the newborn screening kit are rarely successful, and they were invited to submit further evidence at future meetings. It was also clear from the conversations and informal feedback they received after the meeting that important allies were won and that their goals for subsequent submissions had already been refined. With high rates of cardiac defects and hypocalcemia, for which early intervention can undoubtedly save lives and resources, and a test that can be affordably integrated into the existing heel punch, it is certainly possible that 22q11.2DS will one day be added to the newborn screen.

This is a bold but perhaps brilliant claim on state resources by

22q11.2 activists: with 22q's high prevalence and broad phenotypic variability, they have an enormous amount to gain. At the International 22q11.2 Foundation's 2012 conference, its chairperson at the time, Carol Cavana, discussed what a neonatal diagnosis might have done for her severely affected son. Cavana explained how early detection and awareness are two sides of the same coin. She opened her presentation, "Making Newborn Screening a Reality: Why Parents Care," by telling the audience, "Immediate detection is the most important [goal], which will [bring] rapid intervention, optimal care, and global awareness." Donna McDonald-McGinn made the point even more clearly after receiving a kind of lifetime achievement award from the foundation:

So how can newborn screening help us along this journey as we move forward? Because newborn screening will lead to early detection for both deletion and duplication, lead to proper care in the newborn period, lead to early interventions as needed, and *provide accurate prevalence figures* which will lead to *greater awareness by the public, greater understanding by the medical community, more research dollars by government agencies* in search of better treatments and outcomes.

In short, newborn screening for 22q11.2DS would be a game-changer for the 22q movement.

What would it mean if we discovered thousands of seemingly normal or mildly affected people with 22q11.2 microdeletions? Timmermans and Buchbinder (2010, 2012) have shown how positive results for seemingly normal patients in California's newborn screening regime can create "patients in waiting" or force clinicians to engage in ontological "bridging" work between genotype and phenotype. For a genomically designated condition like 22q11.2DS, by contrast, the ascertainment of mild cases holds huge potential. It presents merely an empirical and pragmatic challenge, not an ontological obstacle. Experts and advocates for 22q have no problem with the idea that the full range of the disorder, which would be revealed by screening, may be far broader than its classic clinical profile.

The reasons both for and against including 22q11.2DS in state newborn screening programs actually bear a striking resemblance to the acrimonious debate that swirled around the newborn study of XYY, discussed in chapter 2. A 2010 paper in *Genetics in Medicine* reviewed the benefits and risks of adding 22q11.2DS to the Wisconsin newborn screening kit (Bales, Zaleski, and McPherson 2010:140). The authors discussed the benefits of determining the full phenotypic range of the disorder and the potential for early detection and intervention into a host of 22q11.2DS's associated maladies. Among the risks are the fact that consent will not be required; the interruption of parent/child relationships; the risk of labeling the mildly affected and the creation of "vulnerable child syndrome"; overtreatment and unnecessary anxiety for mild cases. Finally, there is the question of whether the necessary resources would be better spent elsewhere. In sum, the risks and benefits for screening XYY at Harvard in the 1970s and 22q11.2DS today are remarkably similar. And yet, the former attracted the ire of activists concerned about children's well-being while the latter is driven by patient advocacy.[17] These dilemmas are nothing less than endemic to the project of genetic medicine.

There are compelling reasons to question the clinical and public health implications of newborn screening for conditions like 22q11.2DS. For 22q advocates, however, the potential benefits far outweigh the risks. One way or another, there is no question that newborn screening would be transformative for 22q11.2DS and the 22q movement.

Awareness

Increased detection is largely a question of awareness—of having the key fields and publics cognizant of and interested in 22q11.2DS. The International 22q11.2 Foundation's former chairperson, Carol Cavana, summed up how important this goal is at the start of her opening address at the 2012 conference: "I wake up rededicated to the cause, to awareness and early detection."

As the foundation's secretary and one of its founding members, Wendy Rose, put it in a talk entitled "Detection, Care, Cure: A Common Goal," "We have three wide, broad focuses as an organization: *awareness certainly is the first.*" Rose discussed the challenge of raising awareness among the general public. As she explained, "We've focused really on . . . our 22q at the Zoo Worldwide Awareness Day." The first "22q at the Zoo" was originally going to be a local Philadelphia event, but after a dramatic change of plans it wound up being held at sixty-two zoos around the world. The foundation estimated that, as Rose put it, ten thousand people "assembled across the world on that day to celebrate, to meet one another, to support one another, and to tell the world about 22q." The second 22q at the Zoo in 2013 featured events in eighty-two cities across six countries, and in subsequent years it has become bigger still. Nowadays, the foundation aims to have 22q at the Zoo events in thirty countries and all fifty US states.[18] Along with myriad other efforts ranging from fun runs and golf events to calendar campaigns and an annual November awareness month, "22q at the Zoo" sees the foundation engaging in the kind of awareness-raising that we would expect from a disease advocacy organization.

However, 22q advocates were especially focused on the importance of *targeted* awareness-raising among key constituencies. They have heeded the lesson of the Fragile X model described by Robert Miller (above). As Wendy Rose put it in that same speech at the 22q foundation meeting, "We struggle and focus every day on informing the medical community that so many of you focus on as well, whether you are a part of the medical community yourselves or are parents trying to educate your own physicians wherever you are." This is a vital issue for patients, families, and the 22q movement as a whole. There are serious barriers not only to finding people with 22q11.2 microdeletions, but also to translating the detection of that mutation into a 22q11.2 *Deletion Syndrome* diagnosis that can circulate beyond the lab: 22q advocates have to fight against the still-common practice of giving people old diagnoses like DGS and VCFS; they also have to fight to get 22q11.2DS recognized in medical specialties, as well as in fields like psychology and education that are not used to dealing with anything but the most well-known genetic disorders (e.g., Down syndrome). Finally, parents are still likely to be met with incredulity and resistance from physicians and teachers when they invoke 22q to inform a child's treatment or care.

Throughout this chapter and into the next one, I show how hard it often is for 22q advocates to gain traction in pertinent fields like clinical medicine, psychology, and special education. As long as 22q11.2DS remains an obscure and unfamiliar diagnosis to most doctors on the ground, its rates of ascertainment will be both severely depressed *and* biased toward patients with the classic features of DGS and VCFS (tetralogy of Fallot, velopharyngeal insufficiency, etc.). The lack of awareness among neonatologists and pediatricians is perhaps the single biggest impediment to the 22q movement's continued growth and success. After all, it only faces the challenge of rare disease advocacy because 22q11.2DS is so infrequently diagnosed.

Toward this end, Anne Bassett, Donna McDonald-McGinn, and other leading 22q expert/activists spearheaded a 22q11.2 Deletion Syndrome Consortium to produce an authoritative overview of 22q11.2DS and consensus on clinical guidelines. It was published in 2011 in the "Grand Rounds" section of the *Journal of Pediatrics* (Bassett et al. 2011). This was perhaps the flagship achievement of a whole host of projects aimed at raising awareness among medical professionals—it helped to raise 22q's profile among the broadest possible audience of physicians who are in a position to order a test for 22q11.2DS.

The foundation launched an ad campaign around the same time that specifically targeted physicians (e.g., see fig. 5.1). They quickly had the *Journal of Pediatrics* guidelines translated into other languages as well. Through these and many other initiatives that target medical professionals, 22q experts and advocates hope to increase ascertainment and ensure that otherwise nonindicated forms of clinical evaluation and treatment are made available to 22q11.2DS patients.

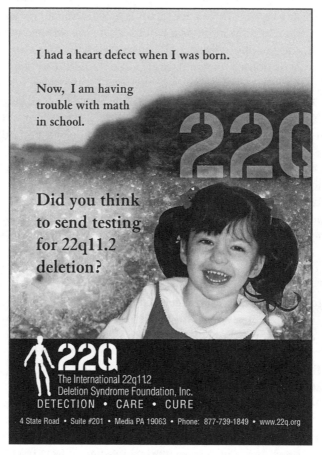

FIGURE 5.1. Ad from a campaign by the International 22q11.2 Foundation (formerly the International 22q11.2 Deletion Syndrome Foundation) to promote awareness among physicians. (Reproduced by permission from the International 22q11.2 Foundation)

Care

Perhaps the most pressing obstacle for people who have been diagnosed with 22q11.2DS, as well as for their families, is access to appropriate care. The published clinical guidelines call for a bewildering array of referrals, tests, and treatments for everyone with 22q11.2DS, even though they may not be indicated by a particular patient's clinical presentation. That topic is taken up in the next chapter. In order to provide access to these kinds services for patients and their families, 22q advocates are following in the Fragile X network's footsteps and trying to build and regulate a network of specialist 22q clinics all over the United States and Western Europe. Indeed, this is often the chief object of the local alliances of parents, genetics experts, and clinicians scattered throughout the country. Once they are established, these 22q groups frequently lobby local hospitals to create multidisciplinary specialist clinics for 22q11.2DS. Given the range of resources and expertise required, these centers tend to be formed at major research hospitals. The foundation is working to promote their creation and to establish criteria to ensure that these centers meet certain minimal standards. The goal, as Donna McDonald-McGinn explained, is that everyone should have access to a dedicated 22q center capable of providing counsel to the newly diagnosed and their families and meeting the many clinical demands of the diagnosis. Referencing the hundreds of families who have traveled from far afield to the 22q and You clinic in Philadelphia to receive such care, she proclaimed, "No one should have to come to CHOP."

There are now more than thirty specialist 22q clinics in cities across North America, and twenty more across sixteen other countries from Japan and Australia to Spain and Chile.[19] The centers guarantee that patients and parents will not be met with responses like "22-what?!" or a refusal to take a 22q11.2DS diagnosis seriously. Ideally, the centers should also be able to provide the full menu of tests and referrals recommended by the established guidelines for 22q11.2DS management, as outlined in the *Pediatrics* article discussed above (Bassett et al. 2011).

However, the reality is far more uneven. It is important to keep in mind that these are not stand-alone clinics with "22q11.2 Deletion Syndrome Clinic" emblazoned above the entrance. At best, there may be a suite of offices and evaluation rooms inside a hospital, as with the 22q and You Center at CHOP. More often, they tend to comprise a group of interested genetics experts and clinicians in a hospital or health care system who are able to work together when it comes to coordinating a 22q patient's care and perhaps holding special clinical sessions once a week or so. Many of these "clinics" simply lack the resources and expertise to meet the consensus-based guidelines for 22q care and management. Others, meanwhile, are biased because of the specialty of the experts who founded them. Three 22q clinics that were started by an immunologist, a cardiac specialist, and a psychiatrist respectively may end up being very different beasts. Not only do they tend to have different forms of expertise and interests, but they are also likely to end up with very different patient populations because of institution and specialty-driven ascertainment bias.

When there is no specialist clinic nearby, 22q parents are encouraged to use foundation resources and even the biomedical literature itself in order to demand the consensus-based evaluations and treatments established by 22q11.2DS experts. They are given binders with information and key articles, as well as fold-out cards with information about treatment guidelines and references to articles that can be used to demonstrate that a given referral or procedure is indeed indicated by the presence of a 22q11.2 microdeletion.

We delve into what this all actually means in terms of practice in the next chapter. For now, I simply want to emphasize the fact that 22q experts and advocates are utterly dependent upon one another when it comes to advancing care. If advocates could not find so much detailed information, so many resources, and even references to the biomedical literature at 22q.org,[20] or if they had not received crash courses in 22q11.2DS and how to interact with physicians at 22q meetings, they would face an even steeper uphill struggle when they try to get local health care providers to follow 22q guidelines. Conversely, if it were not for those same advocates, it would be immeasurably harder for experts to set up specialist 22q clinics and recruit vital research subjects. There would still be lots of people with 22q11.2 microdeletions, of course, but 22q would barely matter at all, either as a medical condition or as a kind of person.

Cure; or, How to Attract Pharmaceutical Research on a Rare Mutation

In contrast to the extensive work being done to detect 22q and create infrastructures for treatment and care, there is relatively little work aimed at curing 22q11.2DS. As Bales et al. succinctly state (2010:138), "Because the missing genetic material cannot be replaced throughout the body, there is clearly no cure for 22q11DS. Once the syndrome is identified, the goal is detection and management of treatable complications." In other words, cure is neither currently possible nor on the horizon; care is the only practicable goal. Nevertheless, we can see the *idea* of a cure as a coordinating device that helps to justify biomedical research on 22q11.2DS, especially studies that require tissue samples and other kinds of interventions. It has helped to create a fast-moving field of research into pharmaceutical compounds that can target 22q11.2 genes in order to get at conditions like schizophrenia and ADHD.

Indeed, we also see elements of the same kind of leveraging that brought the Fragile X and Phelan-McDermid syndrome groups together with autism research and advocacy. The abstract of a recent *Nature Reviews Disease Primers* written by a group of authors that contains many of the most important 22q researcher-activists closed by noting, "22q11.2DS has become a model for understanding rare and frequent congenital anomalies, medical conditions, psychiatric and developmental disorders." They argued that 22q11.2DS "may provide a platform to better understand these disorders while affording opportunities for translational strategies across the lifespan for both patients with 22q11.2DS and those with these associated features in the general population" (McDonald-McGinn et al. 2015:1). Researchers are especially attracted to 22q11.2DS as a model for congenital heart malformations like tetralogy of Fallot, endocrine issues, and psychiatric disorders like schizophrenia, ADHD, and autism.

A recent paper entitled "The 22q11.2 Microdeletion: Fifteen Years of Insights into the Genetic and Neural Complexity of Psychiatric Disorders" (Drew et al. 2011:259; see also, e.g., Karayiorgou, Simon, and Gogos 2010) explained that, "the identification, fifteen years ago, of 22q11.2 microdeletions as a causative factor for schizophrenia was the first demonstration that deletions, or duplications, of chromosomal regions may play an important role in schizophrenia etiology in many cases." Why was that finding so important? They continued,

Such mutations, known as copy number variations (CNVs), result in altered gene dosage, and a rapidly expanding literature shows a high prevalence of such mutations in schizophrenia patients. By allowing the generation of etiological valid animal models, *identification of highly penetrant mutations such as these offer unprecedented opportunities to determine the key neural changes that can lead to psychotic illness. Here we argue that the 22q11.2 deletion can act as prototype for this type of investigation.* That is to say, the rigorous definition of the pathway from mutation to disease phenotype in models of this mutation will provide invaluable insights into the etiology and pathophysiology of schizophrenia as a whole. (259; my emphasis; references omitted)

Others have made similar arguments over the years (e.g., Owen and Doherty 2016; Schneider et al. 2014). In short, 22q11.2DS provided the first association between a copy number variant and schizophrenia, and it went on to offer a model for schizophrenia's underlying molecular pathways as well.

Researchers are now working to leverage 22q11.2 *Duplication* Syndrome to get at schizophrenia. A 2014 study in *Molecular Psychiatry* by Rees et al. reported a striking result that is sure to lead to further research over the coming years. This group of authors from the United States, the United Kingdom, the Republic of Ireland, and Sweden genotyped a sample of 6,882 schizophrenia cases and 11,255 controls. They found a total of zero 22q11.2 duplications in the schizophrenia sample and ten such cases among controls. Meanwhile, they found twenty 22q11.2DS cases among the schizophrenia sample but zero among the controls (Rees et al. 2014:38). After combining their sample with another large data set, Rees et al. advanced a stunning interpretation of their findings: "Our study therefore identifies as *the first putative protective mutation for schizophrenia* duplications of the genomic segment that, when deleted, is the most potent genetic risk factor for the disorder" (39; my emphasis). In other words, their findings confirmed the intuitive idea that the duplication of 22q11.2 had the opposite effect of the 22q11.2 deletion when it comes to schizophrenia risk.

These findings had major implications for future work on the genetics of schizophrenia, and especially for the goal of developing pharmaceuticals to target 22q11.2 genes and their associated pathways. As the authors explained, "The identification of the dosage-sensitive gene(s) at 22q11.2 and the implication of risk and protective mechanisms is therefore an important direction for research—particularly as pharmacological intervention might offer protection from schizophrenia" (Rees et al. 2014:39–40). In short, the 22q11.2 deletion and duplication are set to serve as a pair of genetic models for pharmaceutical research on schizophrenia. Thanks to findings like these, along with the well-established literature on 22q11.2DS and psychosis, a recent commentary in *JAMA Psychiatry* could conclude by stressing "the importance of early recognition of both 22q11.2 deletions and duplications in both research and clinical settings," before noting, "Continued study of these syndromes may facilitate our understanding of pathways from genes to behavior and of the neurobiology of psychiatric disorders" (Harris 2017:E2).

This is why, in 2013, the National Institute of Mental Health awarded $12 million in funding to the International 22q11.2 Brain Behavior Consortium (IBBC). The IBBC brings together 22q experts from twenty-two leading medical research institutions, including most of the major 22q11.2DS research centers and specialist clinics, with the goal of sequencing the genomes of around one thousand 22q11.2DS patients. The IBBC has "ultimate goals of improving detection, treatment and long-term outcomes" for people with 22q11.2DS.[21] However, a broader goal is stated very clearly: "Beyond the potential for yielding a better understanding of a severe manifestation of 22q11DS, *the results will help identify pathways leading to SZ* [schizophrenia] *in the general population in a way that will inform novel treatments.*"[22] Many of the key figures in the IBBC are 22q11.2DS experts first and foremost. Yet just like the various leveraging projects we encountered in previous chapters, this $12 million research initiative would almost certainly not have been funded if it did not have the potential to help unpack the genetics of a common disease. If it does eventually benefit its mutation-bearing study population—people with 22q11.2DS—it will most likely be seen by the NIMH as a secondary benefit. So, once again, 22q experts and advocates like Donna McDonald-McGinn have to forge productive trading zones with experts and institutions geared toward common disorders like schizophrenia.

Both 22q11.2 syndromes are now being leveraged to speak to other psychiatric conditions like autism and especially ADHD as well. In June 2016, a new biotech company, Medgenics, announced the initiation of a phase 2/3 trial of a drug designed to treat ADHD symptoms in patients with 22q11.2DS.[23] Like a lot of 22q11.2 research, this line of investigation was initiated at CHOP—in this case a collaboration between CHOP's Center for Applied Genomics (CAG) and their 22q and You Center. In late 2014 Medgenics paid $5 million for exclusive commercial access to the biobank at CAG and committed to pay CHOP royalties on any drug products developed using the CAG database. Then, in 2016, Medgenics paid a further $2 million to complete the acquisition of a startup founded by CAG's director, Hakon Hakonarson, called "neuroFix Therapeutics, LLC." It was Hakonarson's team, under the guise of neuroFix, that had done the initial work and exploratory trial of NFC-1 on a small group of 22q11.2DS patients recruited through CHOP's 22q and You Center. The International 22q11.2 Foundation enthusiastically reported these initial results in a press release, noting that the treatment was a groundbreaking deployment of "something called precision medicine, . . . an emerging approach for disease treatment and prevention that takes into account individual variability in genes. By focusing on the actual biology of the disease, the aim is to establish more effective treatments." The foundation urged caution regarding these preliminary results, but also promised to keep its members abreast of further developments as NFC-1 makes its way through the trials process for 22q11.2DS.[24]

Medgenics (now rebranded as Aevi Genomic Medicine, Inc.), CHOP, and the International 22q11.2 Foundation are now turning their attention to an even bigger prize: using 22q11.2DS to get at mGluR and autism (see Wenger, Kao, et al. 2016). Hakonarson noted the study's simple finding, that "the *RANBP1* gene is a significant genetic factor in both ASD and 22q.11.2 deletion syndrome," in the industry-based media coverage that followed. By focusing on the subset of autism patients with mGluR disruption, he explained how this work "could be the basis for one of the *first examples of a precision medicine focus in drug development for complex disease*" (quoted in Reynolds 2016). Indeed, it was not long before trials were initiated at CHOP. A 2016 Medgenics release that was picked up by Yahoo! Finance and a number of other financial and biotech news sources explained their plan to "initiate a Phase 1/2 study of psychiatric symptoms in children with 22q11.2 Deletion Syndrome. . . . The study will explore symptoms from three major neuropsychiatric disorders: ADHD, Anxiety and Autism Spectrum Disorders (ASD)" (Marketwired 2016).

In sum, 22q11.2DS is finally being taken up by researchers and highly capitalized biotech interests as a genetic model for much bigger prizes. Experts and advocates for 22q may still be some way from achieving the kind of success that the Fragile X network has had in leveraging their patient population's genomic specificity. Nevertheless, they are starting to reap the rewards that come from 22q11.2 microdeletion's status as a mutation associated with common disorders and medical conditions. A former CHOP researcher who went on to work for the same company, Seaside Therapeutics, that has pioneered Fragile X/autism pharmaceuticals told the crowd at Disney World that genetically specific disorders like 22q are like a "low hanging fruit." This phrase, which came up in chapter 3 and repeatedly during my fieldwork, points to the fact that the primary "translational" goal is often not to cure the rare genetic disorder itself, but to work toward insight and perhaps targeted interventions for more common conditions. Given the range of genes deleted and bodily systems affected in 22q11.2DS, a single pharmaceutical fix is likely impossible. Cure therefore remains by far the most promissory of the "Detection, Care, Cure" trio. It is perhaps best seen as a coordinating device that facilitates research and mobilization rather than as a concrete goal. Still, this new wave of "translational" work means that targeted pharmaceutical treatments are finally being developed for 22q. Only time will tell where this path will lead.

Conclusion

The 22q movement is striving to gain the numbers, awareness, resources, and alliances that will make 22q11.2DS a powerful kind of person. They still have a long way to go.

It is important to keep in mind that 22q11.2DS is *not* yet readily actionable for the majority of people with a 22q11.2 microdeletion. We have seen how geneticists and others are less likely to recognize "funny looking" nonwhite kids and refer them for genetic testing. Furthermore, there are no specialist clinics for conditions like 22q11.2DS, as far as I know, outside of highly developed countries, though there are research reports on diagnosed patients in countries like India (Gawde et al. 2006; Halder et al. 2010), Thailand (Ruangdaraganon et al. 1999), and Chile (Repetto et al. 2009; Guzman et al. 2012). Access to genetic tests that can diagnose 22q11.2DS is enormously uneven both between and within countries. Finally, finding medical practitioners knowledgeable about 22q or visiting a specialist center like CHOP, attending conferences, accessing information online, and so on, all require significant financial, social, and cultural capital on the part of parents.

Nevertheless, a 22q11.2DS diagnosis is being made to matter for more and more people. A local coalition of perhaps a few parents, a genetic counselor, and one or two interested clinical specialists can make 22q11.2DS a very powerful diagnosis in a given locale. As 22q advocates establish more centers and develop an arsenal of tools for swaying local professionals, it becomes far easier for any given family to use 22q11.2DS to shape a child's care. Today, there is even a summer camp just for kids with 22q11.2DS—"a unique and meaningful experience for children with 22q to meet and befriend other kids with 22q, to feel comfortable and understood in terms of their diagnosis, and develop a 'home away from home' with kids and staff who will accept them for exactly the individuals they are."[25] In these and many other ways, the 22q movement continues to make great strides, accruing the resources and forging the alliances that can make 22q11.2DS a powerful category of human difference.

These efforts would be futile, if not impossible, were it not for the biomedical literature on 22q11.2DS. At the same time, social mobilization has profoundly shaped the development of that literature as well as the purposes to which it is put. Cutting-edge knowledge about a condition like 22q11.2DS does not undergo an automatic, even process of diffusion; rather, actors have to forge domains where practice can be guided by it. A condition like 22q11.2DS tends to develop and flourish in scattered bastions—Children's Hospital of Philadelphia, Elwyn Services, Great Ormond Street Hospital in London, the MIND Institute, to name a few examples. That is why a 22q11.2 microdeletion has very uneven chances of being detected, never mind used to reshape treatment and care, even within the same highly developed polity. But those scattered bastions also train young professionals, who then bring their newfound expertise with them to new institutions and locales. As I argue in the next chapter, they can even convert skeptics in far-flung fields like clinical psychology into ardent advocates for the clinical relevance of genetic diagnosis.

Without a doubt, the different actors in these networks have very uneven levels and forms of authority. The preeminent biomedical expert on a genetic disorder is not the same as a parent advocate, nor is a pharmaceutical executive akin to an elementary school teacher. They all bring different resources to the table and get very different things out of their engagement with a genetic mutation. Nevertheless, each depends on the others to realize their goals. This complex mix of unequal authority and mutual dependence is absolutely key to understanding genomic designation today.

In sum, this chapter showed how 22q11.2DS is being assembled as a new kind of person. To be sure, the 22q network was enabled by much broader shifts in biomedicine and society. They consciously draw on the models for organizing, awareness-raising, lobbying, and so on that other disease advocacy organizations have developed to such great effect in recent decades (see Epstein 1996, 2016). But this new brand of disease advocacy is only part of the story. It also took tireless, agentive work by a wide range of actors to make 22q11.2DS really matter in the world. The 22q apparatus has to be assembled one piece at a time—a devilishly hard task when many of the pieces were never intended to fit together in the first place. Advocates for genetic disorders like Fragile X and 22q11.2DS had to develop novel repertoires of collective action in order to redirect practice and resources in fields like clinical psychology and special education that are neither geared to nor accustomed to dealing with genetics. To pursue Foucault's notion of the apparatus, the relations between the many elements involved—the said and the unsaid—had to be pieced together around something as foreign as a genetic mutation.

This is why reiterated fact-making is so useful for studying genomic designation: when new sets of actors came together to mobilize Fragile X and 22q11.2DS, the underlying mutations were all transformed as facts. What it means to have a genetic mutation like the 22q11.2 microdeletion depends on the locale in which you live, the era in which you were born, your race and class, and many other things besides; it depends on a whole host of factors, ranging from societal norms for managing developmental difference to the ability of a mother to wield a journal article during a doctor's visit. Perhaps more than anything, it depends on knowing you have that mutation and gaining entrée to a community of people dedicated to understanding and mobilizing it. In some cases, these groups have even been able to *transform* existing structures (see Sewell 1992) and *realign* practice in seemingly far-flung fields. In this way, these hybrid alliances have turned sociologically thin facts about genetic mutations into full-fledged kinds of people that can transform the experience of being ill or different in the twenty-first century.

SIX

Mutations in the Clinic: Reframing Illness and Redirecting Medical Practice

What happens when we take knowledge about a genetic mutation into the clinic, use it to understand a person's psychology, or organize treatment strategies around it? When it comes to mutations like the 22q11.2 microdeletions or the CGG repeat expansion on the *FMR1* gene, it can be a true game-changer. But why?

For now, at least, the reason has nothing to do with targeted pharmaceutical compounds. Despite some limited progress and an abundance of hope among the Fragile X and 22q communities, no targeted drug treatments have been approved for the conditions discussed in this book. For them, even though we do understand a great deal about the underlying genetics, a pharmaceutical version of "precision medicine" has so far stalled at the trial stage. Perhaps that will change one day soon.[1] As we have seen, pharmaceutical trials for Fragile X and 22q11.2DS are already underway. Still, even if targeted drug treatments for genomically designated conditions do hit the market one day, postapproval trials and issues of access, affordability, and efficacy will loom large in any assessment of their impact.

Instead, this chapter focuses on an altogether different form of precision medicine. Today, in many cases and many places, knowing that a person has a genetic mutation can shift the parameters for clinical judgment and decisively change medical practice.

It is important to note at the outset that this chapter does not provide a representative snapshot of the way people with genetic mutations are understood and treated. Access to genetic testing alone is highly stratified (see Clarke et al. 2003:170), especially here in the United States, where around twenty-eight million people are still uninsured, and many millions more are underinsured. Even once a mutation is found in a patient, it still takes various forms of capital to obtain the sorts of medical care or special education services that groups like the National Fragile X Foundation or International 22q11.2 Foundation recommend. So, while this chapter shows how mutations like the 22q11.2 microdeletion can be mobilized to create small perturbations in the massive edifice of modern medicine, it is entirely possible that genomic designation will remain utterly marginal or even fade away over the coming years.

My goal then is to focus on a vanguard of conditions and actors in order to see the growing impact of mutations on clinical practice. When someone with a complex disorder like 22q11.2DS is fortunate enough to have access to a specialist clinic or resourceful enough to convince local doctors to implement the consensus-based guidelines for 22q, it changes the battery of evaluations and treatments that are made available. In other words, knowing that a patient has a genetic mutation can reshape medical practice by altering what is considered "clinically indicated" in the first place. The specialist guidelines recommend that Fragile X and 22q11.2DS patients undergo a host of clinical evaluations across the life span, regardless of presentation. While experts often stress that interventions should be guided by a patient's presentation, knowledge about a mutation like the 22q11.2 microdeletion can redirect clinical attention and lead to the discovery of medical and psychiatric issues that would have otherwise probably evaded detection. Increasingly, having a condition like XYY or 22q11.2DS can also justify various forms of early intervention and modifications to standard clinical care for young children. Even poorly understood copy number variants, or CNVs, often lead to referrals, tests, surveillance, and interventions, including surgery and new drug regimens (Henderson et al. 2014; Riggs et al. 2014; Tao et al. 2014). In short, knowing the genetic cause of a patient's ills can decisively impact the way medical experts evaluate and treat them.

Finding a mutation can also recast core ideas about disease and difference altogether. It can provide a diagnosis that, because it is rooted in a person's genetic inheritance, is treated as more fundamental than other clinical or psychological diagnoses a patient may have already received. In this way, a diagnosis that is tied to a mutation can often relegate phenotypic diagnoses to mere symptoms of an underlying genetic condition, providing an anchor for patients caught up in a sea of shifting medical and behavioral problems and thereby ending their stressful "diagnostic odyssey." In chapter 7, I show how knowing that a person has a genetic mutation can even destabilize the very boundary between normality and pathology.

In this chapter, I show how some mutations have become key objects of practice in sites far afield from the genetics labs and biomedical journals where they first came to our attention. They have made their way not only into medical centers and doctors' offices, but also into psychologists' clinics and classrooms. If you go to a 22q conference, survey the literature, or explore the resources available on the foundation's website, it becomes abundantly clear that 22q11.2DS has traveled far beyond its point of origin in clinical specialties like cardiology, ENT (ear, nose, and throat), and endocrinology. When mutations are used to guide classification and practice in places focused on cognition, behavior, and development instead of just medical care, they can give rise to even more powerful kinds of people.

Reframing Illness

Receiving a diagnosis like 22q11.2DS can transform the way a family and medical team understand a child. Even when we do not know the pathophysiology of *how* a mutation causes a particular problem, or *which* of its associated phenotypes any given patient will present with, a genetic diagnosis can still provide a powerful perspective on illness. At the same time, these new genetic diagnoses must be made to work in a world still dominated by clinical nosology.

Ending the Diagnostic Odyssey and Providing a Mandate for Early Intervention

One of the most salient features of a genetic diagnosis is simply its capacity to provide an explanation for the medical or psychological challenges a person faces. Take the story of Sheila Kambin—the current chairperson of the International 22q11.2 Foundation—and the "diagnostic odyssey" her family experienced before finally receiving a 22q11.2DS diagnosis for their son. We saw her brief appeal to the committee overseeing recommendations for the US newborn screening kit in the last chapter. But now, let's see how she put it in a speech to a large audience at the 2012 International 22q11.2 Foundation conference:

Our journey began when my son was emergently delivered at term for severe growth restriction. He spent several weeks in the NICU at a very well-known teaching hospital. He was evaluated for thrombocytopenia, hypoglycemia, poor feeding, and temperature regulation. Multiple diagnostic procedures were performed. He was unable to latch for breast-feeding. He had a sacral pit, low set ears, and thrombocytopenia of unknown origin, yet no one recommended genetic testing. He came home at a weight of 4-11. I kept trying to breast feed him and he lost more weight. I had to supplement with formula and pump into a bottle. We saw four doctors and three lactation consultants and no one ever bothered to examine his palate.

At four months of age he underwent a bilateral ingrown hernia repair. Next he was late on every single developmental milestone by at least six months. He finally walked at 18 months. We saw physical therapists and occupational therapists. We saw orthopedics for his ligament laxity and hammertoes at age two. That doctor sent us to a geneticist for an evaluation for Ehlers-Danlos Syndrome. His medical and surgical history were carefully reviewed. He had a full physical exam and a seasoned geneticist looked at my son's bulbous nose, his narrow palpebral fissures, his malar hypoplasia, his retrognathia, his high-arched palate, his bifid uvula, his hypernasal speech, his long tapered fingers, his growth and developmental delays, and his thin appearing skin. He told me no testing is indicated, let's just get a cardiac echo when he turns four to be safe.

Time marched on. We were sent to an orthotist for his anomalous toes and feet. He was fitted for countless braces. His teachers started to raise concerns. We saw a speech pathologist who failed to recognize his anatomy, his hypernasal speech, and the fact that he had a submucous cleft palate. She told me that his speech was normal. When he was four, one of his teachers told his father and I that she thought something was wrong with Aiden. She delicately explained that she had been teaching preschool for over 30 years and she felt that Aiden needed to be evaluated. But by who? We brought him to a world-renowned developmental pediatrician who spent four hours evaluating him. That doctor told us that he might be on the autism spectrum and sent us to 14 specialists. Those specialists included PT, OT, speech again, orthopedics, audiology, back to genetics, psychology for cognitive testing, behavior therapy, and social skills evaluation. Overwhelmed with dampened spirits, his father and I left the office and he said to me, "Aiden does not have autism, and we are not going to make any of these appointments." I said, "I know he doesn't have autism but we are going to see every specialist on this list until we find an answer." And he agreed with me.

It took another six months and fourteen visits. When he was five we saw another geneticist. That doctor also looked carefully at Aiden and again said, "We won't find anything, but I will send a microarray just to be thorough." His diagnosis came back as an incidental finding. That geneticist said to me, "Sheila, this is not the first time I have been burned by 22q. I really need to keep it higher up on my differential."

Aiden is now eight years old. His palate was not repaired until this year because he missed the chance for intervention. His speech patterns are set and most surgeons did not want to touch him. He requires intensive speech and articulation therapy three times per week. It is possible that he suffered from hypocalcaemia at birth. This may play a role in his psycho-social development and cognitive function, but we will never know.

What I left out of this story until now is that besides the 27 clinical specialists that he saw, his two parents are both physicians who practice at major academic institutions in a metropolitan area. His father is an ENT, an ears, nose, and throat surgeon, a very bright and accomplished ENT who did not realize the velopharyngeal deficiency. I am an obstetrician who always thought that her son's ears looked funny, but never put it all together. Furthermore, I am an obstetrician who delivers some of the sickest babies in the world, and to this day I am not certain that I could reliably make this diagnosis in the delivery room.

My story is not one of a child who almost died, but my story is a very common one. I believe in my heart that Aiden would be undiagnosed to this day if he had not been evaluated at CHOP or had parents with the tenacity to keep pushing for evaluations. Newborn screening would have given Aiden a chance for early interventions, which would have improved his prognosis substantially. Newborn screening would have prevented this type of diagnostic odyssey. Thank you.

Why have I chosen to include this speech in its entirety? Kambin's story poignantly illustrates, yet again, the many barriers to 22q11.2DS diagnosis, even for seriously affected patients with access to leading medical specialists. Despite having two parents with pertinent expertise, one of whom worked at the world's leading 22q center, Aiden was only diagnosed as an *incidental* finding on microarray. We see how an unsatisfying autism diagnosis was offered as part of their "diagnostic odyssey" and how the 22q diagnosis resolved that odyssey *not* by obviating the need for further referrals, but by providing an etiological diagnosis that directs evaluation and intervention in new ways.

Indeed, Kambin's story speaks to two crucial, but seemingly countervailing aspects of contemporary genetic medicine: 22q11.2DS is at once highly variable and capable of providing a deep diagnostic certainty to a patient and their family. You may not know what medical and psychological problems a child with 22q11.2DS will face over the course his life, but you will always have an explanation of *why* he is facing them. Her story also provides a sense of just how serious a condition like 22q can be even when the cardinal clinical sign—a congenital heart defect—is absent. The fact that her son did not fit the typical 22q11.2DS profile would not have made him a "patient in waiting," to use Timmermans and Buchbinder's evocative term (2010). Instead, finding the 22q11.2 microdeletion would have prevented years of diagnostic odyssey by providing an explanatory anchor and a lens through which to understand Aiden's manifold challenges.

Kambin's dramatic story, like that of almost every parent of a child with 22q11.2DS that I have met, revolves around the simultaneously trying and empowering process of receiving a diagnosis. That is the one constant, whether it is a prenatal finding that transforms parents' outlooks for the future, an adult diagnosis that brings with it the poignant question of "What if?" or something in between. While some parents receive a diagnosis pre- or neonatally, the experience of a "diagnostic odyssey" is the norm: a range of medical and/or developmental challenges in early childhood and often beyond—from minor and trivial to life-threatening and profound—amounting to a bewildering and stressful experience for both patients and their families.

A genetic diagnosis, it is generally agreed, ends the odyssey by providing a single and encompassing explanation. It also provides the opportunity to meet other families dealing with the same condition, if not the same symptoms. Indeed, the capacity of a genetic diagnosis to put an end to a family's diagnostic odyssey is considered one of the major benefits of genetic testing for children with multiple medical and/or developmental challenges (Ledbetter 2009b; Bales, Zaleski, and McPherson 2010). Take the findings from a piece published in the *Journal of Intellectual Disability Research*, whose last author, Anne Bassett, runs a major 22q11.2DS clinic in Toronto and is highly active in the 22q Foundation: "Diagnostic certainty alone appears closely linked to psychological benefit, even when uncertainty remains about the extent of expression of a particular genetic anomaly in any particular individual" (Costain et al. 2012:648). So even though it may be unclear whether and how a particular mutation will affect a patient, a genetic diagnosis is still thought to provide an important "psychological benefit." However, the authors warn, "This may be overlooked by clinicians who equate diagnostic benefit solely with improved medical management" (648). Doctors should therefore seek out and return genetic results, whether or not they have direct implications for clinical practice. They continue by discussing the example of adults diagnosed with 22q11.2DS: "Identification of a 22q11.2 deletion after early childhood provided many adults with 22q11.2DS and families the satisfaction of an explanation for their lifelong challenges, sometimes after years of fruitless investigations (the 'diagnostic odyssey'). As for autism, genetic findings that explain ID [intellectual disability], schizophrenia or other stigmatised neurodevelopmental conditions may be particularly valued for their explanatory value" (Costain et al. 2012:648; references omitted). A genetic *explanation* of someone's psychiatric and medical problems is therefore considered highly beneficial in its own right. The value of finding a genetic mutation cannot be reduced to its clinical implications.

However, Kambin's speech does not include the chapter that often follows the end of a patient's odyssey: the bemusing experience of reading voluminous material about 22q and its legion of clinical and psychological associations, the obstacles to getting their local clinicians to embrace the 22q diagnosis and its attendant risks and referrals, and then the experience of finding other 22q families who have faced kindred challenges, even when they are, in fact, markedly different. In other words, genetic certainty can bring with it a new world of uncertainty. It prompts the question, Which of this mutation's associated phenotypes and clinical conditions will we have to deal with in the future? As the authors of a 2008 Hastings Report put it, a genetic diagnosis early in life may halt the diagnostic odyssey, but at considerable cost: "The family begins a treatment odyssey—searching the Internet, visiting specialists, running up debt, medicalizing the child's life" (Baily and Murray 2008:29).

One parent recounted the "cycles of grief" he had been through since receiving the 22q diagnosis for his daughter. Over time he came to see it as hugely empowering, even as he admitted he was still grieving the fact that he could never fully fix this problem in his family. He also told me about the huge financial strain of the diagnosis and its associated guidelines. Another described the overwhelming process of reading about 22q, attending her first conference, meeting seriously affected patients, and learning about the various problems that her son may or may not encounter as he grows up. She poignantly described that experience to me as one of *"mourning for the future."* By the time I met her, however, the 22q11.2DS diagnosis and community provided a rubric for understanding whatever lay ahead and a network of support to help her cope with it.

Finally, we see how Kambin imagines a poignant counterfactual past where a 22q diagnosis had been made far earlier, perhaps even at birth, allowing for that most cherished of opportunities: early intervention. Kambin repeatedly expresses the widespread belief that a 22q diagnosis helps practitioners to *see* problems that would otherwise be missed (e.g., the submucous cleft palate and the infant hypocalcemia) and informs interventions that might not otherwise be undertaken (speech therapy, surgical palate repair, calcium infusions, etc.). We return to these issues later.

Even for genetic conditions that are usually very mild, the idea of early intervention looms large. An XYY brochure produced by AXYS, the main organization for disorders caused by sex chromosome aneuploidies, explains, "Infants and very young children may be eligible for early intervention," before going on to list speech therapy, occupational and physical therapy, special education services, social skills training, counseling, behavioral consultation, and regular exercise and upper-body strengthening programs.[2] Although medical issues like acne, tall stature, dental issues, occasional hypogonadism, and hypotonia are associated with XYY, it remains, just as in the 1960s and 1970s, primarily a disorder affecting speech, cognition, and behavior. Now that it has been added to the new wave of noninvasive prenatal genetic tests, more and more of the one in one thousand males with an extra Y chromosome are likely to receive an XYY diagnosis, making them subject to this regime of early intervention before problems even arise. More or less the same goes for the one in one thousand females with an extra X chromosome, or XXX syndrome. Many of these people would have been so mildly affected that they may have never experienced a diagnostic odyssey at all. Nevertheless, finding a mutation recasts their behavior as the phenotype of a genetic disorder and provides a mandate for early intervention.

The all-important point for advocates is this: getting a genetic diagnosis like Fragile X, 22q11.2DS, XYY, 1p36 Deletion Syndrome, or 5p– syndrome very early in life provides a series of cherished opportunities. As Bailey, Skinner, et al. put it in an article discussing Fragile X as a prototype for expanded newborn screening (2008:e694): "Although screening would identify newborns for whom there is no direct medical benefit, it is widely endorsed by parents of affected children, because it could prevent the 'diagnostic odyssey' that most experience, allow access to early intervention during a time of critical brain development, and provide them with important information about reproductive risk." (The authors also discuss a series of serious risks to adding

FXS to the newborn screening regime.) The ultimate goal is to catch things early and intervene before problems can fully take root. Early intervention has become a watchword in fields ranging from newborn screening to autism therapy. When it comes to genomically designated conditions, however, it indexes an opportunity to improve *many* different aspects of a child's development.

In sum, Kambin's speech encapsulates the belief in the enormous power of a genetic diagnosis and the need for screening and early intervention. At the same time, it captures how 22q11.2DS is often invisible to the clinical gaze and how hard it is to mobilize it in most medical settings. Above all, it shows how the very fact of a genetic diagnosis, in and of itself, can provide a sense of certainty and an anchor for patients and their families on their journey through the health care system.

Overcoming the Old Nosology

The biased profile of 22q11.2DS is largely a legacy of its complex relationship to older clinical diagnoses like DiGeorge syndrome (DGS), Velocardiofacial syndrome (VCFS), and several others. As we saw in chapter 1, knowledge about the 22q11 deletion unified research on those conditions into a single field. Then, a new condition emerged: 22q11.2 Deletion Syndrome. The field has now more or less settled on the idea that "22q11.2DS"—both in name and in principle—is the best way to understand everyone with the 22q11.2 microdeletion, regardless of whether their phenotype more closely resembles the old profile of DGS, VCFS, or what have you. With the incidence of 22q11.2DS now thought to be as high as one in one thousand, it is a striking example of the way genomic designation can reshape nosology in ways that are at once radical and complex.

However, that complex history still creates obstacles to the accrual of 22q diagnoses. Even though "22q11.2 Deletion Syndrome" is very much in the ascendancy when it comes to the nomenclature of biomedical research (see fig. 1.1 in chapter 1), DiGeorge and VCFS remain common names for *diagnosis* upon receiving a positive test for a 22q11.2 deletion. Meanwhile, "VCFS" in particular is still used by a number of important organizations, clinics, and advocacy groups. Indeed, until it closed in 2015, the American-based Velo-Cardio-Facial Syndrome Educational Foundation, Inc. (VCFSEF) was still a major player in the field, and the relationship between its leadership and that of the International 22q11.2 Foundation has been strained to say the least.

The key figure in the VCFSEF network was Robert Shprintzen, who published the foundational paper delineating VCFS in 1978. The origins of the dispute are contested, but they go back to an attempt by Shprintzen and the Children's Hospital of Philadelphia (CHOP) team to collaborate on an NIH grant proposal in the early 1990s. Suffice it to say that this attempt at collaboration went awry. In the end, two separate proposals were submitted, and the CHOP team won the day. In the years that followed, CHOP experts and other activists in Philadelphia established the 22q group that has since blossomed into the 22q and You Center at CHOP and the International 22q11.2 Foundation. Each side in this internecine 22q vs. VCFSEF dispute repeatedly accused the other of deception and petty attempts to undermine the other's good work. While some experts have been able to maintain good relations with both groups, key people on either side readily offered recriminating tales and opinions about one another in our conversations.

It is impossible to say how much this fracture cost the broader movement, but most of the parents and experts I spoke to were certain that the effect had been profound. Indeed, parents at both 22q and VCFSEF conferences expressed deep frustration about the unnecessary and costly split in their movement. Here is how one dad of a little girl with 22q11.2DS put it to me:

We're parents, first and foremost; . . . we don't really give a rat's butt what political games are being played. . . . We learned that there are two dominant players in this field. . . . They don't play well together. There's a heck of a lot of good ideas and big brains on both sides of the fence, and it's a damn shame. . . . All we give a crap about is our little girl. It's like, "Put your egos on the shelves guys!" and let's think about who we're serving instead of whose name is on top of a journal article. . . . It pisses me off when people put that above my kid. I think that hurts the awareness, the progression, and the treatment of these kids. Is that too harsh?

Spurred on by this kind of sentiment, there were moves toward rapprochement between the International 22q11.2 Foundation and VCFSEF in the years before the latter folded, with each organization appearing on the other's website and key figures attending each other's events. Shprintzen still runs a 501(c)3 Virtual Center for VCFS that provides medical advice to families and publishes a "journal" (Shprintzen is an author on half of the eight articles published since 2013). But with VCFSEF sunsetting, Shprintzen retiring, and both the biomedical literature and advocacy groups increasingly favoring "22q11.2DS," the International 22q11.2 Foundation may be on the verge of winning the day. Time will tell.

To be clear, this dispute was waged at the level of nomenclature rather than nosology. The VCFSEF Twitter page had the subheading: "VCFS *is the deletion of a small segment of chromosome 22* (specified as 22q11.2 deletion), and is one of the most common genetic disorders."[3] Shprintzen has written an article entitled "The Name Game" (1998), and in a speech entitled "Science Not Politics" at the VCFSEF annual meeting I attended in New Brunswick in 2011, he excoriated the very idea of calling the condition delineated by the 22q11.2 deletion "22q11.2DS." To him, the fact that 22q lacks a clinically descriptive element, and the fact that other conditions that have been associated with a mutation, like Williams syndrome, had not been so renamed, made the use of "22q11.2DS" unnecessary and counterproductive. (However, he was at pains to point out that he held no attachment to VCFS as the name he introduced to the world, or to the once-frequent use of "Shprintzen syndrome.") Others on the 22q side object that, insofar as "VCFS" is descriptive, it is also misleading. They correctly point out that people with a 22q11.2 microdeletion can have neither velopharyngeal insufficiency (V), cardiac defects (C), nor the typical facial phenotype (F). Crucially, even Shprintzen now considers a 22q11.2 deletion to be necessary and sufficient for diagnosis with VCFS.

At a conference on 22q11.2DS and education in Indianapolis in 2011, Brenda Finucane explained to the gathered parents and experts how, before the discovery of the 22q11 deletion, people thought that DiGeorge syndrome and VCFS *"were two completely different syndromes."* In other words, "they are older terms that described specific, clinical— what are called phenotypes or patterns of features." She went on to say, *"We are smarter now,* and genetically we know there's no detectable difference in the microdeletions between people with VCFS versus those with DGS or the other syndromes—*it's the same thing. There's no difference between the child with the DGS diagnosis and VCF."* But without a break in her speech, Finucane goes from "there's no difference," to this: "Now, *could they be very different children? Of course they could* because there's a lot of variability in the syndrome, but genetically it is all just one big continuum or spectrum, all due to the same underlying microdeletion."

So here we have the nosological consensus that relegates clinical observation to the level of symptomatology and carves out the disease strictly according to a genetic mutation. "The one thing they have in common," Finucane hit home, "is the underlying microdeletion." Again, even the VCFS group accepted that two "very different children" can have this condition if and only if they have the 22q11.2 mutation.

Initial optimism that variations in the breakpoint of the deletion would explain the contrasting phenotypes proved to be mostly incorrect, while new ventures to examine gene × gene interaction effects with other genomic regions are in their early phases. Whatever the outcome, the goal is *not* to repartition 22q, and it is certainly not to revalidate VCFS and DiGeorge syndrome as independent conditions. The older, lingering clinical categories are treated as a sort of unfortunate historical efflux.

However, that does not mean that they have no impact on the field today. As Finucane pointed out, having "several different names being used" for people with 22q11.2 microdeletions "creates tremendous confusion not just among families but also the professionals out there. . . . It further divides the resources for an already rare syndrome." And yet, Finucane pointed out, 22q is actually quite common. So why does it get so little attention? Finucane drew a stark contrast with Fragile X, saying that 22q "is so common, and it is even more common than let's say, Fragile X syndrome, which has much more momentum for targeted pharmaceuticals. They're a multi-million dollar organization for kids with Fragile X. We're nowhere near that . . . a lot of it has to do with the name." If the foundation could get families and especially professionals to "think 22q," she argued, then eventually children would cease to be diagnosed with the older names, and awareness, money, and other resources would come more easily to 22q11.2DS. In addition, it would help families and clinicians understand what they are dealing with. The International 22q11.2 Foundation points out how "parents of a baby diagnosed with DiGeorge syndrome may be frustrated by the lack of information about DGS, not realizing that VCFS and 22q resources (including this Foundation!) also pertain to their child." Similarly, even "health care providers may not access all current and available information if they are searching for literature under an older name."

So what does this all mean? Genomic designation has clearly won the day in terms of formal nosology. When it comes to the actual *name* of the diagnosis people receive upon detection of a 22q11.2 microdeletion, however, the old clinical nomenclature continues to represent a major obstacle to 22q's growth as a social movement and development as a kind of person. After all, it is even harder to raise awareness and build a disease advocacy movement—or any kind of social movement—under multiple banners.

The International 22q11.2 Foundation therefore dedicates considerable efforts to its battle against the outdated clinical nomenclature. Consider this announcement: "The Foundation is pleased to launch the Same Name Campaign, an educational effort aimed at professionals and families, with the goal of establishing consistent terminology for the 22q11.2 deletion syndrome."[4] Brenda Finucane heads the foundation's Same Name Campaign, which uses a host of tactics to get clinicians, publishers, parents, media, and everyone else besides to drop the older clinical terms like DiGeorge syndrome and VCFS in favor of 22q11.2DS. They have sent postcards to journals, genetic counselors, and others; lobbied professional organizations; and convinced groups like the Dempster Foundation and the United Kingdom's main group, Max Appeal, to adopt 22q11.2DS in place of their previous use of "DiGeorge syndrome."

The Same Name Campaign adopts different approaches when it comes to families and experts. The foundation's Same Name Campaign pages explain: "As a parent-driven organization, the Foundation acknowledges that families who have lived for years with a diagnosis of VCFS, DGS, CTAF or a related condition may find it difficult to switch to a different name." They simply ask that families mention 22q11.2 along with other names that they may have a long-standing attachment to. When it comes to the professionals who "represent a crucial gateway to diagnosis," by contrast, the foundation adopts a no-holds-barred approach. Every one of the Same Name Campaign's declared tactics targets biomedical experts: presentations at professional meetings, the distribution of literature, the development of a consensus terminology among experts, and lobbying publishers of professional journals to adopt the sole use of *22q11.2DS* instead of the old clinical terms. As they explain, "Over time, as professionals more consistently use the 22q11.2 designation, fewer and fewer people will be newly diagnosed with VCFS, DGS, CTAF or other outdated names; our goal is that eventually, all will be on the same page, moving in the same direction, supporting our worldwide 22q community."

Whatever the outcome of this campaign, the uneasy relationship between 22q11.2DS and the older syndromes shows the deep damage a disease advocacy movement incurs when it is split not only at the level of resources and activists, but also at the level of nosology and nomenclature. It is also indicative of the way genomic designation, as a form of classification, can be impeded by older, clinically derived categories. In order to move forward at full strength, 22q advocates are essentially waging war against the more long-standing clinical syndrome categories like DiGeorge and VCFS that they hope to subsume and replace. They see victory in that battle as an essential step toward many of their broader goals.

Interfacing with Clinical and Psychiatric Nosology

When it comes to conditions like schizophrenia, ADHD, hypocalcemia, and heart malformations, 22q11.2DS advocates adopt a very different approach. Rather than usurpation, they are trying to develop a series of productive relationships between 22q11.2DS and the kinds of common medical conditions and psychiatric disorders that dominate clinical and educational practice. In short, the goal is not to supplant common conditions but to create points of interface with them. This includes everything from the leveraging projects that can lead to targeted pharmaceutical trials discussed in chapters 3–5 to merely probabilistic associations. When it comes to garnering local services, referrals, and resources, researchers and advocates often just use clinical and behavioral categories instrumentally to get what they want.

At the same time, parents are encouraged to reserve a kind of ontological primacy for their child's genetic diagnosis. Indeed, we need look no farther than the same speech by Brenda Finucane at the 2011 conference in Indianapolis (above) to see how 22q11.2DS experts and advocates attempt to achieve commensurability with common diagnoses, even as they relegate them to mere symptomatology. "Psychiatry, psychology, and genetics," Finucane explained to the audience, "have kind of grown up independent of each other and have really developed their own ways of looking at developmental differences." As a result, a child might get caught in the middle of these "different diagnostic systems" and "may get multiple diagnoses depending on who is looking at the child and what their background is." She told the audience that when three kids all present with a learning disability, obsessive-compulsive disorder, and anxiety disorder, "from the school's point of view, these three kids all have the same thing. And yet when you do the math, so to speak, this little boy has Smith-Magenis Syndrome, this child has Williams Syndrome, and this little guy has the 22q11.2 Deletion Syndrome. Three totally unrelated genetic disorders." For schools, she explained, it is primarily the psychiatric diagnoses that determine education plans and eligibility for services. This has meant that, for pragmatic reasons, 22q parents should not eschew psychiatric diagnoses. On the contrary, they should use them for everything they are worth. The same goes for other medical fields as well.

So what does this mean for the way we think about illness, not just in the clinic, but in fields that are even further removed from medical genetics? What is the role of a 22q11.2DS diagnosis when a child is being evaluated and cared for in a classroom or a psychologist's office? This is what Finucane told that group of 22q parents and professionals in Indianapolis: "Psychiatric diagnoses are really important, but they are different from etiological diagnoses; . . . if you pick up the chart on a 17-year-old, you will see six and seven different diagnoses because every time a different symptom constellation comes up, or as the child matures and behavior differences happen, then you are starting to see different diagnoses." When a child is then given an additional 22q11.2DS diagnosis, where does it fit into this already-complex picture? As Finucane explained, "so then you have got, hovering in this [diagnostic] soup here, also the 22q Deletion Syndrome." At first, this may seem like yet another comorbid condition: "The reaction of a parent when she finds out, yet again, that her child would get *another* diagnosis is pretty understandable: after a while you're kind of like, 'What is going on? Every year it seems to be a different thing, every year we are told a different diagnosis.'"

It is not only parents who failed to grasp what was really happening. Finucane explained, "A lot of times parents, and even professionals in education systems will say to me, 'This poor kid, he ended up with seven different things. Oh my gosh, how could you get struck by lightning seven different times?'" At this point, the audience was laughing away, despite the fact that Finucane was recounting a very confusing, trying process that many of them had experienced firsthand. That was Finucane's moment to hammer home her key point. "The bottom line," she explained, "is he *didn't get struck by lightning seven different times. This child has one underlying condition—the 22q11.2 Deletion Syndrome,* which results in patterns of behavior and learning that, [through our] psychiatric and educational diagnostic systems, we can classify by these other names." It may not yet be widely recognized in schools and hospitals, but a genomically designated condition like 22q11.2DS allows parents, teachers, and caregivers to recast a shifting, stressful, and confusing series of developmental behavioral diagnoses into an evolving pattern of *symptoms* caused by a single genetic disorder. It is the real condition—the one constant and the cause of everything a person with a 22q11.2 microdeletion might experience. That is how it resolves a diagnostic odyssey that can span hospitals, schools, and psychologists' offices.

Crucially, the goal is not just to reshape the way patients and their parents think about genetics and difference. Instead, both parents and experts work to get school districts around the country to recognize and appreciate the value of genetic classification. Finucane described how, in her presentations to school districts all over the country, she will often see *"light bulbs start going off over people's heads.* They never realized this, that these genetic diagnoses that are now starting to come in are actually the underpinnings for many of these other behavioral diagnoses."* A genetic disorder like 22q or Fragile X is not just another diagnosis; it means that *"we've gotten down to the bottom line."* Finucane wanted the 22q parents to understand that even schools that had never knowingly dealt with a case of 22q11.2DS before were often able to learn a lot about it and put excellent, tailored programs in place. In practice, Finucane explained to this lecture hall full of parents that "it may be on you to educate education systems" about 22q.

So, for pragmatic reasons, 22q parents should certainly not eschew psychiatric diagnoses. Finucane told this room of 22q parents that they should *"use these diagnoses for everything [they're worth]."* At the same time, she stressed the importance of "realizing and keeping in mind and trying to educate people that *22q is the underlying cause and these other things are all symptoms of it."* Parents should therefore embrace the practical necessity of symptom-based classification, even as they see everything through the lens of the underlying genetic condition. Genomic designation is at its most powerful when conduits of interface and exchange can be established with broader surveillance categories like autism, ADHD, and obesity, as well as fields like clinical medicine, psychology, and special education.[5]

Redirecting Clinical Judgment and Practice

Now more than ever, there is a wealth of evidence and expertise on the way particular genetic mutations should guide clinical practice. In this section, we will see how this works in specialist 22q11.2DS clinics before moving on to less accommodating domains: the psychologist's practice and the local health care providers who may know very little about genetic medicine.

In the last chapter we saw how 22q11.2DS experts and advocates are working to increase numbers of diagnosed patients, garner resources, and court allies in fields that have long been far removed from genetics. For them, no field matters more than pediatric medicine, and no institution is more of a game-changer than a specialist clinic dedicated to their genetic disorder. That is why a key focus of the 22q movement is following in Fragile X's footsteps and building a network of specialist clinics.

Specialist Fragile X and 22q clinics are never independent medical centers with full-time staff. Instead, they are something much more obtainable for a rare disorder: a small group of experts who are familiar with 22q11.2DS and a medical center with the capacity to provide the tests, referrals, and treatments recommended by the consensus-based clinical management guidelines. This might sound quite straightforward. However, when patients find themselves at a specialist center after being diagnosed with 22q11.2DS, there are myriad implications for their clinical evaluation, treatment, and prospect horizons that the clinic must be set up to coordinate and manage. In many cases, 22q clinics are geared toward one or another dimension of the 22q11.2DS phenotype—hence the foundation works to define and regulate what a specialist center should be set up to do.

A range of different medical evaluations and treatments are recommended upon diagnosis with 22q11.2DS. As the 22q11.2 Foundation's newly refurbished website (made possible by a grant from the Robert Wood Johnson Foundation) puts it in their "Healthcare Guidelines" section,

How should individuals with the 22q11.2 deletion be followed medically?
Ideally, children with the 22q11.2 deletion should receive coordinated care from centers that offer multidisciplinary teams of clinicians, often drawn from more than 20 specialties. Centers address each child's individual health problems, as well as issues such as speech or learning delays, in order to help these children and their families lead the best life possible.

Upon initial diagnosis, the standard assessment and work-up for all ages generally includes:

- Cardiology
- Endocrinology
- Immunology
- Speech/Language/Developmental Assessments
- A Renal Ultrasound (to check the kidneys)
- X-rays of the neck (in children old enough to cooperate and where the bones are well ossified—so ~ 3 to 4 years of age)·
- Deletion studies in both parents when available

Thereafter, the work-up is individualized, depending on the symptoms, but may include any or all of the following: . . .[6]

The site then goes on to list "Plastic Surgery/ENT/Audiology; Gastro-enterology/Feeding Team; Hematology; Urology/Nephrology; Ortho-pedics; Ophthalmology; General Surgery; Dentistry; Rheumatology; Neurology/Neurosurgery; Psychiatry." In practice, specialist 22q clinics often provide most of the optional referrals listed above for every new patient. Parents are also encouraged to seek them out from local pro-viders, even when they are not clinically indicated.

The consensus-based guidelines for 22q11.2DS make similar recom-mendations as well. Take this table from a Grand Rounds on 22q11.2DS in the *Journal of Pediatrics* in 2011 (fig. 6.1): we see how no less than twenty-one specialist assessments are recommended for people with 22q, regardless of their presenting signs, usually at several developmen-tal milestones each (Bassett et al. 2011:336). It is important to note the dual role of a paper like this. On the one hand, it provides guidelines for management and care—guidelines that can be used to convince skep-tical clinicians to order the many tests indicated by a 22q11.2 micro-deletion. Indeed, being published in the *Journal of Pediatrics* legitimates the guidelines developed by 22q experts; it helps to constitute all these tests and referrals as valid indications for people with 22q11.2DS. On the other hand, the guidelines represent a signature achievement in the effort to raise awareness among clinicians.

Any given 22q11.2DS patient may require treatment from many or all of these clinical specialties, or they may require none. Either way, with two hundred associated symptoms and counting, there is cer-

Table II. Recommended assessments for 22q11.2 deletion syndrome*						
Assessment	At diagnosis	Infancy (0-12 months)	Preschool age (1-5 years)	School age (6-11 years)	Adolescence (12-18 years)	Adulthood (>18 years)
Ionized calcium, parathyroid hormone†	✓	✓	✓	✓	✓	✓
Thyrotropin (thyroid-stimulating hormone)†	✓		✓	✓	✓	✓
Complete blood cell count and differential (annual)	✓	✓	✓	✓		
Immunologic evaluation‡	✓	✓§	✓§			
Ophthalmology	✓		✓			
Evaluate palate¶	✓	✓	✓			
Audiology	✓	✓	✓			✓
Cervical spine (>age 4 years)			✓‖			
Scoliosis examination	✓		✓		✓	
Dental evaluation			✓	✓	✓	✓
Renal ultrasound	✓					
Electrocardiogram	✓					✓
Echocardiogram	✓					
Development**	✓	✓	✓			
School performance				✓	✓	
Socialization/functioning	✓	✓	✓	✓	✓	✓
Psychiatric/emotional/behavioral††	✓		✓	✓	✓	✓
Systems review	✓	✓	✓	✓	✓	✓
Deletion studies of parents	✓					
Genetic counseling‡‡	✓				✓	✓
Gynecologic and contraceptive services					✓	✓

FIGURE 6.1. Table from the 22q11.2DS guidelines in the *Journal of Pediatrics* (Bassett et al. 2011:336). (Reproduced by permission from Elsevier)

tainly plenty to worry about. Take Sheila Kambin's story, recounted above, where the failure to detect her son's 22q11.2 microdeletion early was blamed for the failure to recognize his submucous cleft palate, infant hypocalcemia, and so on—opportunities for early intervention that were therefore lost forever. Even for mildly affected cases, however, a 22q11.2DS diagnosis realigns clinical attention in such a way that problems are likely to be found even when they may not have been detected or considered problems at all in the absence of a 22q diagnosis. Indeed, as ascertainment broadens and becomes less biased toward patients presenting with cardiac and palatal issues, we can expect 22q to realign clinical judgment in a growing array of people.

After all, when it comes to care for genomically designated conditions like 22q11.2DS, we are confronted with a challenging question: Care for what? The tautological answer—care for the symptoms caused by a 22q11.2 microdeletion—does not get us very far. Unlike other diagnoses that are made according to biomedical observations, genetic mutations do not have any immediately apparent physiological specificity. It is not a question of a clinical sign, nor a combination or subset of signs that necessarily has to be in play. To repeat, as Donna McDonald-McGinn put it to me in an interview (2011): "22q *is* 22q; . . . it's a spectrum from no symptoms to every malformation under the sun." So, while 22q11.2DS has an enormous number of clinical associations, having 22q11.2DS is simply a question of having a chromosomal deletion at 22q11.2. You are at risk for any number of medical or developmental pathologies, but even if you are largely healthy, you are not merely asymptomatic or a carrier—you are just mildly affected. The need for rigorous medical surveillance and perhaps intervention remains. At a specialist center, the 22q population can be treated as a coherent whole despite this extraordinary range in clinical presentation.

The stakes are extremely high. We saw how Sheila Kambin lamented the missed opportunity for early intervention into several of her son's medical issues. Her poignant "what if?" was based on the idea—shared by most 22q experts—that finding a 22q11.2 microdeletion can redirect clinical attention toward issues that are incredibly serious, and yet easy to miss in the absence of the 22q11.2DS diagnosis. Consider a recent paper reporting findings from eleven patients who were neonatally identified with 22q11.2DS only after a positive newborn screening result, but negative diagnostic follow-up, for severe combined immunodeficiency (SCID). The authors point out that many 22q patients are only diagnosed later in life after problems arise like "hypernasal speech due to palatal insufficiency and developmental and behavioral differences including speech delay, autism, and learning disabilities that would benefit from early interventions." Turning to their patient cohort, they report that at least six out of their eleven cases would probably *not* have been diagnosed in infancy were it not for the SCID screening result. Among those six, they explain, the identification of the 22q11.2 microdeletion led to "diagnosis of significant associated features including hypocalcemia, congenital heart disease (CHD), and gastroesophageal reflux disease that may have gone unrecognized and therefore untreated." They conclude by suggesting that all children with a positive newborn screen result but negative follow-up test for SCID should be tested for 22q11.2DS. Better yet, they argue, "direct NBS [newborn screening] for 22q11.2DS . . . would be equally, if not more, beneficial, as early identification of 22q11.2DS will obviate a protracted diagnostic odyssey while providing an opportunity for timely assessment and interventions as needed" (Barry et al. 2017:1).

In sum, the drive for early identification and the redirection of clinical attention go hand in hand—they serve as a dual mandate for increasing the role of 22q11.2DS in patient care.

Mutations in Psychology

Knowing that a child has a genetic mutation can reshape clinical practice in fields like psychology as well. However, it has taken a long time for genetic disorders to gain traction in the "psy" disciplines. No organization illustrates this turn better than Elwyn Services. Elwyn has embodied American norms for managing people with developmental abnormalities for most of the last 150 years. Over that period, Elwyn has embraced prevailing ideas about genetics and abnormality, from early twentieth-century eugenics to the present. Today, it has become a site where genetic mutations have moved to the very core of patient diagnosis and care.

Under Elliott Simon's leadership, Elwyn has moved to the cutting edge when it comes to the integration of genetics into clinical-psychological care for people with developmental disabilities. And yet, Simon himself had very little interest in genetics when he arrived at Elwyn as a young behavioral psychologist in the 1980s. In a 2012 interview, he explained to me, "I wasn't really into that." The genetic diagnoses were there, but Simon did not see much value in them. "I knew what was going on and I knew it was happening. I knew people who had Fragile X Syndrome, I knew people who had Down Syndrome, 5p Minus, I mean all these things, they were diagnosing them. *It was in the chart, but that is where it went—nowhere else. . . . It did not have the status of a clinical condition that was of interest to me as a behavioristic psychologist."* In short, Simon knew about a number of genomically designated conditions, but they remained causal explanations rather than clinical categories in their own right. Simon gave the example of a difficult session with a patient: "This person is throwing crap across the room in his workshop and I have got to deal with that, so I am going to have to look at the behavior." By contrast, the genetic mutations that were sometimes listed in patients' charts simply "didn't factor into my clinical [practice]." Geneticists were using Elwyn to find patients with interesting mutations, but those mutations were not yet objects that could meaningfully inform the clinical evaluation or treatment of psychological issues. They were etiology, and little more.

Nowadays, by contrast, Simon thinks about genetic mutations completely differently. I asked him what a condition like Fragile X or 22q11.2DS means to him when he sees it in a child's chart now. He replied: "Now *it's the first question I ask*. Now it drives—*if there is a genetic diagnosis, it totally changes my clinical approach to the family and to the person."* His description of the contrast between his approach to a patient with a Fragile X diagnosis in her chart thirty years ago, when it would be largely ignored, and his approach today, is extremely telling. He explained, "If I go in there as Doctor Simon from 1983, I would do a functional analysis of the behavior, I would look at the setting variables, I would try to determine what's the function of the behavior" in order to develop a variable-based treatment program. But what about Doctor Simon thirty years later? He continued, "Now let's say I know this guy has Fragile X, right? *Now I know where to start,"* he said laughing. For example, he explained, "people with Fragile X Syndrome don't like noisy places to start with. They tend to be very shy. I can see: do they have this person sitting at a table across from somebody who is looking them in the eye all the time?" A genetic diagnosis can therefore provide a point of entry for behavioral psychology. It allows the practitioner to forgo a series of laborious evaluations and perhaps also missteps. Instead, just seeing a mutation in the patient's chart means they can immediately work with the behavioral phenotype of a condition like Fragile X, whose bearers, to take Simon's example above, are often troubled by direct eye contact and background noise. Knowing about the mutation can profoundly shape psychological understanding, intervention, and prognosis.

Simon recounted the process of coming to Elwyn and discussing genetic disorders with Brenda Finucane and others in an early morning journal club. He explained how "it became somewhat of *a defining moment, clinically,* for me that the [genetic] etiology can be a kind of *synthesizing variable* for these different fields to get involved in around the person." He was adamant that intellectual disability was not such a synthesizing variable. Why not? It just did not tell you all that much. He explained, breaking into laughter midway through his sentence, "If you are a physician, the fact that they have intellectual disabilities is not all that interesting to you because it doesn't tell you anything aside from the fact that their IQ is below 70 and they have got some adaptive behavior needs." He went on to say that even "if you are a psychologist, it is also not all that interesting. If you are a social worker, it may be a little interesting, but not hugely interesting." Intellectual disability is just not nearly as rich a kind of person as Fragile X, 22q11.2DS or Smith-Magenis syndrome. Its meaning is clear, but it is also thin.

By contrast, genetic mutations can yield a wealth of clinically relevant information for a doctor, psychologist, or social worker. As Simon told me,

But now if I tell you this person has Smith-Magenis Syndrome and you are a physician, well now, well that's interesting because people with Smith-Magenis are prone to kidney problems and they have peripheral neuropathy and they have other things, so, I am now interested in this person in a different way. The same if you are a psychologist. They have got a type of self-injury that the developmental courses, this guy is beginning to be ascertained and it is of a particular type and now we are working as a team around supporting somebody with Smith-Magenis Syndrome. And you know, that is how it can synthesize a team.

Although they cannot be *diagnosed* according to clinical presentation, genomically designated conditions can direct clinical attention, judgment, and treatment in more fine-grained, if also more uncertain ways than surveillance categories like intellectual disability. They can also bring together a team—a new network of elements and expertise—according to new jurisdictional formations. That is why a mutation can be a "synthesizing variable" that fundamentally reorients psychological practice around a patient.

Yet a psychologist can never diagnose these conditions. Most of the time they cannot even guess at them. Simon admitted, between laughs, "I am actually pretty horrible at it myself." At a jurisdictional level (see Abbott 1988), it is perhaps surprising that a clinical psychologist would so willingly let his practice be determined by diagnostic categories that cannot, even in principle, be made via psychological expertise. And yet, Simon was almost dismissive of the idea that psychologists should try to learn how to make these new and important psychological diagnoses themselves. "That is their bailiwick," he told me. "Why would I do it when I've got Brenda [Finucane] on my staff? I mean, it would be silly, you know? I don't think psychologists should become experts in recognizing genetic syndromes. That's pointless. . . . *Whether I can pick the people out with Fragile X out of a crowd is immaterial to me.*" For people like Simon, psychology should be willing to cede jurisdiction when it comes to diagnosis in order to gain the ability to work with the distinctive cognitive phenotypes associated with genetic disorders like the ones he deals with in his practice at Elwyn. That is why the loss of diagnostic jurisdiction has become "immaterial" to psychologists like Elliott Simon.

Again, Elwyn is most definitely *not* typical of institutions for managing populations with intellectual disabilities. Still, Simon pointed toward the strides he and others were making in the fields of intellectual disability and special education. He felt that the field's published literature—especially the American Association of Intellectual and Developmental Disability's journals—was moving very rapidly in that direction. Simon suggested, "If you've gotten any journal nowadays, a majority of the articles in there are going to be specific to genetic syndromes, whereas 20 years ago that was not the case." While a cursory look at those journals indicates that may be something of an exaggeration, it is still significant that the field is gravitating toward genetics again. Simon also pointed out that institutional interest in a "gene-first" approach was growing. Elwyn itself has been contracted to provide consultations and guidance on best practice for people with genetic disorders by many different school systems and, among others, the State of California as it moves toward fuller deinstitutionalization.

The major remaining obstacle, he explained, was the resistance of fields like developmental psychology and special education to integrating categories derived from genetics. This resistance, Simon told me, was born largely out of the historical association with eugenics: "Historically the field of intellectual disability's first brush with etiology was disastrous." It was understandable, then, that "for years, the field of intellectual disabilities didn't want to have much to do with genetics at all, and the field of genetics didn't want to have much to do with the field of intellectual disabilities either." Neither behavioral psychology nor mainstream psychiatry's codified diagnostic systems are very amenable to the inclusion of genomically designated syndromes. The *DSM*, in fact, removes diagnoses when a strong etiological finding is made, leaving Simon convinced that Rett syndrome was sure to be excluded in the newest version of American psychiatry's official diagnostic manual, *DSM-V* (he was correct: see American Psychiatric Association 2013). Nevertheless, while Simon may not be representative of behavioral psychology as a whole, he is indicative of the way that genetics is making rapid inroads into fields that did not previously take mutations seriously as categories of clinical practice.

Finally, Simon was adamant that the support groups act back on the professional fields. Support groups, he explained, play "a function to educate the professionals, because, as I said before, a lot of the professionals aren't into this yet, and the support groups all have great materials on the actual disorder." Were it not for the networks forged largely by advocates and genetic counselors, it is hard to see how these complex medical and psychological phenotypes could be developed to the point where they would be useful to someone like Elliott Simon. While the field may be most aware of XYY syndrome from outdated textbooks and the infamy it attained decades ago, genetics researchers, advocates, and insiders like Finucane and Simon are working to turn genetic mutations into meaningful categories of practice in psychology and many other cognate fields.

This turn to integrate genetics and psychology is being taken even further by experts working in academic treatment centers. Tony Simon (no relation to Elliott) is a cognitive neuroscientist with the MIND Institute at UC Davis who now specializes in 22q11.2DS. In our 2012 interview in Orlando, Florida, he described the early work comparing Down and Williams syndromes and explained that it showed how "the early developmental trajectory separates and they are just completely disparate, unrelated genetic populations that create *two different kinds of subspecies of human being*. There's a sort of real developmental emergence of these phenotypes." Those insights presaged crucial lessons about 22q and other conditions.

To be clear, Tony Simon is no genetic determinist. Our conversation took place after a talk about some exploratory research on 22q11.2DS's variable phenotype and the role of the microdeletion's interaction with much smaller genomic variants like single nucleotide polymorphisms and smaller CNVs—that is, "gene × gene" interaction. Simon is close to many of these researchers, but he told me, "I am sitting there going, 'Huh, you know, these people are alive.' Do they not even realize that these people are alive? There are other things in the world." For Simon, it is those other things—like developmental and environmental factors—that shape a mutation's phenotype for any given bearer.

If you can understand a mutation's distinctive developmental trajectory, in all its variability, you are better placed to intervene and alter it through environmental interventions. That is how you can truly shape a mutation's ultimate phenotype and therefore a patient's cognitive outcomes. In fact, it is precisely this kind of detailed attention to the patterns of these living, thinking, environmentally embedded people with genomically designated conditions that makes them potentially so powerful as categories of human difference. That is how the distinctive phenotypes of conditions like Williams syndrome, Fragile X, or 22q11.2DS come into view, and how they can then be mobilized in clinical practice.

Tony Simon first worked on 22q11.2DS at CHOP in Philadelphia. But it was coming to the MIND Institute, with its innovative research programs on autism and Fragile X, that really allowed him to develop a dual research-clinical environment in which new aspects of the 22q phenotype could be discovered. After interviewing Simon at a 22q meeting, a couple of years later I visited him and his colleagues at the MIND Institute, where they had developed cutting-edge clinical and research centers on Fragile X, 22q, and autism. Simon had never imagined that he would end up at a place like the MIND Institute. He was trained as a basic scientist, leading him to ask rhetorically, "Who am I to talk about this stuff? But this is what happens with translation of science, and that is what the MIND did to me." He explained how he developed an "interdisciplinary team [with] a developmental-behavioral pediatrician, a psychiatrist, a clinical psychologist." In other words, his esoteric research on genetic disorders ended up turning Simon into a kind of accidental but now utterly dedicated clinician.

The MIND Institute was creating the same kind of interdisciplinary, hybrid research/treatment space for 22q that it had for Fragile X. Eventually, the significance of all this dawned on Simon: "I suddenly kind of woke up in the middle of the night one night and said, 'Gee, you know, my model is Randi [Hagerman]. . . . Fragile X, *it comes back to the thing it always comes back to: Fragile X being the model. She had a treatment in a research center.* That is what I wanted to develop.'" He was even aided in this endeavor by Nicole Tartaglia, who, as Simon put it, "was really well-trained in doing this kind of work with Fragile X, working with Randi and the sex chromosome aneuploidies." In fact, Tartaglia now leads a specialist clinic in Denver, the eXtraordinarY Kids Clinic, dedicated to the sex chromosome aneuploidies—primarily the XXX, XYY, XXYY, Turner (X), and Klinefelter (XXY) syndromes.

A clinic like Simon's or the 22q and You center at CHOP can mean a lot for 22q patients and their families, just as the eXtraordinarY Kids Clinic in Denver, the eXceptional Kids Clinic at EmorY in Atlanta, or the eXemplarY Kids Clinic in Los Angeles can mean the world to a family affected by XYY or XXX syndrome. Simon described the "life-changing experience" of getting "an evaluation by the very first pediatrician they'd ever seen who didn't go, 'Huh?' when they told them that their kid had 22q. That was wonderful for them." Indeed, one thing that united almost all the parents I have spoken to was the comfort and reassurance they took from finding medical professionals who were familiar with their kid's genetic diagnosis and willing to take it seriously as a driving category of practice.

It is no coincidence that this kind of innovative interdisciplinary team was assembled at the MIND Institute. It was originally founded with funding from three wealthy "autism dads," and for some time it has been the leading center for research on Fragile X syndrome and at the center of the FXS-autism nexus discussed in chapters 3 and 4. Simon was adamant that the MIND Institute "changed [his] career, . . . and now we have a real clinic. We call it the 22q Healthy Minds Clinic." Today, they bring in people who do not qualify for research studies in order to provide treatment, and they are starting to have success in getting people referred to the MIND Institute for 22q assessments through their insurance plans. They combine detailed interdisciplinary workups of every child with an expertise that allows Simon to say, "I've seen several hundred kids with this disorder. The first 20 seconds I go, 'Oh, I think I see roughly where this kid fits.'" They then provide contact details for experts from the family's local area and often conduct follow-ups down the road.

One evening, as I was talking to Simon during a reception at a 22q conference, numerous children with 22q11.2DS excitedly approached and often embraced "Dr. Tony," while their parents told me how wonderful he was. And yet, were it not for 22q11.2DS, he may have never truly worked with a patient in his career. The scientific opportunity represented by a genomically designated condition like 22q11.2DS, combined with the hybrid research/clinical model pioneered by Fragile X researchers at the MIND Institute, have allowed Simon to move in directions he himself says he never could have imagined. Although his early work focused on an esoteric interest in the cognitive basis of the human capacity to deal with numbers (see, e.g., Simon 1997), he now runs a center dedicated to cognition and behavior for children with 22q11.2DS. Simon noted repeatedly that this unforeseen shift in his career trajectory had totally changed his life. He summarized his new, cherished role with what he calls "a sad little joke": "I am not a doctor, but I play one at work."

Although the MIND Institute may provide singular opportunities for patients, it also plays a broader role within the 22q and Fragile X networks. Families visit from far afield to learn about their children and about treatment strategies. They then take that knowledge back to their local care providers, schools, and communities. Simon shows up at almost every 22q conference, and there is a constant stream of trainees from various fields passing through his clinic and other centers at the MIND Institute. Alongside medical centers like the one at CHOP and institutions like Elwyn, these central nodes in the 22q network allow for both the production of knowledge and the proliferation of experts and expertise. What's more, experts who have trained at places like CHOP and the MIND Institute sometimes go on to work with families to set up the *new* interdisciplinary centers of excellence for 22q that are now scattered all over the United States and Europe. To be sure, certain infrastructures need to already be in place—specialist clinics for genetic disorders are almost always found at major medical centers. And yet, in each and every instance, those infrastructures must be reorganized in order to work with 22q11.2DS, just as rubrics for clinical attention and judgment must be recalibrated according to its particular phenotype.

As Simon and his new interdisciplinary team saw more and more children with 22q11.2DS, he recounted, novel discoveries were made. They noticed, for example, that their 22q kids tended to be highly anxious: "The literature says 60%, but fewer than 20% were coming through our doors with any recognition of anxiety. . . . I'm sitting down with the parents and they'll say, 'My child won't go to school, my child has stomach aches and headaches and picking at their skin, and they're OCD, and they can't sleep at night.' It's like, 'OK, that's not seven different things, that's all anxiety.'"

That finding led to far-reaching new ideas about 22q11.2DS's cognitive phenotype and how to manage it. Simon now believes that often-undiagnosed anxiety is itself caused by 22q's differential capabilities: the experience of being at an age-appropriate level for reading and other subjects but potentially several years behind in subjects like math. This stressor can in fact be exacerbated as much by the relative *strengths* as the weaknesses. Simon has found that "we see that IQ is not predictive of adaptive functioning at all in this population. It is almost a 1:1 correlation in regular, typically developing people, and even in other neurodevelopmental disorders, it is high. Here you have a zero correlation." Simon and others even reason that anxiety may contribute to the high rates of schizophrenia seen in later development. It is therefore vitally important to devote time to "training the parents a little bit to *adjust their expectations* and their emotional responses to the kids." As he explained to me, "The parents are a critical part of this [and] can change what we now call the behavioral ecology of the child. *We think we can change the developmental trajectory.*"

Different mutations, with their complex phenotypes, may therefore have profound implications for patient evaluation and care. According to this way of thinking, how you should understand and treat a *symptom* depends on the underlying genetic *disease*. That is how knowledge about genetic mutations can be used to "change the developmental trajectory" of children struggling with behavioral and psychiatric problems both big and small.

Mobilizing Mutations in Alien Territory

What does any of this matter if most local doctors know little or nothing about XXX, Fragile X, or 22q11.2DS? Indeed, when a patient or a parent invokes a Fragile X, 22q, or XYY diagnosis in the course of routine care, they may well encounter a psychiatrist or a pediatrician who is either not familiar with their diagnosis or does not give it much credence. To be sure, parents can also seek out specialist clinics and experts. They often do. Yet the availability of such resources is highly uneven, varying as they do by the mutation in question, locale, medical field, and so on. Meanwhile, differences in wealth, social and "cultural health capital" (Shim 2010), and many other factors mean that some families have a far easier time accessing these kinds of resources than others. Very few families can rely on a cutting-edge center like the eXtraordinarY Kids Clinic in Denver, the 22q and You Center at CHOP, or the MIND Institute for routine care. So what do they do when their local health care centers and schools are devoid of expertise in the genetic disorder that has come to loom so large in their lives?

Most parents do not simply give up or wait for 22q expertise to come to their local city or town. If my fieldwork has taught me anything it is this: when a parent decides that a genetic mutation is the key to understanding and helping their child, they will go to great lengths to make sure that they take advantage of everything that the network built up around that mutation has to offer. They find ways to tap into and actively extend those networks. They access resources online, identify relevant specialists, and join local, national, and even international groups dedicated to their newfound genetic disorder. After one visit to a specialist clinic or one meeting with a dedicated expert, parents and patients can garner referrals to sympathetic doctors in their area or have a credentialed ally intervene with local clinicians who are not familiar with anything but the most well-known genetic disorders.

Parents will often wield the professional literature themselves. In these ways, they can convince local clinicians and teachers that the seemingly weird genetic condition they are talking about is real, well-researched, and perhaps the crucial piece of information for guiding best practice for their child's care. Sometimes, as we saw in the last chapter, an alliance of advocates and experts will even embark on the project of establishing new specialist centers that can meet the steep clinical demands of a complex genetic disorder. In other words, specialist knowledge on a mutation like Fragile X or the 22q11.2 microdeletion can be creatively translated and extended into virgin territory by credentialed and lay experts alike. As those networks have grown in scope and scale, more and more families have sought them out and successfully tied their fate to them.

But what do parents do with all this information when they leave the annual conference or the specialist clinic? While a good geneticist or pediatric cardiologist will likely have some familiarity with 22q11.2DS, most general practitioners, pediatricians, and specialists in other fields do not. Yet on the medical front alone, a diagnosis like 22q11.2DS confers risk for a plethora of ailments spanning a host of bodily systems: scoliosis, cleft palate, endocrine and immunological imbalances, eye and dental problems, constipation, and so on. Parents are actively encouraged to follow the clinical guidelines for 22q11.2DS as faithfully as possible, requiring referrals, evaluations, and sometimes treatments which are not indicated by the usual clinical standards that inform most medical practice.

Parents must therefore work to redirect clinical resources according to 22q11.2DS. In my conversations with parents, this struggle to acquire the evaluations and care they have learned their children need came up constantly. Even though most parents lack medical credentials, they often develop impressive levels of lay expertise. They then engage their local practitioners, with assistance from summary sheets provided by the foundation and the associated biomedical literature on 22q. Consider my interview with three mothers of children with 22q11.2DS (2012). I asked one mom whether she felt that her expertise in 22q, combined with resources provided by the foundation, has meant that she could interact with medical professionals in a different way—as a kind of complementary medical expert. She replied, "Definitely. Definitely. And oftentimes I have walked in with a book and they've said, 'I don't have time to read it,' and I said, 'Fine, here's pertinent information for what we are dealing with now. This is the age range, this is the findings.' When I walked in and told my pediatrician [that] they are now recommending cervical spine X-rays, he looked back in the charts and said, 'Well, we don't have that, we'd better get them then.'" The aforementioned *Journal of Pediatrics* guidelines are a major resource in these kinds of encounters. Another parent told me point blank: "Believe me, when I got a PDF of [those *Pediatrics* guidelines], I shot it to every pediatrician that I knew."

In that same interview, all three mothers agreed when one described her relationship with her local medical team like this: "Well, they trusted me because I knew about 22q, and I would tell them all about that. . . . I usually could walk in there telling them, 'OK, this is what the findings show.' I mean, *I would walk in with literature*, and I did that just on Friday. He had an eye appointment with an eye doctor he hadn't seen before, and I pulled up the website and I said, 'These are common eye problems in children with 22q, here is my smart phone, please take a look.'" Stories like these help us see how parents are able to strategically deploy elements of the 22q network and reshape clinical practice in the process.

A mutation and a mom can redirect practice even when the evaluation or treatment in question is not age-appropriate. This same mother wanted her son evaluated for human growth hormone deficiency. She recalled, "They said, 'Oh, well, he is way too young to have that, it is not soon enough,' and *I said, 'He is not on any growth chart that you have got,' . . . and sure enough, they found two problems.*" Again, this kind of interaction required both the interpersonal skill and lay expertise of the mother alongside the resources produced by the broader network. As she herself put it, "I think that it helped, having the literature showing human growth hormone deficiency is present in children with 22q, and I think it also helped having a good collaborative relationship." In some cases, a credentialed 22q11.2DS expert or a genetic counselor is enlisted to negotiate referrals or courses of treatment. In many others, however, parents armed with the right resources—pertinent biomedical papers, good insurance, cultural capital, and so on—are able to redirect clinical attention and resources according to knowledge about 22q11.2DS.

Of course, this takes capital on the part of the parents. That same mother had been to 22q conferences all over the country, visited specialist clinics, and even traveled from Florida to Sacramento to have her son evaluated at Tony Simon's aforementioned 22q center at the MIND Institute. Still, this is not the preserve of the elite either: I interviewed this group of mothers in a low-budget motel room that one of them was sharing with her three children. At least one of them had driven more than a thousand miles with her kids to be there. Families are often willing to go to great lengths to make it to the latest conference and bolster their 22q expertise. It is anything but a luxury to them.

Her son, who hours earlier had excitedly talked to me about all the books he was reading, did indeed fit Tony Simon's finding that children with 22q experience anxiety as a result of their relative weakness in math. But how did they find that out? "We took him out to Tony Simon, MIND Institute," she recalled, where he was diagnosed with ADHD and generalized anxiety. This came as a total surprise: "I had no clue because the school didn't think that it was relevant that every time math came up, he developed a severe stomach ache and had to go run into the clinic every day." Apparently, the school had told her that they "knew he was just faking it," and they did not want to worry her. It was only when she went elsewhere—all the way to Sacramento—that a 22q specialist referred her son for psychological treatment. As she put it, "Thanks to the MIND Institute, we got him in to see a therapist." This recognition of anxiety, caused by the particular cognitive phenotype of 22q11.2DS, can lead to new expectations on part of parents and entrée into standard psychiatric treatment for anxiety disorders. It is clearly an instance of medicalization-via-genetics, but it was manifestly *not* driven by doctors seeking to extend their professional jurisdiction to cover new kinds of difference. Instead, it comes from a nonmedical expert (even if he does "play a doctor" at work) at an institution founded by "autism dads," and it empowers parents with a new resource as they seek to garner care and support for their children. This particular mother has been able to intervene in almost every aspect of her son's clinical and educational evaluation. She had even been able to garner referrals and treatments that would likely not have been obtained, or even sought, in the absence of a 22q11.2DS diagnosis.

Hers is just one of countless such stories I have heard. As the 22q network grows—accruing knowledge, resources, recruits, and allies—it becomes easier and easier for families to mobilize the 22q11.2 microdeletion with doctors and institutions at the local level. Mobile resources like clinical guidelines, fact sheets, and referrals allow patients and their families to effectively tie their fate to the 22q movement.

For them, lay expertise *is* the ability to effectively use the broader network built up around a genomically designated condition. In this way, a 22q11.2DS diagnosis can reshape the way a person is understood and cared for, even in places devoid of specialist 22q expertise.

Conclusion

Visit by visit and child by child, 22q experts and advocates are making 22q11.2DS a diagnosis that can transform the way we deal with people who are sick, disabled, or different. Against the backdrop of contemporary disease-based advocacy, genomic designation has even gained traction in institutions and fields that have long been resistant to engaging with genetics. Although Fragile X syndrome was the clear trailblazer, specialist clinics for 22q11.2DS, 15q Duplication, sex chromosome aneuploidies like XXX and XYY, Williams syndrome, and others are being opened all over the United States and Europe. Numbers of diagnosed patients are rising, media outlets are taking greater interest, and fields like psychology and special education are starting to overcome their reluctance to take genetic etiology seriously. In short, knowing that someone has a genetic mutation is increasingly shaping treatment and care in a wide range of fields.

A spate of recent ethnographic work in the social studies of science and medicine has examined the impact of genetics on medical practice (e.g., Latimer et al. 2006; Shaw et al. 2003; Timmermans 2015). Moving forward though, it is important to go beyond the small-*n* ethnographic study of particular labs and clinics if we want to see how mutations can become important objects of practice. Take Rabeharisoa and Bourret's (2009) outstanding analysis of the way genetic mutations shape diagnosis and judgment in two research-intensive psychiatry and oncology clinics in France. This book bolsters many of their key findings.[7] Rabeharisoa and Bourret found that, in cancer genetics, a single "bioclinical collective" could render genomic anomalies "clinical entities with enough robustness to be mobilized in medical judgments and decisions" (707). However, in keeping with other work, they argue that, in the case of *"psychiatric genetics, this work remains (almost) entirely in the future"* (707) due to "the absence of a robust corpus of clinical observations on these disorders" (700). To be sure, this is very often the case, and Rabeharisoa and Bourret are undoubtedly correct when it comes to the French labs they studied in the early 2000s. Yet throughout this book, we have seen that the future is now when it comes to psychiatric genetics. Mutations outside of oncology *can* be mobilized in the clinic, with far-reaching consequences.[8]

In order to truly understand how genetic mutations can become bona fide clinical entities in psychiatry and many other fields of medical practice, we have to examine the networks of knowledge production and advocacy that span labs, clinics, repositories, protocols, textbooks, families, and foundations, not to mention far-flung locales. No single "bioclinical collective" could hope to produce the knowledge base for a rare condition like 22q11.2DS. A new kind of person is just not the same as a new kind of cancerous tumor when it comes to the range of fields, interests, actors, and allies that must be aligned and courted. New kinds of people like 22q11.2DS must be assembled using multifarious elements that were not intended to fit together, but were nevertheless made to do so. That is how 22q became a powerful object of knowledge and practice for thousands of patients and their families. Mobilizing mutations in fields like pediatrics and psychiatry may be a much more daunting project, but the effects can be far-reaching. It can change the way we think about identity and difference, development and disability, impacting a person's lived experience from cradle to grave.

However, organizing clinical practice around a genetic mutation sometimes requires an even deeper reorientation of expert judgment. Knowing that a patient has a mutation like the 22q11.2 or 16p11.2 microdeletions can *redirect* clinical attention in novel ways and even shift the very boundary between normal and pathological phenotypes.

SEVEN

Remaking the Normal versus the Pathological in Genetic Medicine

The gene didn't get the memo that 70 is the cut-off for intellectual disability.
BRENDA FINUCANE TO A GROUP OF FRAGILE X PARENTS IN 2014

A quiet revolution is underway in medical genetics. Mutations like the ones discussed throughout this book can be used to reshape the classification of human difference—that is the essence of genomic designation. In this chapter, however, we will see how studying people with those mutations can destabilize the very boundary between the normal and the pathological, forcing researchers to rethink what makes someone a patient in the first place. As this trend gains steam, our rapidly growing knowledge about genetic mutations is going even further beyond questions about inheritance to fundamentally change the way we measure, classify, and approach illness and developmental difference.

This was *not* the intended purpose of human genetics. For more than a century, the overriding goal was to explain the inheritance of traits and conditions that hailed from fields like medicine, psychology, and criminology, not challenge the validity of those categories themselves. Hence the holy grail of molecular biology was a gene for salient categories of people. This way of thinking runs deep. It can be traced back to at least Mendel's seminal nineteenth-century work on dominant and recessive trait inheritance in pea plants. Whether it was with pedigree charts or molecular testing technologies, human geneticists took aim at explananda taken from other fields or just plain old common sense—eye color, height, intelligence, idiocy, aggression, criminality, schizophrenia, or autism, to name a few that have gained prominence at one time or another.

This basic approach is deeply ingrained in the very language of genetic testing. A mutation that almost always results in its associated phenotype is deemed "highly penetrant," and if that phenotype is some kind of medical or psychological malady, then it is also labeled "pathogenic." Conversely, if people with a given mutation are often unaffected or "normal," then it is thought to be of low or moderate penetrance and perhaps even "benign" from a medical perspective. Finally, the possibility that these mutations could express themselves in future generations, especially when paired with a similar "carrier gene" from the other parent, means they often attract considerable interest even when they do not appear to affect their bearers. Terms like these have long played a foundational role in the way we think about genetics and medicine. They help to divide genetic mutations into three highly intuitive bins: ones that confer a particular effect, ones that do not, and others that leave the bearer unaffected but put their offspring at risk. This way of thinking still guides practice at the cutting edge of genetic medicine: clinical genomic reports classify mutations as "pathogenic," "highly penetrant," or "dominant" vs. "likely benign" (or of "uncertain significance"), "incompletely penetrant," or "recessive"/"carrier" variants. This Mendelian paradigm held sway for more than a century, despite myriad changes in our thinking about what genes are and what they do (Keller 2002; Rheinberger 2013).

But this framework for making sense of mutations is beginning to badly fray. A growing body of research on people with mutations like the ones discussed in this book is starting to seriously challenge foundational concepts in the field. As we have seen, it turns out that many mutations are "pleiotropic": they can affect multiple faculties and bodily systems. Complicating matters further still, an avalanche of new findings is undermining the distinction between mutations that are pathogenic and ones that are either benign or merely confer carrier status.

When you look very closely at seemingly normal people who have a known pathogenic mutation like the 22q11.2 or 16p11.2 microdeletions, you often find that they present with a much milder version of the mutation's classic phenotype. Sometimes they have gone through life without ever coming to the attention of a medical geneticist, only to be diagnosed when they pass their mutation on to a more severely affected child. And yet, these parents are not simply labeled carriers: they are diagnosed with the relevant genetic condition, albeit a mild version of it. Does this mean they have a developmental impairment caused by their genetic disorder? What do you do when a person with a mutation is different in some way—perhaps even impeded—but not at a level of severity that would warrant clinical attention on its own? These are the kinds of questions we investigate in this chapter. The emergent answers have sweeping implications for the way we think about genetics, difference and disease in the "postgenomic" era.

Sociologists have drawn on the metaphor of clinical pathology ever since Comte and Durkheim. However, the social and historical studies of medicine began to seriously interrogate what makes a given form of human difference *pathological* with Georges Canguilhem's seminal 1943 work, *The Normal and the Pathological* (Canguilhem 1991; see also 2008). Canguilhem outlined the emergence of the distinction between the normal and the pathological that accompanied the rise of allopathic medicine in the early nineteenth century. But more than that, he explored the historical contingency of what makes something pathological at all. For Canguilhem, the term *pathological* referenced an inability to repel and replace error as well as a failure to thrive in a given environment, not an isolated biological property. The distinction between the normal and the pathological is therefore recast as environmentally and socioculturally embedded. Ever since, scholars of science and medicine have built on the idea that pathology is not an objective biological state but a historically variable concept. In the United States, this line of thought was perhaps most productively developed by sociologists, most notably Peter Conrad (1975, 1992, 2007), who were interested in "medicalization"—the way that forms of human difference are recast as categories of illness and brought under the jurisdiction of the medical profession. More recent work has explored how genetics and other biomedical technologies have transformed our understanding of disease and the experience of illness (e.g., Clarke et al. 2003; Heath, Rapp, and Taussig 2004; Keating and Cambrosio 2006; Rose 2007b), and even the way genetic testing can call established diagnostic criteria into question and challenge our understanding of existing disease entities (Bourret, Keating, and Cambrosio 2011; Hedgecoe 2003; Kerr 2000; Miller et al. 2005, 2006; Navon and Shwed 2012; Timmermans and Buchbinder 2013).

In this chapter, however, I show how genetic medicine is reshaping ideas about health and illness in even more fundamental ways. Knowing that a person has a genetic mutation can call into question the distinction between a normal vs. a pathological phenotype. Drawing largely on the examples of Fragile X, 16p11.2 Deletion Syndrome, and 22q11.2 Deletion Syndrome, I show how a genetic diagnosis can actually change whether or not a given characteristic of a person is understood to be a medical problem at all. More and more, people in medical genetics are pushing the boundaries of what counts as a symptom in the first place. In the last chapter we saw how a patient with a known mutation may still be referred for medical evaluations and treatments even if they are not clinically indicated by their phenotype. Here, I show how some clinical observations—for example, low growth or an ASD scale score well below the cutoff for an autism diagnosis—can be fundamentally rethought because of a person's genotype. What would otherwise be considered a normal finding can be recast as pathological, and vice versa, when you know that the person in question has a genetic mutation. She may, to take the example referenced in the above epigraph, have an IQ that is well within the normal range and yet significantly lower than we would expect based on their parents' and siblings' IQ scores. How then do we make sense of a phenotype that seems affected by a genetic mutation and yet falls far below the usual thresholds of clinical significance? What sorts of treatment, early intervention, and special accommodations should be made available? How might this new approach to developmental difference bias expectations or exacerbate socioeconomic inequalities?

I also show how some "carrier" genes are being recast as mild genomically designated syndromes. The most striking case is the carrier gene for Fragile X syndrome. For decades, researchers have known that Fragile X is almost always inherited from a "carrier" mother. Eventually, the Fragile X "premutation" was identified and incorporated in carrier screening programs. However, it slowly became clear that Fragile X carriers were suffering from a pair of adult-onset conditions later in life. More recently, researchers have begun to explore the developmental impact of the Fragile X premutation. In this way, the Fragile X premutation has gone from a carrier gene, to a gene that confers an extremely high risk of two serious adult-onset conditions, to a mild developmental disorder that expresses itself from infancy onward. Crucially, none of this would have been discovered were it not for the community of families and researchers organized around Fragile X syndrome itself.

So, once again, the CGG repeat expansion on the *FMR1* gene is serving as a vanguard when it comes to our understanding of genetic mutations. The field is finding that, when you look closely, more and more carrier genes have phenotypes that resemble, in milder form, the genetic disorders they can cause in a person's offspring. Making matters even more tricky, many of these "carrier genes" are very common. For example, roughly *1 in 150* women have a Fragile X premutation. As a result, this new wave of findings could dramatically increase the number of people whose lives are transformed by genetic test results, even as it strains the conceptual architecture of modern medical genetics.

Finally, I discuss some of the ethical issues lurking in this turn to see mildly affected people as patients of a genetic disorder. Not only are there major issues regarding tracking, self-fulfilling prophecies, and strained resources—there is also reason to worry that medical genetics could end up contributing to the reproduction of inequality.

Remaking the Normal versus the Pathological

Genomically designated conditions disrupt established nosologies in even more fundamental ways than we have seen up until now. Knowing that a patient has a genetic mutation opens up the possibility that they are dealing with characteristic deficits and tendencies that are both real and patterned, but do not meet existing diagnostic criteria or thresholds of significance. A mutation's phenotype can therefore become far more complex than a simple list of associated medical conditions: it can blur the boundary between what is and what is not a problem at all. How then do we understand the people who have these mutations, the challenges they face, and what should be done about it? In this section, I argue that knowledge about a genetic mutation can shift a normal finding into the realm of the pathological and an abnormal finding back into the normative range. But first, I want to show how experts carve up existing clinical categories in ways that allow for a more variegated understanding of a mutation's developmental phenotype and its bearer's cognitive abilities.

This is part of a much broader trend in medical genetics. "Endophenotyping" and "deep phenotyping" have become key strategies in the study of mutations and their effects. The prefix "endo" flags something that lies within or makes up a smaller part of a phenotype. Increasingly, by attending to more subtle forms of human difference, researchers have been able to establish stronger correlations between genetic mutations and what people are actually like. After gaining traction in genetics research on schizophrenia (Gottesman and Shields 1972), endophenotyping has now been adopted across a variety of disorders and fields. This strategy is by far the most advanced in psychiatric, behavioral, and neurogenetics. Rather than autism, schizophrenia, or even intellectual disability, researchers in these areas are shifting their strategy to look at more specific *parts* of these important but genetically intractable kinds of people. In other words, conditions like autism are increasingly rethought of as deficits in several interdependent but distinct domains. Its constituent elements can then be parsed out into a series of endophenotypes that can be more powerfully connected to genetic variants (Abrahams and Geschwind 2008; Betancur 2011; Gottesman and Gould 2003; Insel and Cuthbert 2009; Waterhouse 2013:77–91; on "deep phenotyping," see, e.g., Delude 2015).

Crucially for us, endophenotyping allows researchers to identify traits that are more fine-grained than established categorical diagnoses as well as impairments that do not meet standard thresholds of significance. Researchers are therefore able to develop an understanding of a condition like 22q11.2DS that is far more nuanced than "*x* percent have autism," "*y* percent have intellectual disability," and "*z* percent have schizophrenia." Instead, you can identify different autistic behaviors, particular cognitive strengths and weaknesses, and varying forms of "schizotypy." In this way, we will see how an IQ of 87 in a child with 22q11.2DS can be disaggregated into a normal verbal IQ score and a performance IQ score that represents cause for concern, early intervention, and special educational accommodations. It is also how the Fragile X carrier gene can be shown to cause its own, albeit very mild, genetic disorder (e.g., Goodrich-Hunsaker et al. 2011).

Tony Simon, who runs the cutting-edge 22q11.2DS clinic at the MIND Institute discussed in the last chapter, described the optimal approach to dealing with genetically specific disorders like this in our 2012 interview: "It is all about *endophenotyping* as widely and broadly, as interdisciplinarily, as wide as you can possibly get." In order to really help, you need to understand everything that makes people with genetic disorders different, no matter how nuanced or how mild that difference may be. Whether the term is used or not, the strategy of attending to endophenotypes is now commonplace for making sense of genetic mutations. It allows researchers and clinicians to understand a mutation's effects on a person in far more nuanced ways, even as it also strengthens that mutation's tie to important categories like intellectual disability and autism. It means that a child does not have to meet the diagnostic criteria for a psychiatric condition in order to be understood as suffering from important autistic, intellectual, or other cognitive deficits.

When genetics and medicine meet, in other words, things get complicated. Either you accept genetic complexity and leave it at that, or you let long-standing clinical categories break up into constituent parts and float in ways that blur existing distinctions between illness and health. As a field, medical genetics is understandably gravitating toward the latter approach. More and more, experts in other fields and even patient advocates are following them down this path. In a way, this follows quite naturally from the basic logic of genomic designation: if a deleterious mutation does not line up with existing phenotypic categories, rethink the phenotypes. If that means reevaluating the boundary between normal and pathological phenotypes altogether, then so be it.

Parsing Phenotypes and Redirecting Clinical Attention

Take the case of IQ in 22q11.2 Deletion Syndrome. One commonly noted feature of 22q11.2DS's cognitive phenotype is the frequent divergence of scores in different intellectual domains (see, e.g., Jacobson et al. 2010; Woodin et al. 2001).[1] This divergence is thought to *invalidate* full-scale IQ scores for people with 22q11.2DS. I saw Donna McDonald-McGinn address this issue in a talk to an audience of parents at a conference geared toward development and education in 22q. She explained how IQ scores in 22q11.2DS tended to be quite high for a genetic disorder: "[U]sing the appropriate Wechsler IQ test we found out about 18% of kids had an IQ that was in the average range, 20% below average, 32% borderline, and then 30% in the mentally retarded range, . . . and so these are not really too bad in terms of numbers."

But the point she really wanted to make was not about these general scores, but about the particularity of 22q11.2DS's cognitive phenotype: "But we found that the *full-scale IQ generally doesn't reflect the individual's cognitive ability.* So how so? Well, for instance in this child, he had a full-scale IQ of 87, but his verbal IQ was 111 and his performance IQ was 65. So verbal are things like reading and rote memorization, and performance is math and abstract reasoning, things like that. So this is an incredible split which really *renders that 87 invalid.*" After finding the verbal/performance IQ split in this particular child, McDonald-McGinn and her colleagues went back and looked at the larger population of patients they were studying and treating. They found that 65% had a >12-point split between their verbal and performance IQ scores (see Woodin et al. 2011 for a report of this research). McDonald-McGinn explained their finding like this: "The full-scale IQs don't necessarily represent these patients accurately." This was no mere research oddity either. She told the assembled experts and parents that *"this has direct ramifications for cognitive remediation in this population* because only 1% of the general population has that kind of split."

Parents were then encouraged to delve deeper into a child's IQ score on the basis of the fact that they had a 22q11.2 microdeletion. Even a full-scale IQ of 87—well within the otherwise normal range—can be disaggregated in order to reveal a serious deficit in a more specific phenotype: performance IQ. McDonald-McGinn implored the parents to make sure that educational and remedial services were reoriented around this deficit in contradistinction to the usual focus on language deficits. As she put it, "Schools are not generally prepared to deal with this, and so it is important that you *know whether your child has this kind of split or not, and that the remediations are set up specifically for your child* and not for the whole classroom."

In short, 22q11.2DS is mobilized to redirect clinical judgment toward a specific deficit that would have otherwise evaded expert attention. In this way, an observation that would have put a child squarely in the normal range of variation can be recast as a serious cognitive deficit requiring individualized intervention. And yet, were it not for the 22q11.2 microdeletion, this unusual cognitive profile would have most likely gone unnoticed. The verbal-performance IQ split is not nearly as extreme as it is in Williams syndrome (Campbell et al. 2009), which we encountered in chapter 3. Nevertheless, it has become a key part of the 22q11.2 microdeletion's cognitive phenotype and therefore part of 22q11.2DS as a kind of person.

What's more, this relative strength in language stands in contrast to the usual developmental trajectory of 22q11.2DS. As McDonald-McGinn explained in the same talk, "Across the board [22q] kids have delays in emergence of language, with a mean age of talking at two-and-a-half. . . . We have had kids who were seven who didn't say a word and then suddenly were speaking in full sentences." This raises an intriguing question about children with 22q11.2DS: *"Why do we have these delays in language and then it becomes a strength because the kids, when they are older, are really eloquent speakers?"* So, experts are not only seeing this specific cognitive phenotype, where language becomes a relative strength by school age, but also a particular *trajectory* that goes from delayed speech to relative strengths in reading and language.

This sort of observation has complicated implications. On the one hand, parents should not worry too much if their child is late in hitting key language-acquisition milestones, because they are likely to catch up more than similarly delayed kids. On the other hand, there is

"No question: *all [22q kids] benefit from early intervention strategies*, and the sooner we can get kids into speech therapy and OT [occupational therapy], PT [physical therapy], etc., the better things will move along." After all, McDonald-McGinn explained, there is "a subset of [22q] kids with frank autism or autistic-like features." Despite its enormous variability, the 22q11.2 microdeletion provides grounds for careful and highly nuanced scrutiny, a source of hope for rapid language development after a delayed start, and a mandate for multiple forms of early intervention.

The verbal-performance IQ split in 22q11.2DS is but one example of the way distinctive cognitive and behavioral phenotypes are identified in genomically designated syndromes: the aversion to eye contact in Fragile X, the anxiety associated with 22q11.2DS, the spasmodic upper-body squeeze in Smith-Magenis syndrome, to mention just a few. Indeed, the "spasmodic upper-body squeeze" is particularly illustrative. In our 2012 interview, Finucane explained to me that she published a paper detailing that particular phenotype (Finucane et al. 1994) after *teachers* became aware of their Smith-Magenis students (i.e., which ones had a 17p11.2 deletion) and reported what they described as "this adorable self-hugging thing they do when they're happy" (a phrase that Finucane still uses in conversation). While their characteristic destructive outbursts would certainly get a person with a 17p11.2 microdeletion into a psychologist's practice even absent a genetic diagnosis, these subtler traits have become important parts of what it means to have Smith-Magenis syndrome. When these nuanced forms of difference are observed in high proportions of people with a particular genetic mutation, they can become part of its published phenotype and then redirect clinical attention, expectations, and intervention. In short, subtle forms of difference can become important parts of the kind of person fixed to a mutation.

In this way, deep phenotypic commonalities are observed even among very different patients with the same genomically designated condition. A key example is facial phenotypes. One constant refrain is that kids with 22q tend to "look like siblings"—perhaps even more so than their actual siblings. The 22q11.2DS craniofacial phenotype is variable, mild, and unlikely to be picked up even as a diagnostic indicator by anyone without dedicated 22q11.2DS expertise. In the community, however, it is enormously salient. The same goes for many other genomically designated conditions. Some craniofacial phenotypes are considered highly specific, like the "elfin" appearance of people with Williams syndrome, while others are far less distinct. Still, as we saw in chapter 5, a patient's facial features, or "craniofacial phenotype," are often the basis for referral for a genetics evaluation—a fact that contributes to the underrepresentation of racial and ethnic minorities in the populations of people actually diagnosed with genetic disorders. Subtle phenotypic differences are just easier to spot in certain settings and among certain groups.

Normalizing the Pathological

Building up knowledge about a genetic disorder can recast a worrying sign of illness as a normal part of a mutation's particular phenotype. Take the example of growth patterns. Comparing children with 22q11.2DS to the standard Centers for Disease Control and Prevention (CDC) growth charts is considered to be *invalid*. For while children with 22q11.2DS tend to fall into the very low end of the standard distributions of height and weight in their first years, often qualifying them for a very serious "failure to thrive" diagnosis, they also tend to catch up before they reach adulthood (Habel et al. 2012).

A 2012 paper in the *American Journal of Medical Genetics* went so far as to provide separate growth charts for people with 22q11.2DS (Tarquinio et al. 2012). Consider weight in females with 22q11.2DS. Over the first thirty-six months of life, girls with 22q11.2DS lag well behind their normative counterparts at every percentile, with half falling below the tenth normative percentile. Meanwhile, more than 25% of girls with 22q11.2DS are below the *second* percentile for population growth (2673). A failure to thrive diagnosis, meanwhile, usually only requires two measurements that place a child below the fifth percentile. For parents, a child's failure to grow or gain weight can be incredibly trying, especially as it may seem to portend more problems down the road. This is a huge issue for families dealing with 22q11.2DS. Several 22q parents told me that their child's inability to gain weight was even more trying than the acute medical challenges like neonatal cardiac surgeries that children with 22q11.2DS often face in their first months and years.

But, when we switch our perspective from the first thirty-six months of life to the first twenty years, a very different picture emerges. Hence a second chart shows that the 22q kids catch up with and, at many brackets, even overtake their normative counterparts by adulthood (2676). The authors of the study explain that these mutation-specific growth charts allow clinicians and parents to "avoid needless investigation of growth deficiency in those who are exhibiting a growth profile which is typical for this condition" (2680). In other words, many of these kids who would have been evaluated in an effort to explain and perhaps treat their low weight should simply be left to develop according to the natural growth trajectory of people with a 22q11.2 microdeletion. Put simply, "Growth curves specific to the 22q11.2 deletion will assist the pediatric clinician in deciding which children with this syndrome need further investigation of their growth deficiency" (2672).

This point is made again and again at 22q/VCFS meetings. The International 22q11.2 Foundation features no fewer than twelve growth charts on its website.[2] The goal is to assure parents that their children's low growth in their early years, at least compared to the standard CDC chart, is not necessarily a cause for concern: kids with 22q are likely to catch up, given the divergent growth trajectory observed in 22q11.2DS. Experts are therefore at pains to put those same kids' growth in the proper perspective: growth patterns for the 22q11.2DS population. Here is how Robert Shprintzen put it at the annual meeting of the main VCFS foundation for parents and professionals in New Brunswick in 2011:

Now, remember, in growth issues, *children with VCFS have a different growth velocity.* I have had conversations with a number of parents during the course of this meeting, all of whom are having their children compared to the CDC growth charts. *The CDC growth charts are normed against the general population, the normal population.* People with Down Syndrome, people with Williams Syndrome, people with achondroplasia [a common form of dwarfism], *people with VCFS should not be compared with the CDC growth charts,* all right? . . . *I know hundreds of adults with VCFS and they are all in the normal range of height and people with VCFS, they get there on a different path than other children.* So their group velocity is different but their eventual growth goals are essentially the same as the general population, and we have data that supports that.

Again, even Shprintzen considers VCFS to be coextensive with the 22q11.2 microdeletion. He also gestures to the same point about divergent growth patterns in other genetic disorders like Down and Williams syndromes. His point was clear: people with genetic disorders should not be compared to the general population because, at least when it comes to growth, doing so can lead to undue worry, testing, and intervention. Like other 22q experts, he assures parents that their kids will reach healthy weights and heights in the end as they follow the 22q11.2DS phenotype's distinct growth trajectory.

Like other genomically designated conditions, 22q11.2DS is not diagnosable or even strongly indicated by low growth. Still, the post factum observation of different growth *patterns* in probands can become part of a mutation's distinctive phenotype. Perhaps the most remarkable aspect of the example of growth in 22q11.2DS is that it does *not* represent an instance of "medicalization" through geneticization, but precisely the opposite: knowing that someone has a 22q11.2 microdeletion can normalize a clinically significant observation of low growth or even a serious failure to thrive diagnosis. In this way, a finding that is pathological in the general population may just be part of the normal developmental trajectory for people with a particular genetic mutation.

Pathologizing the Normal

By far the greater tendency in genetic medicine, however, is to include subclinical traits and deficits in a mutation's phenotype. In other words, knowing that someone has a mutation can recast otherwise normal observations as pathological findings that require further evaluation and perhaps treatment.

Conditions like 22q11.2DS and 16p11.2DS are highly variable, with some patients confronted by dozens of serious medical issues and others with few or even none at all. But why treat people with a 22q11.2 deletion who do not even have *any* of the major clinical associations as anything more than carriers or asymptomatic cases? How can the penetrance of the 22q11.2 microdeletion be 100% if some patients seem to be mostly fine? A major part of the answer has to do with the way that genomically designated conditions serve to *realign* clinical judgment and undermine the very boundary between the normal and the pathological.

At the 22q conference held at Disney World in 2012, I saw a highly instructive talk by an eminent medical geneticist. He was reporting unpublished results from a major prenatal study that tested 4,400 fetuses using chromosomal microarrays (Wapner et al. 2012). Crucially, 3,000 of the 4,400 had *not* been referred for testing on the basis of a clinical indication. In other words, this was one of the only 22q studies whose sample was not based on biased ascertainment. What did they find? Of around twenty-five anomalies observed at 22q11.2, ten were in the form of the "classic" 22q11.2DS 2.5mb deletion. Of those ten, three were in otherwise normal pregnancies. They were *not* clinically indicated. That meant there was "an incidence, in this study, of 1 in 1000" *normal pregnancies* as well as the 7/~1,400 where an anomaly had been detected. As we saw, a similar study reporting comparable findings based on a large European sample came out a few years later (Grati et al. 2015). The geneticist explained, "There's a great deal of variability [in most copy number variations]. And they are obviously found sometimes in apparently normal [people]."

What would this mean for our understanding of the syndrome itself and for genetic disorders more generally? He went on to explain that there is a term "that geneticists use for this, incomplete penetrance, if you can't really find anything clinically that you would say is affecting the individual." However, this group of 22q experts wanted the audience to think about incomplete penetrance differently, as "just *a lower-hand of a variation of expression which goes across a spectrum.*" He implored them, and the field more generally, to adopt a new approach to subclinical traits in people with genetic mutations: "instead of looking at qualitative dichotomous traits—either you have it or you don't," he argued, we should "*look at continuously* [and normally] *distributed quantitative traits.*" Incomplete penetrance should give way to spectrums of variation and impairment. The distribution of IQ scores, he explained, is "artificially centered" on one hundred, and we "arbitrarily" define intellectual disability as an IQ that is at least two standard deviations below that mean. Then, he showed a curve of IQ scores for people with 22q11.2DS, where the mean was just a little above seventy—the cutoff for intellectual disability. In other words, mean IQ in 22q11.2DS is almost two standard deviations below the normal mean. Hence, he concluded, "*the gene deletion effect probably operates all the time, but with variable consequences,* which is up to us to understand."

The fact that a 22q11.2 microdeletion may well leave a person on the normal side of certain thresholds of clinical significance has broader implications. For one thing, it means 22q11.2DS may be far more common than the usual 1 in 2,000–4,000 prevalence estimate—a fact that is now reflected in major reviews (e.g., McDonald-McGinn et al. 2015) and the 1 in 1,000 figure often cited by advocacy organizations like the International 22q11.2 Foundation. For another, it pushes us to rethink the relationship between mutations like the 22q11.2 microdeletion and long-standing clinical categories, ranging from intellectual disability and autism to growth hormone deficiency and hypocalcemia.

So, with the example of IQ, we begin to see how knowledge about a genetic mutation can trump our usual definitions of clinical significance. It can lead caregivers to see an actionable deficit or symptom in place of normal variation. This turn was captured quite poignantly in a line that Brenda Finucane often deploys in speeches at meetings of the International 22q11.2 Foundation and the National Fragile X Foundation: *"The gene didn't get the memo that 70 is the cut-off for intellectual disability."* The point was very clear: children with a genetic mutation should not be excluded from support and services just because their deficit fails to meet some arbitrary cutoff point based on what they are actually like.

The Mildly Affected

Most patients that have been diagnosed with 22q11.2DS do face serious medical and/or psychological problems. The same goes for most other genomically designated conditions. Some 22q patients, however, are so mildly affected by their 22q11.2 microdeletion that no one would ever suspect that they have a genetic disorder on the basis of their clinical presentation. In fact, the most mildly affected 22q11.2 microdeletion bearers are usually only picked up because their more seriously affected child or sibling is diagnosed with 22q11.2DS.

In my fieldwork, and in my conversations and interviews with experts, I have met and heard stories about several of these 22q patients.[3] One woman had been fairly successful and healthy throughout her life, with a graduate degree, a good job, and no major medical problems. Nevertheless, when she found out she had the 22q11.2 microdeletion, just like her more severely affected son, it made her rethink her past. She took it to explain her relative lack of success, shorter stature, and dark complexion as compared to her high-flying, tall, blond siblings. Another parent who had struggled in high school and had nasal speech felt a sense of relief and exoneration when she found out about her 22q status. For both women, it helped to explain their pasts and who they are today. I heard about the older sibling of a seriously affected child who was absolutely delighted to learn that he too had 22q11.2DS, because it meant he could be an even more powerful advocate as a mildly affected case than he could as a mere sibling. Their parents, however, did not want to find out which one of them had passed on the deletion. (The experts who were there when this story was related had little doubt as to which one it was after seeing a family picture.)

Incidental findings like these,[4] along with evidence from prenatal studies like the one discussed above, give 22q11.2DS advocates even more reason to believe that the real prevalence of the disorder is in fact significantly higher than the standard estimate of 1 in 2,000–4,000. They also provide further impetus to pursue newborn screening. In order to find most people with a mutation like XYY or a 22q11.2 microdeletion, you cannot assume that they will all conform to a particular clinical phenotype, or even that their "symptoms" will meet standard thresholds for clinical significance. You not only have to "cast a wide net," in the words of an important article about the diagnosis of 22q11.2DS (McDonald-McGinn et al. 2001); you must also use a netting that is tightly woven enough to catch traits that would usually evade the clinical gaze altogether.

All of these people considered themselves 22q patients, rather than just carriers, even though they usually did not have any clinical signs that would have led to a referral for a 22q11.2DS test.[5] So again, this is *not* a question of Timmermans and Buchbinder's "patients in waiting" (2010, 2013), where there is a biomarker but not the disease it is supposed to index. In cases like this, experts are not simply waiting for a disease to present. Instead, they see a presentation in a person with a genetic mutation where they otherwise would not.

In this way, 22q11.2DS further challenges the idea of "incomplete penetrance." Conditions like the XXX and XYY syndromes, 16p11.2 Deletion Syndrome, and 22q11.2 *Duplication* Syndrome present even more forceful challenges to that older, dichotomous orientation to genetics and disease. A genetic mutation may not always result in any of the clear-cut clinical issues it is associated with, but it still might cause a series of milder impairments that resemble them. Once again, incomplete penetrance is rendered a spectrum of variation that cuts across established clinical categories and thresholds of significance. With mildly affected people, subclinical traits can therefore represent "penetrance" even in the absence of *any* of the serious medical problems associated with a given mutation.

Rethinking Normality; or, "Shift Happens"

In a 2015 *Annual Review of Medicine* piece on genetic mutations and autism, William Brandler and Jonathan Sebat discuss mutations like the 16p11.2 microdeletion. "Each mutation," they explain, "is associated with a variety of clinical diagnoses and can also be found in a small percentage of individuals with no clinical diagnosis." People with the 16p11.2 microdeletion "have a mean IQ that is 32 points lower on average than their first-degree relatives who do not carry the deletion, but only 20% are below the threshold IQ of 70 for intellectual disability" (491). Meanwhile, around 15% are not diagnosable with *any* of the conditions like ASDs, motor delays, and so on that are associated with 16p11.2DS. Nevertheless, they argue, "Those CNV carriers without a diagnosis may not be entirely unaffected," because even "controls" who have a mutation associated with intellectual disability, autism, or schizophrenia "typically present with *intermediate cognitive phenotypes* or fecundity compared to neurodevelopmental cases and population controls" (491; my emphasis).

What are we to make of this? Brandler and Sebat (2015) are very clear that the answer has everything to do with your genetic starting point—that is, your family background. This broader genetic inheritance, along with the environment, shapes the expression of de novo mutations. The very same "disease mutation" exerting the very same effect, they argue, might produce different clinical outcomes that can "be explained by the starting conditions (genetic background)." If the genetic background "predisposes an individual to be socially responsive but of below average intelligence, the clinical outcome of a mutation may be intellectual disability." If, on the other hand, a person's family/genetic "background predisposes an individual to above-average intelligence but low social responsiveness, the individual may meet criteria for an ASD" (494). With two different "starting points" based on family background, a mutation may result in two very different clinical diagnoses.

That same year, in a *JAMA Psychiatry* article, a group of leading medical geneticists and childhood development specialists begin by noting the range of psychiatric disorders associated with the 16p11.2 microdeletion. However, Moreno-De-Luca et al. quickly turn to the murkier cases where there is no obvious clinical diagnosis to be found: "The 16p11.2 deletion," they point out, "has also been reported in apparently healthy individuals, a finding frequently *interpreted* as evidence of incomplete penetrance" (Moreno-De-Luca et al. 2015:120; my emphasis). However, even these apparently normal people still "exhibited a variety of cognitive and neuropsychological deficits despite the fact that none reached traditional clinical diagnostic thresholds for a neurodevelopmental or a neuropsychiatric disorder." These kinds of findings have huge implications. Like Brandler and Sebat, Moreno-De-Luca et al. invoke people's broader genetic inheritance to explain the wide variability seen in many genetic disorders. "Many of the traits that constitute the phenotypes of genetic syndromes," they explain, "are distributed continuously in the general population, and trait variability may be greatly influenced by the parental genetic background" (120). In other words, even if heritable traits like height, IQ, and sociability are affected by a de novo mutation, it is the inherited genetic background plus the "hit" of the mutation that will best explain variable outcomes. The impact of the mutation may be the same, but two people with the mutation may end up on either side of the normal/pathological divide depending on their family background.

The authors therefore undertook a study of fifty-six people with de novo 16p11.2 microdeletions and their immediate families. They presented their findings in a series of charts that show a "gene-effect" at work even when a person with the mutation does not meet clinical thresholds of significance. Each chart shows three separate normal distributions of scores: one for probands and one each for unaffected siblings and parents. (See fig. 7.1 below for a similar, but more schematic chart.) In each case, the probands' scores are much further *toward* the pathological range even though, in a large majority of cases, they do not actually meet the relevant clinical cutoff. So, while a large majority of these kids with 16p do *not* have an IQ under 70, and therefore do not have an intellectual disability, their IQs are an average of 1.7 standard deviations lower than those of their unaffected family members. (We will come back to the fact that, in this study population, the unaffected family members had a mean IQ of 112.) Likewise, when we look at the Social Responsiveness Scale in the right panel, where a score of 76 or above is usually considered necessary for an ASD diagnosis, we see that most of these kids do *not* have autism per se. And yet, they are a full *2.2* standard deviations higher on the SRS scale than their unaffected family members (Moreno-De-Luca et al. 2015:123). One finds similar charts for conditions like 22q11.2DS (Klaassen et al. 2016) and the even milder "hit" conferred by XXX syndrome as well (Tartaglia et al. 2010:3).

Moreno-De-Luca et al. argue that their findings support the NIMH's move away from the traditional categorical diagnoses of the DSM toward "dimensional approaches to mental health research." As they put it, "A dichotomous all-or-none approach to diagnosis has long dominated the fields of medical genetics, psychiatry, and psychology, in which the penetrance of a disorder in a population is determined by dichotomizing a quantitative trait and applying somewhat arbitrary thresholds to classify individuals as affected or unaffected. Although such approaches may appeal to our tendency to adopt simplified heuristics, they fail to recognize *the complexity of a more nuanced, quantitative underlying biological reality*" (Moreno-De-Luca et al. 2015:123; my emphasis). Their findings led them to explicitly reject the common argument that the 16p11.2 deletion displays incomplete penetrance. "Simply because arbitrary diagnostic thresholds are not met," they argue, "does not indicate that a particular proband is unaffected or that a given mutation confers no deleterious impact in some individuals"

(125). If we can overcome our dichotomous classificatory tendencies and embrace "a more nuanced, quantitative biological reality," incomplete penetrance starts to melt away into spectrums of variation for people with mutations like the 16p11.2 and 22q11.2 deletions.

In a 2016 "Special Article" in the leading journal, *Genetics in Medicine*, a team from Geisinger that included many of the same authors provided perhaps the most clear and forthright articulation to date of this new approach to genetics and difference. Brenda Finucane was first author (2016). The last and senior author was leading medical geneticist, David Ledbetter, who is now both executive vice president and chief scientific officer of Geisinger Health System. The article was playfully entitled "Shift Happens" (the subtitle was more descriptive), but its point was both serious and far-reaching. Throughout the paper, the authors contrast their approach to the Mendelian logic and its central tool: the pedigree chart and its strategy of recording inheritance patterns for categorical diseases and traits. Oftentimes, they argue, what seems like a family with more than its share of unrelated psychiatric challenges scattered over several generations—depression, anxiety, autism, epilepsy, intellectual disability, and so on—turns out to be one genetic mutation giving rise to different phenotypes of "brain dysfunction." The point is clear: by focusing on categorical diagnoses, we may miss the fact that the family is affected by a single genetic issue. When we turn our attention to genetic mutations, "[t]he traditional pedigree that separates autism, ID, bipolar disorder, and schizophrenia as distinct and unrelated conditions in a family *can no longer be considered valid*" (302; my emphasis).

Finucane et al. directly confront the relationship between the deficits caused by genetic disorders and existing thresholds of clinical significance. They explain how recent findings "have revealed the inadequacy of using a categorical model to describe neurodevelopmental outcomes in genetic disorders" (2016:302). The reality, they argue, is "that neurodevelopmental outcomes in children with this CNV represent a predictable 'shift' from expected functioning, based in part on parental background across multiple domains" (302). So even though a 16p11.2 microdeletion "confers a 2.2 standard deviation deleterious effect on social behavior, a highly heritable and continuously distributed trait" (303), only around 15% of known cases actually have autism.

A child's risk for any given behavioral or neurodevelopmental condition, in other words, depends on an *interaction* between de novo mutations and the family background. Studying the family is therefore key to providing a prognosis for many genomically designated conditions.

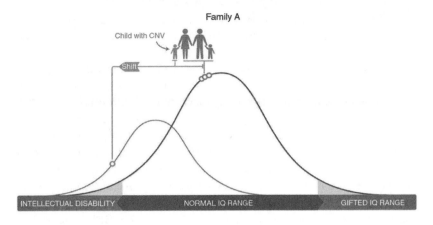

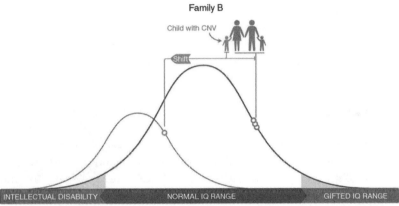

Figure 3. The blue curve represents the normal distribution of intelligence quotient (IQ) in the general population. The smaller, orange curve shows the IQ distribution for individuals with a particular copy-number variant (CNV). Circles on each curve indicate IQ scores for specific family members. In both family A and family B, this CNV confers the same magnitude of deleterious impact ("shift") on a child's IQ. In family A, the CNV shifts the affected child's IQ into the range of intellectual disability. In family B, because the family IQ starting point is higher, the CNV shift does not reach the defined threshold for intellectual disability. Even in family B, however, the shift has an effect, lowering the child's IQ from where it would have been without the CNV.

FIGURE 7.1. Chart on the "shift" caused by CNVs in *Genetics in Medicine* (Finucane et al. 2016:303). (Image reproduced under the Creative Commons Attribution-NonCommercial-NoDerivatives 4.0 International license; http://creativecommons.org/licenses/by-nc-nd/4.0/)

As we see in figure 7.1, the "shift" caused by CNVs like the 16p11.2 or 22q11.2 microdeletions may or may not put a child in the pathological range—it all depends on the family baseline.

This represents a fundamental reorientation in medical genetics. Finucane et al. close by arguing for a wholesale rethinking of heritable psychiatric disorders: "Traditional models of pedigree interpretation and categorical description are no longer adequate to explain the neurodevelopmental aspects of genetic disorders. . . . Gone are the days when an empiric prevalence figure for ID or autism can simply be listed in the same breath as a cleft lip or a club foot" (2016:304). Instead, we need to understand how autistic traits and measures of intelligence are distributed, and especially how genetic mutations leave some seemingly normal people worse off than they otherwise would be.

This "shift happens" approach captures the logic that often guides clinical judgment for genomically designated conditions, especially in fields like psychiatry and clinical psychology. It is the same logic that sees "an IQ of ~10 points lower than an unaffected sibling" become a key feature of a condition like XYY or XXX syndrome (see chapter 2; Leggett et al. 2010; Tartaglia et al. 2010). An IQ that is comfortably in the normal range can therefore be put into stark relief compared to where it *would* have been, absent the genetic hit of a mutation, and therefore recast as a symptom.

The Fragile X Premutation: From a Carrier Gene to a New Kind of Person

The focus on mutations and their milder, later-onset, or even subclinical effects is poised to become far more widespread. More and more, experts in medical genetics are rethinking the very idea of "carrier" genes. Mutations can attract a great deal of attention when they confer risk of an offspring inheriting a serious disease. Screening for and reporting carrier genes for reproductive risk is not considered particularly controversial as long as consent has been granted. However, it also opens the aperture for learning about and acting on carrier mutations. If you start to find symptoms in people with a carrier variant—even if they are markedly different than the known genetic disorder itself— then perhaps you are simultaneously dealing with a milder pathogenic mutation. Once that happens, the genomic designation of a new, less severe disorder is likely.

Of course, this is not entirely new. To take a famous example, it has long been recognized that people with one HbS allele are not necessarily *just* carriers for sickle cell disease: they can sometimes suffer from symptoms as well, and may even be at risk of exercise-related sudden death (Goldsmith et al. 2012; see also Fullwiley 2011:197–220; Wailoo 2001:169, 216–19). More and more, medical genetics is starting to turn to the mild phenotypic impact of certain carrier variants—a development that could potentially impact huge swaths of the population (Bastarache et al. 2018; see below).

Still, emerging knowledge about mutations associated with developmental abnormalities blurs the boundary of the normal and pathological in even more fundamental ways. The group built up around Fragile X has taken this line of thinking further than perhaps anyone else. They are turning the long-recognized Fragile X carrier mutation into a complex set of genetic disorders that now includes two late-onset conditions *and* a childhood-onset genomically designated condition associated with mild developmental difference.

To cut a long story short, it turns out that Fragile X "carriers" may in fact have a mild neurodevelopmental disorder themselves. What's more, with a prevalence of around 1 in 450 men and 1 in *150* women, the Fragile X "premutation" may affect many millions of people throughout the world. This raises an intriguing question: will Fragile X represent, once again, a kind of vanguard for the way genomically designated conditions can impact our approach to human difference? More broadly, as researchers find that more and more carrier genes and variants actually have subtle phenotypes that sometimes resemble their more straightforwardly pathogenic brethren, will medical genetics take on a new relevance for the population as a whole?

Fragile X Families and the Family of Fragile X–Related Disorders

To people familiar with the field, it may come as something of a surprise to read that the Fragile X mutation represents something new in the history of medical genetics. It is one of the most long-standing genetic syndromes in the literature, and it was also the subject of one of the first successful applications of genomic testing to identify carrier status. Yet when it comes to spinning off new kinds of people, Fragile X finds itself serving yet again as the vanguard of revolutionary developments in medical genetics. The sprawling network assembled around Fragile X has allowed a number of other "Fragile X–related disorders" to be identified, studied, and turned into new kinds of people in their own right. These Fragile X *pre*mutation conditions open up entirely new dimensions of genetic risk and illness for families affected by the original object of mobilization, Fragile X syndrome itself.

In contrast to most of the conditions discussed in this book, Fragile X is usually inherited from a carrier mother rather than de novo (of unknown cause). This wrinkle in the underlying genetic mechanism that causes Fragile X has now been pried open, revealing a panoply of biosocial complexity in the process. To recall, most of us have around thirty cytosine-guanine-guanine or CGG trinucleotide repeats in the *FMR1* gene on the long arm of our X chromosomes. Around 1 in 4,000–5,000 people have more than two hundred CGG repeats—they have Fragile X syndrome. For more than a couple of decades now, it has been recognized that mothers who have a "premutation" of around 55–199 CGG repeats on their *FMR1* gene are at extremely high risk of having children with the full Fragile X mutation. In general, the longer the premutation repeat sequence—and it tends to grow with each passing generation—the more likely that the next generation will have full-blown Fragile X syndrome.

This has several huge implications for Fragile X as a kind of person. First of all, it means that a Fragile X diagnosis is rarely just a one-off for a family. Very often, diagnosing a Fragile X proband leads to the identification of other cases of Fragile X in the extended family. In some cases, especially in larger extended families, a whole host of people can be identified through this kind of "cascade" testing, often explaining patterns of behavioral and intellectual difference that have been informally recognized by the family for many years. This leads to higher rates of detection than other genetic disorders and a greater salience for the diagnosis among families. As Robert Miller put it in our interview, he has always stressed the importance of the fact that "Fragile X is a family disorder" in everything the National Fragile X Foundation does.

Second, even when other full-blown cases are not identified, Fragile X has important reproductive implications. Knowing that a woman is a Fragile X carrier entails risk for her future pregnancies, for those of her daughters (even if they do not appear to be affected), and for other women in the extended family. The premutation tends to expand every time a woman passes it on, so the risk of Fragile X syndrome grows throughout an affected family with every passing generation. In sum, the Fragile X inheritance mechanism creates complex recurrence and risk patterns throughout a pedigree, impacts reproductive decision-making, and places a new form of "genetic responsibility" on families (Raspberry and Skinner 2011a). In practice, this scrutiny falls mostly on women. Women are much more likely to carry the Fragile X premutation, thanks in large part to their two X chromosomes. Thus, while males will generally have a more severe phenotype if they have full-blown Fragile X, women are around three times more likely to have the premutation than men: 1 in 151 vs. 1 in 468, according to a recent CDC estimate (Seltzer et al. 2012). Perhaps even more importantly, only carrier mothers can pass on Fragile X syndrome itself.

(Males' X chromosomes do not recombine during meiosis—the moment when the instability conferred by the premutation can lead to the further expansion of the CGG repeat sequence into the 200+ range that causes Fragile X syndrome.)

Fragile X therefore implicates and involves families even more than the other conditions discussed in this book, creating a powerful rationale for testing parents and family members for both the full Fragile X mutation and the "carrier" premutation. This is why the Fragile X mutation and the premutation that causes it were two of the earliest and most important instances of applying genomics to identify carriers for a serious condition. Because of the Fragile X premutation's extremely high prevalence of 1 in 151 women, commercial screening is now being made available and marketed even to people who do not have a history of Fragile X syndrome in their families.[6]

However, Fragile X's inheritance mechanism has also led to the recognition of something new and even more perplexing for the social studies of science and medicine. In fact, it has created three new things. What we have long thought of as the "carrier" gene for FXS has been transformed a couple of times since the Fragile X support groups and foundations started bringing families and researchers together en masse.

A Pair of Novel Adult-Onset Disorders

The first novel disorder associated with the Fragile X premutation entered the literature in 2001. It all began when Randi Hagerman's work on Fragile X led to the intriguing identification of several patients' grandfathers who had succumbed to tremors and ataxia (losing control over bodily movements). As she explained, "We decided to look into this issue because I kept hearing the same story about a lot of the grandfathers. . . . After seeing 6 of these grandfathers, we realized that they all had the same behavioral phenotype and tremor/ataxia." It was at a National Fragile X Foundation meeting in Los Angeles in 2000 that Hagerman realized her anecdotal findings might portend the discovery of an entirely new disorder: "I presented the 6 cases to a roomful of families and asked whether any other people had seen these kinds of issues in the grandparents. About one-third of the people in the room raised their hands, and I suddenly realized this could be a very common problem" (quoted in Partridge 2007).

In a 2015 interview at the MIND Institute in Sacramento, Hagerman told me that she was stunned by this turn of events. However, she immediately knew that she was really on to something. With teams of Fragile X researchers already in place at the MIND Institute and elsewhere, Hagerman and her colleagues quickly assembled their findings. Still, they faced pushback in the field. Hagerman told me that their first paper was rejected by the *American Journal of Human Genetics*, and then only accepted by *Neurology* because the editor decided it was important enough to override the two negative reviews the manuscript received. Thus the first paper on this new Fragile X premutation disorder was published in 2001 (Hagerman et al. 2001; see also Berry-Kravis et al. 2003), with another paper formally delineating Fragile X–associated tremor/ataxia syndrome or FXTAS a few years later in the *American Journal of Human Genetics* (it seems they had finally come around) (Hagerman and Hagerman 2004).

The second premutation disorder entered the literature a little later than FXTAS, but its origins can be traced back even further. Beginning in the mid-1990s, researchers began to realize that there were high rates of early menopause or primary ovarian insufficiency among women with the Fragile X premutation (Conway et al. 1995; Schwartz et al. 1994; Sherman 2000). However, this discovery was not the product of a carefully designed study of premutation carriers. Instead, it was the result of *informal* conversations within the Fragile X community. Hagerman recounted the story to me in our interview. She said that it was at

a meeting that we had, I think in 1990, I remember at one of the luncheon tables several women were sitting around along with professionals. One woman said, "Well,"—they were all carrier mothers—and one woman said, "Well, I've had early menopause, and I'm only 36." Then two other women at the same table said, "Well, the same thing's happened to me." It was really nice, 'cause it was an informal exchange of information, so that . . . basic researchers, clinicians, and families could talk about some of the problems that they've experienced. It really helped to guide some of the research.

When Hagerman and her colleagues followed up by looking for more Fragile X premutation carriers with early onset menopause, they found them in large numbers. By 2008, a new disorder had entered the literature: Fragile X–associated primary ovarian insufficiency or FXPOI (De Caro, Dominguez, and Sherman 2008). Over the last few years a small but vibrant literature on FXPOI has emerged.

Thus, FXPOI has joined FXTAS and Fragile X syndrome itself among, as the National Fragile X Foundation calls it, the "Fragile X–Associated

Disorders."[7] In fact, the foundation has significantly recalibrated its mission in order to address these two adult-onset conditions along with its original raison d'être, Fragile X syndrome. Attending an NFXF annual meeting, one quickly realizes that the movement and the teams of researchers are now dedicated to a set of related disorders, not just Fragile X syndrome itself. That said, it is certainly not a coincidence that the more serious, more typical genetic condition came first: these carrier adults were identified *after* the diagnosis of children with full Fragile X. It was only in the setting created by social mobilization and community formation around Fragile X itself that FXPOI and FXTAS were made visible.

To be clear, FXTAS and FXPOI are *not* genomically designated in the strongest sense—you need to show a particular sort of phenotypic expression (tremor/ataxia symptomatology and premature ovarian insufficiency, respectively) along with the premutation in order to be diagnosed. However, the story did not stop there.

A New Developmental Disorder?

In recent years, FXTAS and FXPOI have proven insufficient to capture the phenotype of the premutation. Researchers and carriers alike have begun to recognize a diffuse and subtle phenotype characterized by a range of medical issues from sleep apnea, thyroid disease, and migraines to cognitive abnormalities, anxiety disorders, and autistic traits that resemble those of FXS in much less severe form (see, e.g., Bailey, Raspa et al. 2008; Bourgeois et al. 2011; Clifford et al. 2007; Kenna et al. 2013; Roberts et al. 2009; Rodriguez-Revenga et al. 2009; Wang et al. 2012). There is now evidence that this Fragile X premutation phenotype is present even in families unaffected by Fragile X syndrome itself,[8] and from the neonatal period onward.

In 2008, a team of researchers led by a leading Fragile X parent/researcher, Donald Bailey, published a major paper in the *American Journal of Medical Genetics* (Bailey, Raspa, et al. 2008). They had recruited a national survey of families affected by *FMR1* mutations from three leading Fragile X foundations, including the NFXF. Along with results for 1,235 children with Fragile X, they included findings for 57 male and 199 female child *premutation* carriers. Crucially, they were able to compare premutation bearers to controls taken from the same population of families affected by Fragile X. They found statistically significant rates of the following problems among premutation bearers as compared to the matched controls: "Developmental delay," "Attention problems," "Aggressiveness" (significant for males only), "Autism" (males only), "Seizures" (males only), and "Anxiety and Depression" (significant for females only) (2064–65).

Discussing their results, Bailey and colleagues note the "striking finding" of prevalent "co-occurring conditions in premutation carriers, reinforced by within-gender comparisons matched on age and family income" (Bailey, Raspa, et al. 2008:2067). A full third of male carriers had been diagnosed with developmental delay, and "as a group they were more likely to have experienced problems with attention, aggression, autism, seizures, and anxiety." For females, there were also higher rates of developmental disorders than seen in controls and "significant differences" in "attention problems, anxiety, and depression" (2067). The authors went on to argue that their data supported earlier findings, bolstering the notion that *FMR1* premutation carriers had significantly increased risk for autism and ADHD, along with a bevy of other physical and behavioral challenges. In short, this study provided the most authoritative evidence up to that time that the Fragile X premutation was far more than a mere carrier gene—it might index a mild, childhood-onset genetic disorder.

A great deal of research on the premutation has appeared since 2008. A review in the *Journal of Neurodevelopmental Disorders* noted how the premutation was "historically" understood solely as a carrier gene that conferred risk of Fragile X in future generations, but with no effect on the "carriers" themselves. "However," they go on, "research on the premutation phenotype over the last 10 to 15 years has demonstrated clear health risks associated with *FMR1* expansions in the premutation range" (Wheeler et al. 2014:1). They point toward "a continuum of involvement with mild anxiety or shyness in some children or adults with the premutation to more severe psychiatric problems and as carriers age, appearance of neurological problems that may eventually result in FXTAS" (2). The authors note the following problems as being possibly, probably, or definitely related to the Fragile X premutation: thyroid disease, hypertension, fibromyalgia symptoms, migraine, neuropathy, vestibular difficulties, ovarian insufficiency, estrogen-related conditions, fertility issues, obstetric and perinatal difficulties, postpartum depression, arithmetic difficulties, executive dysfunction, attention deficits, verbal memory, verbal working memory, visual memory, language, anxiety, autism traits, psychosis, ADHD, and sleep issues (see tables 1–4 on pp. 4, 5, 7, and 10). Hence, they conclude, "Females with an *FMR1* premutation may be variably at risk for multiple medical, reproductive, cognitive, and psychiatric difficulties, . . . [which] should be considered whenever a premutation carrier presents to a clinic" (10).

In short, there is plenty for these hitherto "carriers" to worry about vis-à-vis their own health and psychic well-being. Even more recent evidence that I have seen discussed at research conferences indicates that there are cognitive differences between Fragile X premutation bearers and matched controls *from birth*. Failing to meet the diagnostic criteria for serious disorders like autism, neuropathy, or an attention disorder does not mean that a mutation will be relegated to the realm of "low penetrance." Instead, researchers can turn to endophenotypes and subclinical cognitive processing features of the mutation's phenotype. This is exactly what is happening with the Fragile X premutation.

It is important to keep in mind that the status of the Fragile X premutation is far from settled. It is yet to be formally or widely recognized as a disease entity. Nevertheless, things seem to be heading in that direction. In our 2015 interview, Hagerman told me that she had encountered skepticism about the "reality" of both FXTAS and FXPOI, as well as the association between Fragile X and autism, only to be proven right as the evidence grew. She was convinced that the Fragile X premutation would soon be recognized as an important new genetic disorder. So far, the developing literature on the topic seems to strongly support Hagerman's position. Still, Hagerman said that there was no agreement yet on a name, and that the NFXF and the NIH require consensus in the relevant research community before admitting a new disorder into their official nosologies.

Crucially, and far from coincidentally, the National Fragile X Foundation may be poised to support the turn to recognize the premutation as a fourth member of the family of Fragile X disorders alongside FXS, FXTAS, and FXPOI. For now, the NFXF website remains somewhat guarded about the status of the premutation beyond the risk for FXTAS and FXPOI. However, Hagerman is still one of the central actors in the NFXF, and family interest in the whole range of premutation effects is extremely high. At the NFXF annual meeting I attended in 2014, Hagerman delivered a plenary session on the premutation and its complex phenotype. She told a rapt ballroom full of Fragile X families and experts what they had learned about the premutation and its myriad, if often subtle, effects across the life span. Hagerman also noted that female premutation bearers appeared to have *higher* than average IQ scores compared to the normal population and outlined a slew of measures that could be taken to improve their health and cognitive outcomes.

In fact, the NFXF cosponsored the First International Conference on the *FMR1* Premutation in 2013. In a 2014 report on the conference, Tassone, Hagerman, and Hagerman summarized the history of the premutation, FXTAS, and FXPOI before discussing some recent findings about adult premutation bearers. Then, they went on to discuss "a growing awareness of neurodevelopmental problems in early childhood" for people with the premutation, even though "such features remain woefully underrecognized." Unsurprisingly, these problems appear to especially affect males: "Boys have higher rates of attention deficit hyperactivity disorder (ADHD), shyness, social deficits, autism spectrum disorder (ASD) and, less commonly, intellectual disability (ID)." Still, new data from studies that screened newborns found "patterns of differences in developmental trajectories are present as early as 24 months in premutation carriers" in both sexes. The authors also noted a finding of "visual motion processing deficits" that demonstrated "an intrinsic early deficit caused by the premutation." Finally, they called for further research that can overcome questions about clinically biased samples (Tassone, Hagerman, and Hagerman 2014:2–3).

Robert Miller, while he was still executive director, published a more hesitant report on the conference on the NFXF website. Miller included an important caveat for Fragile X families: "With the exception of consensus around FXPOI and FXTAS, at this time there was only limited consensus about possible additional disorders related to the premutation, **and many attendees expressed the critical importance of communicating that point to families!**" (emphasis in original). Nevertheless, the report includes the following "takeaway points that may be of interest to families":

- Those with the premutation may be more susceptible to the effects of environmental and lifestyle stressors such as smoking, excessive alcohol consumption and environmental toxins. Although the evidence is inconsistent at this point with respect to specific stressors, all individuals should be encouraged to live healthy lives and continue to use preventive health care measures.
- A recent survey suggests that some children with the premutation may have developmental problems. The effect appears to be much milder than that caused by the full mutation. If this finding is borne out in future studies, it will have implications for early diagnosis and intervention. . . .
- Some studies found that medical conditions unrelated to FXPOI and FXTAS, such as irritable bowel syndrome, restless leg syndrome, migraine headaches, social phobias, panic disorder, hypertension, anxiety, depression,

sleep apnea, fatigue, joint pain and other seemingly unrelated problems such as autoimmune conditions, may be associated with the premutation. (Miller 2013)

Miller also discussed growing evidence of "an increased risk for autistic behaviors and other 'neuro-dysfunctions,'" plus research on differences in MRI studies as well as the epigenetic and proteomic impact of the premutation.

By way of conclusion Miller argued that, despite the lack of consensus among researchers, "certain beliefs about the premutation are already held to be true simply because they are repeated often enough on the web and in social media." Like the report from Tassone and the Hagermans, Miller closed with a call for further research, arguing that "researchers need to provide accurate new information as it becomes available to the estimated 20 million carriers worldwide who struggle with, at best, the uncertainties that come with being a carrier." In sum, the jury is still out. Still, it is clear that the existing evidence has already had a profound impact on people who know they carry the premutation.

The risk of having a child with full-blown Fragile X is no doubt still an extremely salient part of having the Fragile X premutation, but it has also come to mean far more than its "carrier" status. Fragile X's unusual inheritance mechanism, combined with the capacity of the network built up around it, has led to the creation of a new kind of person: the Fragile X premutation bearer. People with the Fragile X premutation are now thought to be at extremely high risk for two serious adult-onset disorders *and* most likely affected by a mild neurodevelopmental disorder from cradle to grave. Finally, we have seen how looping processes among premutation bearers are already underway in the Fragile X community with expectations for development, treatment recommendations, and a knowledge base that are all still very much in flux. Again, none of this would have been recognized were it not for the incredible work the Fragile X community has done to bring patients, their families, clinicians, and researchers together around the goal of understanding and mobilizing CGG repeat expansions on the *FMR1* gene.

With so much research still to be done and so many people with the premutation out there, this is surely a topic that needs to be followed closely over the coming years by social scientists interested in the intersection of genetics and medicine.[9] After all, the premutation is *not* rare at all. This may be a novel genetic disorder, but it is by no means rare: the recent CDC estimate cited above implies that there are around 1.3–1.4 *million* people with the Fragile X premutation in the United States alone. As Wheeler et al. put it, "Understanding the phenotype associated with the premutation is important from a public health perspective, given its prevalence" (2).

Cause for Concern?

With "incompletely penetrant" mutations being discovered all the time, this new way of thinking about genetics and pathogenicity has huge implications. Consider again the 2013 paper from *Lancet Neurology* discussed above (Moreno-De-Luca et al. 2013). It was also the subject of an accompanying editorial, and the inspiration for that issue's cover art (see fig. 7.2). The image captures this realignment quite poignantly: we see a child who is not necessarily sick per se, but just a few steps behind where he *should* be relative to his family background.

A few years later, the paper by Brenda Finucane, David Ledbetter, and their Geisinger colleagues (discussed above) explained how this reorientation represents nothing less than an opportunity "to expand 'precision medicine' beyond cancer treatment to other areas of medical practice" (Finucane et al. 2016:304). They conclude with a remarkable passage—at once cautionary and promissory—that situates this new focus on the quantitative neurodevelopmental "shift" caused by mutations in the broader history of genetics research on human difference:

Genetics has a well-documented and checkered past with regard to family studies that resulted in errant social policies, including involuntary sterilization, based on naive notions about the heritability of intelligence, criminality, and antisocial behavior. The future goal of family studies in the context of neurodevelopmental disorders should be to enhance prognostic focus and maximize the appropriateness of interventions to improve outcomes. Regarding family studies for intellectual and behavioral traits, medical genetics now has a rare opportunity for a "do-over," with the benefit of hindsight in a (hopefully) more socially enlightened era. Meticulous research on clinical applications of neurodevelopmental "shift," in close collaboration with families and with careful consideration of social consequences, may allow us to get it right the second time around. (304)

In other words, this new approach represents nothing less than an attempt to bring genetics back into the systematic study and treatment of human difference across generations. These authors are committed, in their work and in their practice, to helping families effectively

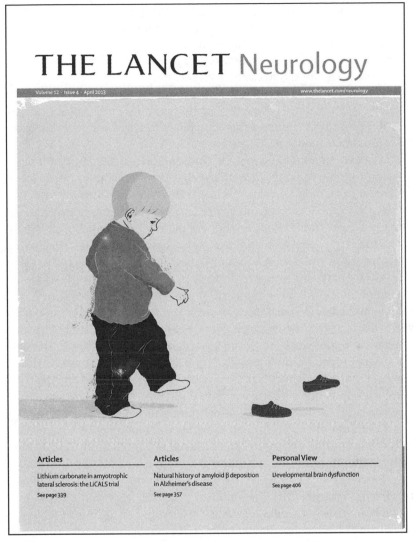

FIGURE 7.2. Cover of *Lancet Neurology*, April 2013, accompanying Morena-De-Luca et al.'s paper in that issue: "Developmental Brain Dysfunction: Revival and Expansion of Old Concepts Based on New Genetic Evidence." The editors also wrote an enthusiastic editorial on the way genetics is reshaping the classification of "neurodevelopmental disability." Art by Carlo Giambarresi. (Reproduced by permission from Elsevier)

confront the medical, psychiatric, and developmental challenges they face. Nevertheless, the specter of eugenics looms large over this kind of work. The authors' decision to tackle it head on is a testament to their commitment to the patients and families they work with.

But there is still serious cause for concern. The eugenic nightmare of confinement, forced sterilization, crass prejudice, and grotesquely distorted ideas about the heritability of human difference probably *should* forever loom over human genetics. However, there are other genomic dystopias that should be avoided as well.

Consider this: in the research on people with the 16p11.2 microdeletion discussed above, the unaffected family members had a mean IQ of 112 (Moreno-De-Luca et al. 2015). What does this suggest? We know that genetic testing and participation in this kind of research are highly skewed toward families that are middle-class and above. We also know that privilege and privation both have a profound effect on a person's ability to perform on an IQ test. In fact, the much-discussed *heritability* of IQ declines precipitously as you move down the socioeconomic scale (Turkheimer et al. 2003): it turns out that people need the right physical and social environment to realize their "genetic potential" on an IQ test (whatever it even measures). Finally, there is a long history of middle-class advocacy and research participation in the field of developmental difference—dating back at least as far as the rise of the autism movement (Eyal et al. 2010)—geared toward maximizing children's potential. When you put these pieces together, it is all too easy to see how this new emphasis on maximizing the "genetic potential" children inherit from their families will end up mostly benefiting the children who, despite the "hit" of a de novo mutation, already benefit from multiple forms of advantage.

"Precision medicine" may therefore be on the verge of biologically vivifying long-standing inequalities in health care and education—imparting new responsibilities and conferring new means of advancement on families who already enjoy considerable social and economic privilege. Consider once again the meaning of the phrase "The gene didn't get the memo": if you have a child with a genetic mutation, you have a mandate to act, even if they appear normal by older disciplinary standards. It is entirely understandable for parents to bring all their material, social, and cultural capital to bear to help a child with a genetic mutation maximize her potential. Who could argue with that? However, the biological arbitrariness of a threshold like <70 IQ points for a diagnosis of intellectual disability belies a crucial social exigency: we have scarce resources for early intervention, educational remediation, and care. This new approach to the genetics of developmental difference may provide a rationale for giving more to the most privileged families.

We therefore need to take stock of the way genomic designation may lead to lowered expectations, self-fulfilling prophecies, overtreatment, and perhaps even the reproduction of social inequalities. Indeed, with the rollout of a new generation of noninvasive prenatal genetic tests (discussed at length in the next chapter), knowledge about genetic mutations can still, and probably *will*, have eugenic outcomes. As Finucane et al. themselves point out, we need to grapple with the way knowledge about mutations is actually being used in practice *before* we stumble into new versions of old tragedies. In this case, we need to think carefully about what it means to judge human difference based on what we know, or think we know, about a combination of their family backgrounds and the genetic mutations they bear.

Conclusion

It turns out that studying a population of people with a specific genetic mutation can reveal subtle forms of developmental and psychiatric difference which often fail to meet existing diagnostic criteria. And yet, the failure to meet clinical thresholds of significance does *not* necessarily mean that people with a particular mutation are deemed unaffected or simply "carriers." Instead, traits that are within the clinically normal range can still be thought of as *symptoms* of an underlying genetic disorder like Fragile X, 16p11.2DS, or 22q11.2DS. We saw how clinical judgment and expectations can be recast when it comes to both IQ and growth charts—the quintessential tools of twentieth-century surveillance medicine, according to David Armstrong (1995:396–97). From dangerously low growth that is actually normal for 22q to an IQ of 87 that masks an important cognitive deficit, having a genetic mutation can do far more than indicate risk factors: it can change the way we observe and understand childhood abnormality.

Perhaps even more strikingly, we saw how the Fragile X premutation has begun to challenge other fundamental assumptions in human genetics. Although it began its career as a carrier gene that could lead to full-blown Fragile X in someone's offspring, the Fragile X premutation has metamorphosed into a mutation that can cause two serious adult-onset conditions. Now, a growing body of research suggests it is also associated with a host of ailments and a mild cognitive phenotype that is observable from infancy. In short, the premutation is beginning to be thought of as a childhood-onset *developmental* disorder. What does this mean for the staggering 1 in ~450 males and 1 in ~150 females who have this Fragile X premutation? The jury is still out. However, at the risk of speculation, it seems like only a matter of time before Hagerman and her allies are "proved right" once again by the formal recognition of a new Fragile X premutation syndrome. Given its prevalence and generally very mild clinical presentation, not to mention a social movement already working to mobilize it, a new genomically designated condition based on the Fragile X premutation has far-reaching implications.

However, it is important to keep in mind that this mild disorder—this very subtle kind of person—was only made visible in the context of the network built up over many years by experts and advocates dedicated to Fragile X. Likewise, the often very mild 22q11.2 *Duplication* Syndrome discussed in chapter 5 would not be nearly as widely recognized or well understood if it had not been picked up and catapulted to salience by the network build around its genomic sibling, 22q11.2DS. Today, FXTAS, FXPOI, and Fragile X premutation differences are all growing topics of research and concern for organizations like the National Fragile X Foundation.[10] The same goes for 22q11.2 Duplication Syndrome and the International 22q11.2 Foundation. In fact, now that the NFXF is dedicated to the umbrella topic of Fragile X–associated disorders, rather than just FXS, and the 22q foundation has dropped "Deletion" from its name, they are both well placed to absorb these new syndromes into their constituencies. The Fragile X movement provided what Foucault (2002:41) would call the "surfaces of emergence" for the *FMR1* premutation to be recast as a disorder in its own right. By bringing patients and their families together, groups like the National Fragile X Foundation made it possible for experts to discover that carriers were suffering from two late-onset conditions and a series of generally mild neurodevelopmental symptoms from birth onward. This community, organized because of Fragile X syndrome itself, allowed for what Wailoo (2001) deftly terms the social and clinical *visibility* of the mild premutation phenotype. In this way, we begin to see how testing technologies are just one component of the larger project of making genetic disease visible.

Increasingly, many geneticists are starting to question the very notion of "carrier genes" and "incomplete penetrance" altogether. Hence the Fragile X premutation could be a harbinger of things to come as we move further into the age of genomic medicine. Today, new surfaces of emergence are making the effects of carrier mutations visible on a much broader scale: electronic medical records, whole genome screening, huge public databases, and algorithmic matching are combining to unearth the mild, late-onset, and diffuse symptoms that can be associated with previously overlooked variants in disease genes. So, the other big question here is this: How many other carrier genes will turn out to have milder or late-onset phenotypes?

The surge of interest in "semi-recessive" mutations and affected carriers is not confined to the sorts of conditions discussed in this book. More and more, researchers are finding that heterozygous carriers deal with less severe or late-onset symptoms that resemble the classic genetic disorder they are carriers for. A recent study in *Science* by a team from Vanderbilt shows just how widespread the turn to looking at the pathogenic effects of carrier variants could become. They considered around 1,200 Mendelian disease genes. In a cohort of 21,701 adults, 807, or around 3.7%, had a statistically significant relationship between a gene variant and their phenotype. Only *eight* had been diagnosed with the relevant genetic disorder. A large majority of the seemingly affected people, they reported, "were heterozygous for variants in genes with a presumed recessive inheritance and yet still had symptoms consistent with the Mendelian disease pattern." That is, they were carriers for serious genetic disorders. "These individuals," they continue, "tend to have disease that is mild compared with the classic presentations but severe relative to the general population. . . . This work adds to the evidence that Mendelian and complex disease are not dichotomous, but rather exist on a spectrum" (Bastarache et al. 2018:6). Yet again, we see how mutations point toward phenotypes that just do not line up with established disease categories. Instead, they index symptom patterns that would be invisible to the clinical gaze. If this sort of framework were applied to much larger cohorts and a longer list of genes, who knows how many people would find themselves with an uncertain genetic diagnosis?

This reevaluation of carrier genes, if it does become widespread, could completely transform the proportion of the population that has an actionable genetic finding. After all, carrier variants and mutations tend to be orders of magnitude more common than their clearly pathogenic counterparts. In short, the discovery of mild phenotypes in people with carrier genes has the potential to transform the scope and practice of medical genetics.

It is increasingly clear that genetic mutations have no fealty to prevailing disciplinary boundaries, thresholds of significance, or categories of human difference. They "didn't get the memo" that we have long-standing systems of classification and practice that we would rather not disrupt. It is far from unclear what this will mean for patient identity, health care delivery, education, inequality, and many other issues. Perhaps it will not amount to much. Moving forward though, we should pay close attention to the way genomic designation can remake boundaries between pathology and normality across a host of important fields.

EIGHT

The Future for Genomic Designation and the New Prenatal Testing Landscape

In this final chapter, we take stock of how far genomic designation has come over the last sixty years before turning a cautious eye toward the future. Conditions like XXX syndrome, 5p– syndrome, and 22q11.2DS have gone from obscure categories of biomedical research to robust categories of human difference backed by small but vibrant social movements. And yet, for all the enormous progress that researchers and advocates have made in recent years, they cannot fully control how the mutations they care so much about are mobilized. What then, can we expect of genomic designation moving forward?

I begin with a potted history of Elwyn Services—an institution that has been at the forefront of the genetics of developmental difference since the eugenics era. Nothing better illustrates the way mutations have gone from objects of esoteric genetics research to ones that can shape a person's social life, education, and psychological treatment.

Then, looking at clear and emerging trends, we turn our attention to the future for these kinds of genetic mutations as well as the groups of patients, parents, advocates, and experts for whom they have come to mean so much. There is good reason to believe that the rise of clinical genomics, the affordances of social media, and the repertoires of collection pioneered by groups like the National Fragile X Foundation will see a bevy of new genomically designated conditions emerge and achieve salience quite rapidly over the coming years.

At the same time, new developments in prenatal genetic testing have the potential to upend the field. The rollout of a new, noninvasive prenatal genetic testing technology means that many of these mutations could become salient to an unprecedented number of people, but not necessarily in the way that advocates have fought so hard for.

The Illustrative History of Genetics at Elwyn Services

Alongside sweeping change, many of the institutions and actors that are so key to genomic designation—not to mention several of the mutations themselves—have endured since the heyday of the XYY-criminality nexus. Reiterated fact-making helps us understand this combination of deep continuity and radical transformation. Nowhere illustrates this better than Elwyn Services.

Founded in 1856, Elwyn lies less than fifteen miles from downtown Philadelphia. As a large and long-standing institution for people with intellectual impairment (see Trent 1995), it serves as a kind of microcosm of the history of genetics and people with developmental disabilities in the United States. Geneticists' long-standing interest in people with developmental disabilities led them time and again to places like Elwyn. This has been one of the great constants of human genetics from the eugenics era through to postgenomic medicine. What that interest meant for patients, however, has varied dramatically. Over the last century-plus, Elwyn has been, in turn, a major center of eugenics research (Hansen 2005:14–19), a source of biological samples for esoteric human genetics, and, as we saw in chapter 6, a leading center for using genetic mutations to inform patient diagnosis and care.

One of the central figures in this transformation was Brenda Finucane, who spent the bulk of her career to date as a genetic counselor at Elwyn. She worked there from the time she completed her training in the early 1980s until 2012, and spearheaded Elwyn's emergence as a leading site for treating people with genetic disorders like Fragile X and 22q11.2DS. Over that period, Finucane went from the traditional genetic counseling she had trained for to being one of the world's foremost experts and advocates for genomically designated conditions. Finucane also used her position at Elwyn to help foster support groups and professional awareness—making Elwyn a key node within and between many of the networks dedicated to genomically designated conditions. Tracing Elwyn's history therefore helps us understand both the historical conditions and forms of collective action that have transformed the scope for mobilizing mutations.

Long before Finucane came along, Elwyn was home to one of the leading XYY researchers in the United States, Mary Telfer. During a visit to Elwyn, I interviewed Elliott Simon (2012)—the behavioral psychologist encountered in chapter 6, who serves as Elwyn's executive director of research and health services, as well as their unofficial institutional historian. Comparing Telfer's work from the 1960s and 1970s to Finucane's work in the early 2000s, Simon laid out the contrast quite clearly. Telfer, he told me, "was actually drawing blood, doing research, bench-type stuff. She was not a genetic counselor; I mean, she was a genetics person. And she was doing research on XYY. I mean, she was like *the* person in the country for this." Yet even though Elwyn was perhaps the leading center for XYY research in the late-1960s United States, it barely mattered to the actual boys with an extra Y chromosome. Simon explained, "[W]hether it changed how people here were treated, I don't think so. . . . *It was not part of the support services of Elwyn during that time period.*"

As a behavioral psychologist, Elliott Simon had been aware of genetic diagnoses for years, ever since he had worked in a state developmental center in the 1980s, and Elaine Zackai had come out from Penn to diagnose children for research purposes. Zackai is a major figure in medical genetics research, director of Clinical Genetics at the Children's Hospital of Philadelphia, and the medical director of their 22q and You Center. But that is the Elaine Zackai of today. As Simon put it, "If you're Elaine Zackai back in 1980, '81, you are interested in places like Emeryville, which had 400 people with intellectual disabilities in them." The interest, Simon made clear, was not mutual: the institution's subjects fascinated geneticists, he explained, but the institution was not particularly interested in the geneticists' findings.

So, while early twentieth-century eugenics researchers did gain substantial traction at places like Elwyn, the early decades of research on abnormal human chromosome complements did not. Telfer made some waves with her XYY research at Elwyn, infamously claiming that serial killer Richard Speck was a prototypical XYY proband (it turned out that Speck had just one Y chromosome). However, geneticists tended to treat institutions like Elwyn simply as a repository of biological samples. Put simply, institutionalized populations yielded many of the most fruitful pedigrees and chromosomes for basic genetics research. Those geneticists did not, however, see any great clinical or social potential in working with those populations—they were there to collect biological samples and perhaps some phenotypic data, nothing more. Genetics had very little impact on clinical practice.

Even Finucane, who now epitomizes the turn to mobilizing mutations, was originally hired as little more than an intermediary charged with providing biological samples for human genetics researchers.[1] This was in the early 1980s. As Finucane explained to me in our 2011 interview, this was not only her first job in genetic counseling, but also a new initiative for Elwyn: "They didn't have a genetic counselor there. They were just starting to think about genetics and people with developmental disabilities." Finucane found herself with a sizeable population to work with as well: "Elwyn had, at that time, like 750 residents there with intellectual disabilities plus thousands of other people in our school programs and other programs." However, we should not assume that Finucane was hired with the goal of turning Elwyn into a leading center for treating and managing patients with genetic disorders. Here is how she described the role she was hired to fill: "There was a job opening for a genetic counselor and *it was actually lobbied for by a geneticist* who was from a local institution. . . . [The local geneticist] *was trying to have a liaison to the institution to try to get blood samples for research on genetics.* So that was ostensibly the purpose of the genetic counselor at Elwyn and why I was hired." Finucane was hired as a genetic counselor at Elwyn to facilitate the identification of people with mutations for use in genetics research, not for what we would now call "personalized medicine" or anything of the sort.

More broadly, very little thought was dedicated to the way knowledge about genetics could inform clinical practice, at least after birth. Things were just starting to change in a few places, but for the most part, this was all in keeping with the picture of immobile mutations painted in chapter 2: geneticists were fascinated by people with intellectual disabilities and congenital abnormalities, especially "funny looking kids," because they were hoping to find interesting mutations and pedigrees; meanwhile, those patients and their caregivers still had very little reason to care about genetic etiology. There is little evidence that anyone at places like Elwyn even *tried* to use mutations to inform treatment or build communities. Stated in terms of reiterated fact-making, the chromosomal abnormalities found at Elwyn well into the 1980s remained almost entirely in the domain of esoteric genetics; they were clearly *not* seen as the kind of facts that could inform treatment and care.

By the mid-1980s, however, things began to change quite rapidly. New genetic testing techniques became available, and new repertoires for dealing with developmental difference came into view. Meanwhile, Elwyn moved away from institutionalized care and began providing more and more nonresidential support services for patients and families. This was the context in which Elwyn became one of the first large institutions to integrate genetic test results into patient treatment and care. Finucane was at the very forefront of these stirrings in medical genetics, having become involved with the new Fragile X group a year after its formation in 1984. For her, finding people with genetic mutations was not just a means to a journal article, but also a tool to advance care and, later on, the basis for the formation of support groups.

Within six months of arriving at Elwyn, Finucane found herself at a crossroads. The geneticist who had pushed to hire her as a kind of liaison to help identify interesting subjects for research had moved on. As Finucane put it, "[It all] changed . . . I was left with a position without its original role." What did she do with this newfound freedom? This is how Finucane described the shift at Elwyn to me: "We did diagnostic testing of lots of individuals in the Elwyn system. Within five years we found literally over 150 individuals with Fragile X, which was this new thing that we were being able to test for. *We found all sorts of different genetic conditions and so it was really a heady time*, I have to say, where you had all these people with these symptom diagnoses, with these behavioral and psychiatric diagnoses, and *now we were diagnosing all these specific genetic conditions*." These genetic diagnoses could now supplement and eventually begin to supplant the existing behavioral and psychiatric ones. Armed with her experience with the Fragile X organization, Finucane helped to establish and develop support groups and foundations for several of those "specific genetic conditions." She also used those genetic diagnoses to provide referrals, guide care, and help patients and families understand their situation and their likely future.

That is why Simon is so proud that, under his leadership as executive director of Research and Quality Improvement, Elwyn became one of the first institutions of its kind to send every patient to a genetic counselor. As its website explains, "Elwyn is a nationally recognized leader in genetics research and education, specializing in the practical implications of genetic disorders in people with developmental disabilities." Elwyn has been at the forefront of research on these kinds of genetic disorders since at least the 1960s, but, even for them, targeted treatment is a much more recent development: "For over 20 years, we have provided a range of services to individuals, families, providers, and educators involved in caring for people with genetic conditions."[2]

During our interview at Elwyn in 2012, Simon left no doubt about his newfound belief in the importance of these diagnoses: "Every single person, in my opinion, with intellectual disabilities, should have a look-see by a genetics counselor to determine etiology." Almost every child who comes through Elwyn Services—it is primarily nonresidential now—is given a genetic workup by Finucane's former department. Suffice it to say that this process yields a high volume of genomically designated diagnoses. As the website explains, "Genetic factors play a major role in causing developmental disabilities. Down syndrome is widely recognized, yet there are hundreds of lesser-known genetic conditions that can cause intellectual, behavioral, and psychiatric symptoms." In contrast to previous decades, however, those results do not remain confined to the lab and the field of human genetics. Not only does finding an explanatory genetic mutation "help individuals and family members to better understand why it occurred and the chances for a recurrence in future generations," but it also "enable[s] families and providers to access syndrome-specific interventions relevant to an individual's unique needs."[3] In places like Elwyn, a genetic diagnosis is now integrated into almost every aspect of the *clinical* care the patient receives. As we saw, this is true even in Elliott Simon's own field of clinical psychology.

Institutions like Elwyn can also become gateways to the broader network formed around a mutation. After receiving a genetic diagnosis, patients and their families are likely to be put in touch with the relevant support group. "[O]ne of the things I impart" to clinicians-in-training at Elwyn, Simon told me, "is if you have somebody with a genetic disorder, you as a team have an obligation. Let's get to know about it, get to know is there a local support group? Should your person be going? Should you be involved in that?" A genetic diagnosis, he explained, "can greatly inform your approach and open up areas of free support that wouldn't otherwise be accessed." Simon also thinks that it is important to direct families toward support groups for genetic disorders and perhaps even become involved with them as allied professionals. As he said in our interview, "You now can go into the Smith-Magenis support group. And yeah, before you could have gone to the Arc,[4] and you could have gone to other places, but it's different, because it is more specific." He also pointed out that they provide the research subjects for clinical trials, meaning that support group members will get access to the most cutting-edge treatments—a topic of increasing relevance as Fragile X and 22q pharmaceuticals make their way toward the market. In short, patients and experts alike have a lot to gain from these new mutation-centered networks.

Elwyn is certainly not representative, but it is also far from an anomaly. For as much as Elwyn may have been an early mover when it comes to genetics and developmental disability, it was also a harbinger of things to come. In fact, Elwyn offers consultative and training services to help other organizations and far-flung families make the most of a genetic diagnosis. This is how they explain that kind of work in a brochure about 22q:

Many professionals first hear about the 22q11.2 deletion syndrome when they begin working with a student who has this diagnosis. At Elwyn, we have extensive knowledge and expertise with this special population. We offer consultative services for individual students, as well as staff training to help schools address the complex needs of children and adolescents with the syndrome. Our staff travel throughout the US and Canada to provide on-site consultations at a child's school and/or home. Let us show you how Elwyn's expertise can make a lasting difference in the lives of these students.

The list of services includes "Individual evaluations of students with 22q11.2[DS] at their schools"; staff training; "Objective and expert assistance to aid in the development of IEPs [individualized education plans], behavior plans, residential and day programs"; "Anticipatory health guidance"; and genetic counseling.[5]

In sum, Elwyn represents a kind of microcosm of the way people with developmental disabilities have been understood and managed in the United States during the last century-plus—from eugenics and mass confinement though deinstitutionalization, the development of nonresidential assistance programs, and now the deep integration of genetic testing into clinical practice. In this one institution, mutations have gone from immobile objects of esoteric research to powerful categories of practice. Elwyn helps make a diagnosis like 22q11.2DS truly matter in places where it would otherwise struggle to gain traction. Through these and similar processes of outreach and translation, knowledge about genetic mutations is being integrated into education and patient care in more and more places.

Whither Genomic Designation?

There are a lot more genetic mutations out there than anyone realized. Recent research shows that we all have numerous mutations in genes that have been associated with disease, and most of us have rare copy number variants as well (Harel and Lupski 2018; Sebat et al. 2004; The 1000 Genomes Project Consortium 2010). It is probably not an exaggeration to say that new mutations are reported on a daily basis, and in the vast majority of cases they do not line up well with long-standing clinical entities. The question is, What is to be done with all these mutations?

Nowadays, clinical teams do not need a robust understanding of the way a mutation is likely to impact a patient's health, never mind a notion that it is a gene for an established clinical disorder, in order to put it in their medical chart. All they need is a reasonably strong belief that the mutation is pathogenic, not for a well-defined clinical phenotype, but just for *something*.

In recent years, there have been more and more calls to start with a novel mutation and then piece together the condition it delineates post factum. For example, a 2007 study published in *Genetics in Medicine* by leading geneticist Lisa Shaffer and colleagues argued that the move *away* from a reliance on phenotypic features represents a key advantage. The "traditional" discovery of microdeletion syndromes, they pointed out, "depended on the serendipitous ascertainment of a patient with established clinical features and a chromosomal rearrangement." For them, this process was hampered by the "assum[ption] that the clinical features are distinctive enough to establish phenotypic relations among patients"—an assumption that "is limited by human subjectivity" (Shaffer et al. 2007:607, 610). Instead, this team examined ten thousand subjects with developmental delay using chromosomal microarray and found seven who had "a novel microdeletion syndrome of 1q41q42." Although no clinical features other than developmental delay (the basis for sample selection) were shared by all seven cases, they argue that their "genotype-first" approach introduces "an objective means" of delineating a syndrome (611).

Just a couple of years later, a debate about the "genotype-first" approach to the discovery of syndromes unfolded over a series of articles and letters spanning the *New England Journal of Medicine* and *Genetics in Medicine*. The exchange represents one of the most explicit discussions of genomic designation in the medical literature. It began with a 2008 paper outlining the discovery of recurrent abnormalities at site 1q21.2 with highly variable phenotypic implications (Mefford et al. 2008), but quickly moved to address the role of genomic testing in clinical practice (Cody 2009; Ledbetter 2008, 2009a, 2009b; Saul and Moeschler 2009). As David Ledbetter put it, new syndromes tend to be discovered on the basis of genetic markers following technological breakthroughs, and "this 'genotype first' method of syndrome identification is currently undergoing an exciting new renaissance because of cytogenetic arrays" (2008:1728).

Ledbetter, long a leading figure in medical genetics, goes on to discuss the implications of all this: "The total number of disorders is now far too large for a pediatrician, or even a pediatric geneticist, to make a specific clinical diagnosis before genetic testing." With the rollout of whole genome arrays, he argues, "*Clinicians, like researchers, can now shift to a 'genotype first' model of diagnosis for children with unexplained developmental abnormalities.*" They can also "expect a much higher yield of clinically significant results" than ever before (2008:1729–30; my emphasis). Having discovered several genomically designated conditions earlier in his career, Ledbetter now directs Geisinger Health System's Autism and Developmental Medicine Institute—the center responsible for several of the key studies discussed in the last chapter. Moreover, he is also the executive vice president and chief scientific officer of the entire Geisinger health care system. Ledbetter is spearheading an unprecedentedly ambitious initiative to sequence the genomes of one hundred thousand Geisinger patients in order to see how this process, along with its results, affects their clinical diagnosis, care, and cost. This is just the sort of site where we should pay close attention to the role of genetic mutations in patient care over the coming years.

The emergence of behavioral neurogenetics, which "starts with a known biologically validated gene or chromosomal abnormality and uses it to define the study cohort" (Feinstein 2009:1050), further suggests that genomic designation will increasingly be used to pry open questions related to the brain, behavior, and cognition. We saw how the NIMH is directing funding toward research aimed at moving psychiatry away from the symptom-based classification of the *DSM* and toward a new, biologically grounded nosology. As the director put it, "Biology never read [the *DSM*]" (quoted in Belluck and Carey 2013). His agency therefore decided to fund research that will help "transform diagnosis by incorporating genetics, imaging, cognitive science, and other levels of information to lay the foundation for a new classification system" (Insel 2013). The *New York Times* reports past and present directors of the NIMH and others saying that they hoped psychiatry would follow cancer research in the move to reclassify disease according to genetic markers. They even quoted one former director as saying that the *DSM* had become a "scientific nightmare." He explained how "many people who get one diagnosis get five diagnoses, but they don't have five diseases—they have one underlying condition" (Steven E.

Hyman, quoted in Belluck and Carey 2013). Of course, this is precisely the rationale in favor of genomic designation that I saw time and again at 22q11.2DS and Fragile X conferences: your kid did not get hit by lighting seven different times, she has one real genetic disorder that can cause a range of symptoms. In the NIMH then, genomic designation appears to have won a major institutional ally.

Several other important trends suggest that genomic designation may be poised to play a much larger role in patient care and identity formation. Innovation in genomic testing technologies is continuing apace, making it easier, cheaper, and faster to test for mutations. The days when testing kits had to target particular genes or chromosomal regions on the basis of clinical suspicion about this or that genetic disorder are quickly coming to an end. When a child is screened using a nontargeted test like chromosomal microarray or whole genome (or exome) sequencing, unexpected results regularly come back.

With so many thousands of potentially pathogenic mutations in play, no one expert can possibly hope to be familiar with every possible genetic disorder. Thanks to publicly available databases like OMIM, DECIPHER, ClinVar, ExAC, and others, when researchers and labs find an unfamiliar variant in a patient, they have a series of tools at their fingertips for finding information about existing cases and likely pathogenicity. Gone are the days when identifying multiple patients with the same novel mutation requires some combination of phenotypic overlap and serendipity (see Check Hayden 2013a, 2013b). Even the rarest of rare genomic variants can be checked in a few minutes, and other cases from all over the world can be identified. As more and more people have their genomes screened for mutations, we should expect a new wave of genomically designated conditions to spring up along with a flood of new patients diagnosed with older ones.

More broadly, the genetic intransigence of most common conditions, the continuing public fascination with the human genome, and the new push for "precision medicine" all seem favorable to the development of genomically designated conditions as objects of research and care. Genomically designated conditions are more likely than ever to be taken up by biomedical researchers and pharmaceutical companies as models for more common conditions. On top of that, there is a growing chorus calling for the integration of genetic diagnoses into previously hostile fields and institutional spaces (see, e.g., Berg, Potocki, and Bacino 2010; Griffiths and King 2004; Miller et al. 2010; Reilly 2012; Robin 2006). Meanwhile, the forthcoming revision to the World Health Organization's *International Classification of Diseases* shows how far genomic designation has come in official nosologies. While 1992's *ICD-10* references just a very small handful of genomically designated conditions, the draft of *ICD-11* includes dozens, including nearly all of the conditions discussed at any length throughout this book.[6]

Perhaps most important of all, the repertoires of collective action established by HIV/AIDs, breast cancer, and especially autism advocates paved the way for groups seeking to mobilize genetic mutations. There is even a proven model—largely pioneered by Fragile X syndrome advocates—for turning rare mutations into new kinds of people backed by expansive programs of research, care, and activism. They are giving rise to clinical protocols and specialist interdisciplinary centers. Social media and other communication technologies make it ever easier for far-flung families to find each other, build communities, and turn mutations into objects of bona fide social action. All in all, things can move much more quickly now than they did just a decade or two ago.

Genomic Designation in an Era of Clinical Sequencing

In April 2017—just as I was working on this concluding chapter—a paper was published in the *American Journal of Human Genetics* by an international team of researchers. They had pooled their data and contacted seven subjects from previous studies in order to arrive at a sample of fourteen unrelated people with either intellectual disability or developmental delay and a particular genetic mutation. Based on this sample, they were able to "report on an ID syndrome caused by de novo germline mutations in the last and penultimate exons of *PPM1D*." All but one child had mild to severe intellectual disability. One child had an IQ of 96 but did still "need extra tutoring at school and showed an anxiety disorder and attention problems." How this child ended up being referred for genetic testing is unclear. By "deep phenotyping" these fourteen subjects, they expanded the phenotype of this mutation—and therefore the profile of this novel genetic disorder: "11 individuals (79%) had behavioral problems, such as anxiety disorders, attention deficit hyperactivity disorder (ADHD), obsessive behavior, sensory integration problems, and autism spectrum disorder (ASD)," as well as hypersensitivity to sound (50%), high pain threshold (90%), vision problems (64%), small hands (91%), short stature (62%), feeding difficulties (71%), hypotonia (71%), broad-based gait (50%), facial dysmorphisms, and periods of fever and vomiting (62%) (Jansen et al. 2017:650–51). The authors even established a website to help researchers add to our knowledge of this novel genetic disorder tied to de novo mutations in the penultimate exons of the *PPM1D* gene.[7]

Meanwhile, that very same issue of the *American Journal of Human Genetics* included papers like "Mutations in *TMEM260* Cause a Pediatric Neurodevelopmental, Cardiac, and Renal Syndrome" (Ta-Shma et al. 2017); "Biallelic Variants in *OTUD6B* Cause an Intellectual Disability Syndrome Associated with Seizures and Dysmorphic Features" (Santiago-Sim et al. 2017); and a correction entitled "De Novo Disruption of the Proteasome Regulatory Subunit *PSMD12* Causes a Syndromic Neurodevelopmental Disorder" (Küry et al. 2017). In short, we see a handful of novel conditions in one issue of one major journal whose table of contents happened to hit my inbox as I was trying to make this point about the role of genetic mutations in the field today. In a sense, this is hardly surprising. Genomic designation has made enormous gains in the literature over the last half century. We have gone from the *Lancet*'s 1960 injunction to search for phenotypes associated with trisomy of all twenty-two autosomal chromosomes to the delineation of new genetic conditions on the basis of chromosomal deletions, duplications, copy number variations and single-gene mutations that are not visible under even the most powerful microscope.

In the new era of clinical sequencing, genomic designation seems poised to play an ever-greater role in both esoteric and applied biomedical research. There is a growing acceptance of the idea that children with developmental delays, behavioral abnormalities, and congenital anomalies should be referred for genetic testing as a matter of course.[8] Patients are increasingly likely to be referred for whole exome or genome sequencing rather than targeted tests or panels. The animating idea behind these moves is clear: people with unexplained neurodevelopmental and congenital abnormalities should receive the sort of test that is most likely to provide the real genetic diagnosis.

It is hardly surprising, then, that we are seeing the emergence of new condition after new condition. The three novel syndromes reported in the aforementioned issue of the *American Journal of Human Genetics* are just the tiny tip of a massive iceberg. Recent high-profile work suggests that sequencing technologies may provide molecular diagnoses for a considerable proportion of patients with neurodevelopmental disorders, even when they have already undergone an older form of genetic testing (Soden et al. 2014). This has already led to a new wave of novel genomically designated conditions entering the literature. For now, most still just take the form of "such-and-such gene associated with developmental delay and other congenital symptoms." Many others, like

Smith-Kingsmore syndrome (a point mutation in the *MTOR* gene that is associated with macrocephaly, developmental delay, and dysmorphic facial features, etc.) have been the subject of further research and renamed after the researchers who discovered them (Moosa et al. 2016; Smith et al. 2013). As Ledbetter predicted (2008), new genetic testing technologies are bound to lead to the identification of novel genetic conditions. Online databases and "deep phenotyping" then allow researchers to see and report complex medical and behavioral profiles for these new genomically designated conditions—a process that once took years and decades.

It is also clear that *some* of the novel conditions discovered using sequencing technologies are already being mobilized. Take the recent case of *NGLY1* mutations. Although it was first reported in the *Journal of Medical Genetics* just a few years ago (Need et al. 2012), and even though it appears to be exceedingly rare, *NGLY1* has already received considerable attention from researchers, families, and popular media outlets. It was first discovered in a boy named Bertrand Might, who had a debilitating glycosylation disorder. Bertrand and his family had participated in a project at Duke that used whole exome sequencing to try to provide molecular diagnoses for seriously ill patients. After they discovered an inherited mutation in both copies of Bertrand's *NGLY1* gene and consulted a leading expert in glycosylation disorders, a diagnosis was made. This novel disorder was included in Need et al.'s 2012 paper on exome sequencing in twelve patients with undiagnosed disorders. The research team told Bertrand's parents, Matt and Christina Might, that little could be done until other *NGLY1* cases were identified. Christina had even identified a promising compound available from Genzyme that may one day be able to serve as a replacement for the N-Glycanase enzyme that is missing due to Bertrand's *NGLY1* mutation. However, there was no chance of getting FDA approval to use it, or the funding necessary to move forward, without additional cases. The Mights, it seemed, would just have to wait.

But simply waiting around for another patient with such a rare disorder to be identified was not acceptable to the Mights. Matt Might—a well-known computer programmer and author from a very wealthy family—set out to compose a blog piece detailing his family's diagnostic odyssey, the discovery that their son had a novel genomic disorder, and their current plight as a family who finally knew their child's real condition but found themselves as true disease orphans. That piece, entitled "Hunting Down My Son's Killer" (Might 2012), went extremely viral. The piece begins with the evocative line, "I found my son's killer.

It took three years." A few short sentences later, he explains, "My son Bertrand has a new genetic disorder. Patient 0."

Within days, researchers who had read the piece about Bertrant identified a new pair of siblings with *NGLY1* mutations. The piece also found its way into the hands of Matt Wilsey—heir to one of the elite families in San Francisco and a major Silicon Valley entrepreneur. Wilsey's daughter, Grace, was also suffering from a glycosylation disorder. At first, they thought the phenotypes were just far too different for Grace and Bertrand to actually have the same condition. Unlike Bertrand, Grace was developing considerable language skills and did not appear to be suffering from seizures. The blog piece was just a poignant and cognate story. In the end, it was a geneticist at Baylor who finally decided to delve into Grace's *NGLY1* mutation (it had been noted, but ignored, by other geneticists), and a quick internet search brought him to Matt Might's blog piece. The Mights and Wilseys connected just days later.

In just over a year, the blog piece had led to the identification of nine *NGLY1* mutation cases. By 2014, a new paper was published in *Genetics in Medicine* describing the phenotype of eight of those patients and declaring that "*NGLY1* deficiency is a novel autosomal recessive disorder" whose "phenotypic spectrum is likely to enlarge as cases with a broader range of mutations are detected" (Enns et al. 2014). They also explain how "the rapid ascertainment of cases occurred over a period of several months and was assisted by strong advocacy from families and connections made possible by the Internet and social media" (756). A new genomically designated condition had been born and rapidly catapulted into action.

The *NGLY1* story was widely covered in outlets like CNN (Wilson 2014) and most notably in an outstanding piece in the *New Yorker* by Seth Mnookin (2014). Because of a blog, two elite families, and the high rate of a poignant shared feature—hypolacrima, or difficulty producing tears—*NGLY1* attracted the kind of attention that many other rare disorders spend years striving for. A registered 501(c)(3) foundation called NGLY1.org is already working to advance research, treatment, and advocacy for this new condition. With millions of dollars of donations from the Wilseys and Mights and a great deal of attention from researchers and the media, they have made rapid progress. A mouse model has been developed, research on targeted treatments is underway, and new study of twelve *NGLY1* patients that further broadened the phenotype was recently published (Lam et al. 2017). Matt Might was even invited to the White House for the announcement of the

Precision Medicine Initiative in January 2015, where he and a handful of other advocates for medical genomics met privately with President Obama. In sum, with the right kind of capital at their disposal, the tiny *NGLY1* community has been able to mobilize their mutation to a remarkable extent in just a few short years.

Another recently identified mutation similarly shows how quickly genomically designated conditions can develop in the age of clinical genomics. As with *NGLY1*, this story also begins with a family enrolling in a research study that aimed to use whole exome sequencing to identify undiagnosed diseases. This ongoing study is called Idiopathic Diseases of Man, or IDIOM. The very first patient tested by the IDIOM team was a girl named Lilly Grossman—a sixteen-year-old who had suffered from painful muscle tremors since early childhood. While most experts had suspected a mitochondrial disorder, the IDIOM team found a mutation in Lilly's *ADCY5* gene.

The *ADCY5* story goes back to 2001. It begins with a clinical report on a multigenerational family with eighteen people affected by "familial dyskinesia [impaired movement] with facial myokymia [muscle quivers]" or FDFM. The authors argued that their results "suggest that a novel gene underlies this new condition" (Fernandez et al. 2001). Eleven years later, a follow-up study on that same family published in *JAMA Neurology* proved them right: a mutation in Adenylyl cyclase 5 (*ADCY5*) appeared to be the cause of FDFM (Chen et al. 2012). However, the identification of the *ADCY5* mutation has led to a clear case of genomic designation. In 2014, a group that included members of the IDIOM team published a paper on Lilly and one additional, sporadic *ADCY5* case. As they put it, "Significant phenotypic overlap with FDFM was recognized in both cases *only after discovery of the molecular link*" (Chen et al. 2014:542; my emphasis). The following year, a major paper on *ADCY5* came out in *Neurology*. Reporting on twelve new families and three new sporadic cases along with the previously reported cases, the authors had a total sample of fifty patients to draw on (Chen et al. 2015). This allowed them to speak to the *ADCY5* mutations' phenotype with unprecedented authority. It had become clear that the label "FDFM" cannot capture the phenotype of this disorder. Hence, the authors of the 2015 piece write, "To encompass the broader phenotype, we suggest changing the name from FDFM to *ADCY5*-related dyskinesia" (2033).

Tying the disease to *ADCY5* mutations appears to have considerably altered not just its clinical range, but also its prevalence: "With 18 families described herein and 3 other published families, it appears this disorder is less rare than initially thought. As additional families are found, the full spectrum of mutations and their relationship to phenotype will be elucidated" (Chen et al. 2015:2033). Indeed, another recent paper found that *ADCY5* should be considered in patients with benign hereditary chorea, even when there is no evidence of facial myokymia at all (Mencacci et al. 2015). In other words, this new disorder falls somewhere between the ideal types of genomically designated recalibration and de novo genomic designation discussed in chapter 1: tying the condition to the *ADCY5* mutation recast a clinical disorder and ended up creating something qualitatively new. Finally, the authors point toward the opportunity to *leverage ADCY5* mutations to understand and perhaps one day treat other forms of dystonia as well: "Increased understanding of the pathogenesis of *ADCY5*-related dyskinesia will facilitate development of pharmacologic treatments for all forms of dystonia that involve the same or related pathways" (Chen et al. 2015:2033). It is plain to see that there are many parallels between *ADCY5* and the more long-standing cases of genomic designation discussed throughout this book.

ADCY5 has already been the subject of several pieces in major news outlets as well. As a piece in the *Atlantic* about Lilly and *ADCY5* put it, "Before, there were isolated pockets of people around the world, dealing with their own problems, alone for all they knew. Now, there's a community" (Yong 2015). The piece notes that, when researchers "started identifying more people with *ADCY5* mutations," they also began to recognize new cases and were able to "finally gauge the full breadth of symptoms caused by those faults." Hence, the condition is now known as "*ADCY5*-related dyskinesia." The piece provides a quotation from one of the leading IDIOM researchers, Ali Torkamani: "[T]his is something we can expect to see more of. . . . You'll see people get an initial diagnosis based on genome sequencing. Then, the patients themselves proactively establish a network and identify additional individuals with the same mutations. If it wasn't for [the Grossmans] and their willingness to take this beyond just a diagnosis, to get the word out and identify new subjects, I don't think we would have been nearly as successful as we have been" (Yong 2015). So far, knowledge about *ADCY5* has not led to any targeted treatments. Still, everyone involved knows that it is likely to be a long journey. For them, the endeavor has already reaped great rewards. An earlier *National Geographic* article about Lilly, her family, and the *ADCY5* mutation put it like this: "Genomics gave them something arguably more important—hope. It turned the nameless, unknowable ailment that had stolen years of sleep from their daughter into something tangible—a condition with a cause that can eventually be addressed" (Yong 2013).

It also gave them a cause and, now, a growing community of *ADCY5* patients and families. ADCY5.org has a board of directors and a scientific advisory board, each composed of researchers and advocates. They describe their group like this: "From citizen scientists to world-renowned Ph.Ds., the ADCY5.org team has expertise in precision medicine, neurology, genetics, genomics, bioinformatics, statistics, clinical research, drug discovery, genetic counseling, neonatal care, biology, chemistry, IOT, wearables, web development, software development, finance, training, non-profit management, and most importantly, patient support."[9] Matt Might of NGLY1.org is even on their scientific advisory board. They host hybrid meetings for families and researchers from around the world, run an international patient registry to help facilitate research and keep *ADCY5* research open and moving.

The many parallels between these newly discovered genomic diagnoses and conditions like 22q11.2DS and Fragile X could hardly be clearer. Above all, a genomic diagnosis ends the long diagnostic odyssey, unites families, and catapults a rare mutation and the people affected by it to the center of a new network of research and care.

At the same time, there is a striking sociological contrast here: the families united by *ADCY5* and *NGLY1* mutations have achieved so much so quickly, despite the fact that their conditions are almost certainly orders of magnitude less common than 22q11.2DS. The same could be said for conditions like *ADNP* syndrome, first reported just a few years ago (Helsmoortel et al. 2014), and the ADNP Kids Research Foundation.[10] When it comes to mobilizing rare mutations, times have changed almost beyond recognition since the 22q11 deletion was first identified in the 1980s. In sum, new movements seeking to mobilize mutations find genomics databases, social media, avid interest in human genetics, and repertoires for mobilizing novel mutations already at their disposal. What surer sign could there be that genomic designation is primed for rapid growth on multiple fronts?

Still, despite these and other gains by researchers and advocates, genomic designation remains a mostly marginal feature of modern medicine. In an era of spiraling health care costs and widespread inequality in access to care, there may be little appetite to embrace a raft of new and confusing genetic disorders. However many syndromes are delineated in the literature, the number that actually matter outside of human genetics may well remain confined to just a couple dozen cases. Indeed, genomic designation could ultimately amount to little more than a biosocial oddity that peters out if and when the genome loses its aura as a privileged site for understanding the origins of abnormality. Either way, the fate of these mutations as social and scientific facts will always be beholden to broader forces. As we are about to see, just such a new force in medical genetics may well scramble the map when it comes to mobilizing these kinds of mutations: widespread, noninvasive prenatal detection.

Noninvasive Prenatal Screening for Mutations

Mutations are being mobilized with unprecedented frequency in *prenatal* settings. Prenatal testing for genomically designated conditions is nothing new. We saw in chapter 2 how it has been perhaps the only consistent form of biomedical intervention on the basis of genetic mutations since the late 1960s and early 1970s. While there was the occasional call to use prenatal testing to materially reduce the population prevalence of conditions like XYY or Down syndrome, such proposals fell on deaf ears in a post-eugenics era. These days, no one of any seriousness is calling for a centralized eugenic program. Nevertheless, the disquieting prospect of prenatal eugenics has loomed larger and larger over the last few years. Why?

A long-hypothesized but only recently proven technique now allows for noninvasive prenatal genetic screening early in pregnancy. This new wave of noninvasive prenatal tests (NIPT) allows genetic screening to be performed on a fetus via a simple blood sample from the mother. (A positive NIPT screen can only be confirmed via a diagnostic test like amniocentesis or chorionic villus sampling [CVS].) Uptake has been rapid, and competition between the companies offering NIPT kits has been fierce. While most of the discussion of NIPT thus far has understandably centered on trisomy 21/Down syndrome,[11] the other mutations included in NIPT kits are mostly clear cases of genomic designation.

This revolution in prenatal testing therefore has huge implications for the kind of genetic disorders discussed in this book. On the severe end, one finds the almost always fatal 13 and 18 chromosome trisomies included on these new screening kits. However, NIPT kits also include highly variable, often mild mutations like the 22q11.2 microdeletion and the XXX and XYY sex chromosome aneuploidies (SCAs). The explosion of the NIPT industry therefore means that many thousands of would-be parents will have to grapple with positive results that are at once undoubtedly serious and deeply uncertain. Would-be parents will also have to navigate the added uncertainty created by a prenatal diagnosis—in many cases there will be little or no information on how the fetus's phenotype has been affected by the mutation in question. To top it all off, they will face a profound dilemma: what to do about the ~10-week-old fetus with a genetic mutation that may or may not lead to serious illness or disability? Finally, noninvasive prenatal genetic screening raises enormous issues for the networks built up around these mutations.

Before we see how, let's take a step back and see how we arrived at this particularly complex juncture in prenatal genetic screening.

A Lonely Clinical Constant

The termination of fetuses with genetic abnormalities is perhaps the most long-standing form of clinical intervention in the history of genomic designation. With the development of techniques for karyotyping fluid extracted through amniocentesis in the mid-1960s and the legalization of abortion in the United States in 1973 (Steele and Breg 1966; see Rapp 2000 for the authoritative social scientific account of amniocentesis), syndromes like Edwards syndrome, Patau syndrome, and sex chromosome aneuploidies like XYY became routine objects of prenatal diagnosis and intervention by the mid-1970s (see Harper 2006:162; Reinhold 1968).

For obvious reasons, reliable figures for termination following a prenatal genetic diagnosis are not available. Figures prior to the 1990s are particularly hard to come by.[12] The best American study comes from Verp et al. (1988), who combined an analysis of all pregnancies in which a fetal chromosomal abnormality was found between January 1977 and June 1986 at Northwestern Memorial Hospital with a systematic review of existing studies available at that time. They begin by saying, "Although when faced with the diagnosis of a fetal abnormality most couples do choose pregnancy termination, we have found that parental behavior is by no means uniform" (613–14). In their combined meta-analysis of studies from the late 1970s and 1980s, covering more than a hundred thousand pregnancies, 96% of 554 of autosomal trisomies detected using amniocentesis were terminated compared to 67.3% of 281 SCAs. In the smaller volume of studies on CVS testing, 109 of 110 (99.1%) autosomal trisomies were terminated as were 15 of 17 (88.2%) SCAs. Verp et al.'s explanation of this discrepancy is openly speculative but, I think, cogent: different patients choose CVS, and there is likely "less reluctance to undergo pregnancy termination in the *first trimester* than in the second trimester. First trimester abortion procedures are simpler, safer, less expensive, and presumably emotionally easier" because parents are not yet attached to the fetus, and they likely have not yet told many friends and relatives about the pregnancy (620; my emphasis). A much more recent study reached similar conclusions.[13] As we will see, the new noninvasive kits can be used to identify fetal mutations as early as *nine weeks* into a pregnancy.

More recent studies make it clear that both testing and termination rates vary considerably according to individual-level characteristics, national and institutional contexts, time period, and the genetic mutation in question (Hamamy and Dahoun 2004; Jeon, Chen, and Goodson 2012; Mansfield, Hopfer, and Marteau 1999; Shaffer, Caughey, and Norton 2006). Rates for trisomy 18, 13, and 21 (i.e., Edwards, Patau, and Down syndrome) are consistently very high. The sex chromosome aneuploidies are more mixed. For example, in a meta-review of eight studies published between 1987 and 2004, Hamamy and Dahoun (2004:61) found that XYY pregnancies where no anomaly was identified on ultrasound were terminated between 20% and 54.5% of the time, while XXX fetuses were terminated at a rate of 17%–70%. In a larger study conducted at UC San Francisco, Shaffer et al. (2006:669) found that of the more than eight hundred prenatally detected cases of chromosomal aneuploidy following amniocentesis or CVS, termination rates for conditions discussed in this book were as follows: trisomy 21 (Down syndrome), 87%; trisomy 18 (Edwards syndrome), 81%; trisomy 13 (Patau syndrome), 90%; X (Turner syndrome), 65%; XXY (Klinefelter syndrome), 70%; XXX, 57%; XYY, 40%.

What then, if we could noninvasively screen for fetal chromosome abnormalities both large and small even earlier in pregnancy?

Extracting Fetal DNA

On October 21, 2011, a press release from Sequenom and articles in major media outlets like the *New York Times* (Pollack 2011) reported the availability of Sequenom's new MaterniT21™ test. The validating findings of a Sequenom-funded study had been published a few days earlier by Palomaki et al. in *Genetics in Medicine*. MaterniT21™ was based on Sequenom's SEQureDX™ technology, which uses genomic sequencing to identify extra material from chromosome 21 in the fetal DNA that is found circulating in a maternal blood sample.[14] In short, this first NIPT kit could screen for trisomy 21 (Down syndrome) in the fetus simply using a normal blood sample from the mother as early as ten weeks into pregnancy. The screen represented a significant advance in prenatal genetic testing because, unlike amniocentesis or CVS, it is noninvasive, carries no risk to the fetus, and can be reliably conducted in the first trimester. As CBS news put it just months before MaterniT21™ launched (Edwards 2011), "If San Diego–based Sequenom could bring a non-invasive prenatal test for Down syndrome to market it would likely be a blockbuster: Every pregnant woman would want to take it." The *New York Times* (Pollack 2011) quoted one expert who described this new wave of screens as "a game-changer" in prenatal testing.

Sequenom's early returns were swift, with 148,500 MaterniT21™ PLUS screens ordered in 2013 alone.[15] Uptake was bolstered by quick success in getting insurance companies and twelve state Medicaid programs to begin reimbursing for MaterniT21™ screening for high-risk pregnancies (see Heger 2014; see also Hollmer 2014). As we will see below, the obvious demand for NIPT meant that rival companies quickly jumped into this burgeoning new field. Ever since, progress has been rapid (see, e.g., Belluck 2014; Bianchi et al. 2014; Heger 2017; Tirrell 2014), and millions of women have undergone NIPT screening.

MaterniT21™ has rightly received extensive attention for its likely impact on prenatal testing and termination rates for Down syndrome. It is entirely understandable that Down syndrome dominates discussions of NIPT. However, all the rival offerings in the NIPT market—Ariosa Diagnostics' Harmony Prenatal Test, Verinata's verifi®, Natera's Panorama, and others—have gone far beyond Down syndrome. They now offer NIPT platforms that screen for many of the mutations that we have dealt with time and again throughout this book.

NIPT for Genomically Designated Conditions

At the at the sixteenth International Conference on Prenatal Diagnosis and Therapy in 2012, Verinata Health reported results demonstrating that they could detect sex chromosome aneuploidies using NIPT. On November 6, 2012, a press release from Verinata announced that they were "expanding the verifi® prenatal test capabilities to include detection of the most common sex chromosome abnormalities. Clinicians will now be able to select the sex chromosomes option on the verifi® test to access this addition." As they explained, XXX, XYY, XXY and monosomy X are actually quite common, and "Subtle neurodevelopmental, language and learning difficulties, as well as anatomical changes result from most forms of sex chromosome aneuploidies"

(Verinata Health 2012c). In another press release on December 3, 2012, Verinata Health, Inc. announced "the launch of [our] expanded verifi® prenatal test to detect the most common fetal sex chromosome abnormalities." This time, they included a supportive blurb from the executive director of the leading SCA advocacy group, KS&A (now known as AXYS), Jim Moore:

Today, SCAs are severely under-diagnosed. In fact, one in 500 babies born in the United States has an X or Y chromosome variation, with less than a quarter of the population diagnosed today. . . . We are pleased to see Verinata Health expand its verifi® prenatal test to include detection of sex chromosome aneuploidies during pregnancy. *Early identification and subsequent intervention could end the "diagnostic odyssey" and lifetime of struggle that so many face as a result of never being diagnosed. KS&A stands ready to serve this community through educational resources and support.* (my emphasis)

Then they invite the reader: "For more information on KS&A, please visit www.genetic.org" (Verinata Health 2012b).

Not to be left out, Sequenom announced that they would also include the major SCAs on all test samples received from February 4, 2013. Sequenom's chief medical officer explained the rationale for their inclusion in the associated press release. He explained that the SCAs "may be recognized at birth, as part of the spectrum of less severe chromosome abnormalities," but they are also often "found in adults, many being incidentally discovered in the course of evaluating patients for infertility or endocrine problems." Using MaterniT21 PLUS to screen for these often mild disorders, he explains, "will *allow the health care provider and patient to discuss the medical issues associated with these conditions as well as to develop both short- and long-term care plans*" (Sequenom 2013a). The history of prenatal genetic testing makes it very clear, however, that selective termination is also a common course of action after the identification of a sex chromosome aneuploidy.

Still, it makes all the sense in the world for advocates to focus on the potential for early intervention. The recently renamed Association for X and Y Variations, or AXYS, is surely right in trying to shape the information given to parents about SCAs. The National Down Syndrome Society, which has dealt with these kinds of issues for decades, took similar steps after MaterniT21 was first released.[16] There can be little doubt that these new tests have the potential to lead to a significant increase in terminations, perhaps seriously impacting the total SCA population moving forward. At the same time, the new wave of noninvasive screens could lead to a huge increase in the number of people actually diagnosed with SCAs like XXX and XYY. This is why AXYS devotes considerable attention and effort to the issue of prenatal testing. As their website puts it, "At AXYS, we consider providing information and support to parents who receive a prenatal diagnosis of an extra X and/or Y chromosome in their fetus to be one of our most important tasks. Our Help Line volunteers and support parents give priority to providing information to expectant parents." They emphasize the fact that "Children with sex chromosome aneuploidy are unlikely to have severe developmental disabilities." In addition, they direct potential parents to one of the multidisciplinary specialist SCA clinics scattered around the United States, as well as the numerous support groups, a YouTube channel, and a series of educational brochures.

The AXYS site's pages on prenatal diagnosis also include a letter from a mother to would-be parents wrestling with a prenatal SCA finding. She empathizes with the "indescribable shock" and the "great apprehension for your child's future," paired with the fact that "you may even have been told that you need to make a decision, quickly, about whether or not to continue with this pregnancy." She tells the reader about her son who, despite some learning difficulties, now lives independently at the age of twenty-five and hopes to complete a college degree, marry, and have a successful career. She explains, "There is enormous variation in how these children and adults present. In perhaps one-third of kids, there are no learning disabilities and few other complications or signs of the syndrome. In the other two-thirds, there can be mild to moderate learning disabilities, but intellectual disability (mental retardation) is rare. Most adults with SCA establish themselves in careers and live independently. Many have satisfying relationships and become parents." Finally, she tells potential parents that "these conditions are not devastating, either to the child or to his or her family," and that if "you know about the condition before birth, you have a great advantage." Knowing about an extra sex chromosome at an early age is key, because kids "with SCA often are remarkably responsive to early intervention therapies. . . . When you are aware of the specific deficits that SCA may cause, you can more quickly qualify your child to receive the services that he or she needs."[17] In other words, many children with SCAs are so mildly affected that they would never be referred for genetic testing in the first place. Prenatal testing therefore provides not only the opportunity for termination, but also the chance for parents to know that their baby has a genetic disorder from the outset and prepare accordingly.

NIPT is not, however, limited to the aneuploidy syndromes. Indeed, the key patent in the field, "Noninvasive Diagnosis of Fetal Aneuploidy by Sequencing," was issued to Stanford University bioengineer and Verinata founder Stephen Quake, and his student Hei-mun Christina Fan. In it, they specifically note deletion syndromes like 5p–, 22q11.2DS and 16p11.2, "and other deletions or imbalances, including those that are presently unknown" (Fan and Quake 2010:6). In other words, the ability to detect genetic mutations both large and small was seen as an important element of NIPT's commercial potential from the very beginning. Commercial research on this front was already attracting significant attention by the end of 2012.[18]

By late 2013, that potential was already being realized. Beginning in October 2013, 22q11.2DS was included in Sequenom's MaterniT21™ PLUS test along with other conditions touched on in earlier chapters like 5p– syndrome and 1p36 Deletion Syndrome (Sequenom 2013b). Most of the other major companies soon followed suit. Given the hundreds of disorders already offered on existing invasive prenatal genetic screening kits—many if not most of them being clear cases of genomic designation—we should expect the range of disorders offered on NIPT kits to continue to grow quite rapidly.

Newly released guidelines, especially from the American College of Medical Genetics and Genomics (ACMG), took the important step of recommending that NIPT screening be offered to *all* pregnant women (Gregg et al. 2016). Until recently, NIPT was only recommended for high-risk pregnancies—either because of advanced maternal age, family history, or some kind of finding on ultrasound or another form of prenatal screening. The guidelines cover the autosomal *and* sex chromosome aneuploidies as well as CNVs. As the ACMG's executive director, Michael S. Watson, put it, "Ultimately, we believe that a patient, with guidance from her provider, should be able to make an informed decision on the current use of prenatal screening options including NIPS and understand the ramifications of a positive, negative or 'no call' result" (quoted in American College of Medical Genetics and Genomics 2016). Similarly, the American Congress of Obstetricians and Gynecologists (ACOG), the Society for Maternal-Fetal Medicine (SMFM), the International Society for Prenatal Diagnosis (ISPD) and the National Society of Genetic Counselors (NSGC) have all recently released similar recommendations. In sum, there is something approaching an expert consensus that every pregnant woman in the United States should be offered noninvasive prenatal genetic screening.

Much will depend on questions of reimbursement and consumer

demand. As Sequenom's CEO put it, "I'm sure there is a huge demand [in the low-risk market], but the question is who is going to pay for it, if and when will they start paying for it, and what price will they pay for it?" (Heger 2014). The UK's National Health Service already provides NIPT for a limited set of conditions. Prenatal testing is now offered to expectant parents in the United States under the terms of the Affordable Care Act and other state-level insurance programs, and NIPT companies are working to ensure their kits are made available through government-funded health care initiatives. Sequenom is continuing its already successful work with government insurance programs to ensure low co-pays, pledging that insured consumers never pay more than a few hundred dollars. Ariosa's test is only $795 and is covered by California's Medi-Cal—a state program providing prenatal health for low-income women (see Agarwal et al. 2013). Meanwhile, private insurance reimbursement will be essential to further market penetration in the United States. The early signs look extremely promising for the NIPT industry. In a recent report, Natera CEO Matt Rabinowitz explained that 105 million Americans were already covered by insurers who reimburse for average-risk NIPT kits (though there have been hurdles in getting tests for microdeletions covered). He was probably only slightly exaggerating when he said, "Ubiquitous coverage is inevitable" (Heger 2017). After all, many genomically designated conditions require very expensive forms of care. For example, although a child with 22q11.2DS may require little medical attention whatsoever, many require hundreds of thousands of dollars' worth of care in infant heart surgeries alone. Sequenom's and Natera's success in ensuring low co-pays for their tests suggests the inevitable: insurance companies will do the math.

NIPT screening is big business. In January 2013, a major genomic sequencing company, Illumina, Inc., acquired Verinata for $350 million, with a commitment to invest a further $100 million to help them expand their reach (Reuters 2013). It is easy to see why there have been several patent lawsuits between the various companies, as well as an acquisition by a biotech behemoth like Illumina. One report cited an investment analyst who said that the noninvasive prenatal genetic testing industry could soon be worth more than a billion dollars a year. The same report also noted that observers expect the advantages of noninvasive screening to increase the annual uptake of prenatal genetic testing "from fewer than 100,000 to as many as 3 million" (Check Hayden 2012).

It took qualitative technological innovation to turn the discovery of fetal DNA in maternal blood in 1997 (Lo et al. 1997) into a biomedical and commercial reality. But now the race is on to make quantitative improvements on several key fronts: price/coverage, accuracy (sensitivity and specificity), how early a fetus can be tested, and especially the conditions covered by the screens.

That last point is key. Competition over the number and range of mutations included in NIPT kits has already led to rapid expansion. In principle, the endpoint is nothing short of whole genome sequencing. In fact, the team that developed the original patent for cfDNA testing published a paper in *Nature* in 2012 demonstrating that this project is already well underway in the realm of basic research (Fan et al. 2012). One lab claimed to have already sequenced an entire fetal genome in 2012 (Kitzman et al. 2012). Meanwhile, a news article in *Nature* explained, "Companies are trying to stand out by expanding the number of conditions their tests check for. Microdeletions and microduplications—genetic defects that can be millions of base pairs long—are seen as the first step, although some companies have designs to sequence the entire fetal genome" (Check Hayden 2014:19). In keeping with that prediction, Sequenom now offers every whole chromosome duplication or deletion, including all of the sex chromosome aneuploidies like XXX and XYY, several microdeletion syndromes like the 22q11.2 and 1p36 Deletion Syndromes, and *any* copy number variant seven megabases or longer (regardless of what we know about it, if anything). These screens are now available beginning nine weeks into pregnancy. This new MaterniT® GENOME test,[19] released in 2015 and refined to improve 22q11.2 microdeletion detection the following year, is clearly not the end of the road for NIPT innovation. Just recently, in fact, Natera announced a new NIPT product that can screen for single-gene mutations, which they hope to bring to the market before long (Heger 2017). In sum, hundreds of pathogenic mutations, many of them indexing genomically designated conditions, could be part of the near future for NIPT.

All the interests appear to be aligned for the continued expansion of noninvasive prenatal genetic screening. In fact, a Coalition for Access to Prenatal Screening (CAPS) has even been formed to advocate for the continued expansion of NIPT. CAPS is no patient advocacy group: it was formed and funded by five major genetic testing companies: Illumina, Counsyl, Progenity, Natera, and LabCorp's Integrated Genetics. With this balance of astroturf advocacy, market competition, and expert acceptance—combined of course with prospective parents' understandable desire to learn about the genomes of their potential children—noninvasive prenatal screening for mutations is fast becoming a routine part of pregnancy. What are the implications of this revolution in prenatal testing for genetic disorders like the ones discussed in this book?

Uncertain Dilemmas and a New Back Door to Eugenics?

Almost as soon as amniocentesis was developed in the mid-1960s, there were those who saw it as an important opportunity for society.[20] Thus we saw Bentley Glass speculate in his 1970 presidential address to the American Academy of Arts and Sciences (1971:28) that humanity might embrace the power of scientific progress and use "perfected techniques of determining chromosome abnormalities in the developing fetus to rid us of the several percentages of all births that today represent uncontrollable defects such as mongolism (Down's syndrome) and sex deviants such as the XYY type." Thankfully, this vision of a new prenatal eugenics has remained a fringe position in the field.

And yet, disability rights advocates, critical scholars of science and medicine, and right-wing ideologues alike have pointed toward the emergence of a new prenatal eugenics. Abby Lippman even argued that it is "disingenuous" to avoid discussions of eugenics when it comes to prenatal genetic testing (1991a:24–25). After all, if prenatal genetic testing is based on ideas about which forms of inheritance are compatible with a life worth living, and if it has population-level effects, why not call it a new eugenics? Perhaps, some argue, it is eugenics through and through, whether those effects on our "gene pool" are driven by coercive policy or merely the aggregate outcome of thousands of individuals making decisions based on current thinking about genetics and disability. (For recent, thoughtful engagements with this debate, see, e.g., Comfort 2013; Entine 2013; H. Rose 2007.) As Nathanial Comfort has forcefully argued (2014:xii), there is no escaping eugenics when we apply the science of heredity to human health: "The promises of genetic medicine *are* the promises of eugenics." These are important definitional issues, but not ones I can address. What I do want to argue, rather, is that paying attention to genomic designation allows us to see how noninvasive prenatal genetic screening could have far-reaching population-level effects, and soon.

Coverage of MaterniT21™'s launch immediately turned toward the impact on the Down syndrome population (e.g., Pollack 2011). These concerns built upon issues that Down syndrome advocates have been facing for decades—hence their immediate response to the rollout of NIPT. It is widely recognized that prenatal testing has already had a substantial impact on Down syndrome populations: even as rising maternal age should have led to a huge increase in Down syndrome births, all else being equal, termination rates following a positive test have prevented this from happening in most OECD countries.[21] A number of scholarly studies have therefore examined the eugenic implications of prenatal testing for Down syndrome (e.g., Dixon 2008; Epstein 2002; Harmon 2007b; Kerr, Cunningham-Burley, and Amos 1998; Lippman 1994; McCabe and McCabe 2011; Shakespeare 1998; Skotko 2009). Meanwhile, commentators on the right have made not entirely dissimilar arguments, though with a strikingly different orientation and tone (for perhaps the most thoughtful, remarkably, see Carlson 2012).

Down syndrome, however, is only the tip of the iceberg. Most of the conditions included on the major NIPT kits are precisely the same conditions discussed in this book. Some are always severe, like trisomy 13/Patau syndrome, and others, like 22q11.2DS and XYY syndrome, are highly variable or often very mild. Making matters even more complicated, almost all of these conditions' clinical profiles are undoubtedly shaped by a systemic ascertainment bias: as we have seen throughout this book, genetic testing is still mostly reserved for patients with congenital abnormalities or developmental and/or intellectual deficits. To top it all off, each condition brings its own set of very real concerns and deep uncertainties.

Thousands upon thousands of would-be parents are going to be confronted with positive screening results for these genomically designated conditions. After all, these conditions are *not* rare at all in cumulative terms. The history outlined above gives us reason to think that termination rates will be high, even for mild genetic conditions like XXX and XYY. What's more, termination rates will also be highly socially patterned by socioeconomic status, country or region, religiosity, and many other factors. In short, we need to think seriously about genomic designation in order to make sense of the coming flood of NIPT findings.

Parents facing reproductive dilemmas need skilled genetic counseling and accurate information about the mutations discovered via NIPT. Given the paucity of both—almost all our knowledge about these mutations is ridden with ascertainment bias, and there is already an acute shortage of qualified genetic counselors—meeting those needs will require years of investment, training, and research. As it stands, rapidly growing numbers of parents every year will be told, just months into a pregnancy, that their fetus has a genetic disorder that may or may not cause serious developmental and medical problems. This will of course be enormously trying for expectant parents. At the same time, it may have profound implications for the way we deal with abnormality and developmental difference as a society. Finding abnormal genomes is becoming relatively easy. Helping people understand and make decisions based on prenatal genetic testing results with uncertain implications, by contrast, represents a largely overlooked challenge.

There are of course compelling, ethically sound reasons to offer prenatal genetic testing to expectant mothers: above all, the right to make informed reproductive decisions and the ability to prepare for the care of a child with a genetic disorder. Still, it is imperative that we avoid the trap of allowing discussions about NIPT to be subsumed by broader debates about abortion. That might not be easy, especially when it compels us to recognize an important sliver of truth in a common anti-choice argument. Rick Santorum, who has a child with trisomy 18/Edwards syndrome, took up the prenatal testing provision in the Affordable Care Act during the 2012 presidential election campaign. To him, that provision was included "because free prenatal testing ends up in more abortions and, therefore, less care that has to be done, because we cull the ranks of the disabled in our society" (quoted in Rafferty and Montanaro 2012). It should go without saying that the attribution of eugenic *intention* in this particular piece of right-wing electioneering was wholly misplaced (or contrived).

But the liberal response, perhaps best expressed by esteemed University of Chicago public health professor Harold Pollack (2012), has its blind spots as well. Pollack has a brother-in-law with Fragile X. To him, Santorum's comments were "indescribably insulting," and "only made uglier by their utter lack of foundation. . . . The proliferation of genetic diagnostic technologies coincides with great progress in public acceptance and support for people with disabilities." Pollack is undoubtedly correct that the authors of the Affordable Care Act had no desire to "cull the ranks" of the disabled. He is also right when he writes, "Certainly liberals are willing to spend more money on disability services." Pollack is also correct about today's unprecedented support for people with disabilities, much of it due to "liberal" policy-making.

However, even a stopped clock is right twice a day, and in this case Santorum and his fellow travelers might actually be on to something. Why? Despite the emphasis on anticipatory care following a positive NIPT result, there is a strong empirical basis to the claim that many fetuses prenatally diagnosed with genetic disorders, even mild ones, will be terminated. Even in the complete absence of any centralized plan, the aggregate effect of parents exercising the right to know about and act on genetic mutations detected using NIPT may have population-level effects. Twenty-first-century eugenics, if it happens at all, is likely to be the secondary effect of millions of deeply personal decisions.

This is why we need to chart a productive middle path between the existing discussions of prenatal testing for conditions like Down syndrome or cystic fibrosis and bioethical debates about "designer babies." As Steinbock put it in the *Lancet* (2008:1295), "Genetic enhancement is, for the present, science fiction." Even with the development of CRISPR system technologies, we will not be designing babies anytime soon. If genetics is going to change the population in the foreseeable future, it will not be through making smarter, stronger, more attractive children, but through many thousands of parents making the hard choice to terminate pregnancies when some kind of genetic mutation is identified cheaply, easily, and early.

The new, noninvasive prenatal genetic screening kits therefore bring a profound ethical question to the fore—one that does not conform to our usual binary of "pro-life" or "pro-choice." The potential scope and scale of NIPT challenges those of us who believe in the rights of women and parents to make informed reproductive decisions to consider a near future where legitimate individual decisions have significant eugenic effects at the population level. It is therefore worth asking whether, borrowing from Troy Duster ([1990] 2003), this new wave of prenatal genetic screening might combine with genomic designation to create a new "back door" to eugenics.

Conclusion: A New Challenge for Advocates

Researchers, caregivers, and advocates for genomically designated conditions will inevitably be dragged along by powerful currents that they cannot truly control. A lot depends on when, where, and how we test for mutations. Who gets tested in the first place and what for? How easy is it to detect genetic mutations? Does it become routine to screen for them? And at what point in development—when problems manifest or early in pregnancy? More broadly, how do we think about disability and difference? What makes a life worth living, and what steps are we willing to take to help make a life affected by a deleterious mutation worth living? How might NIPT change that calculus?

I offer these questions, in part, to dispel a teleological interpretation of my account of genomic designation. For while it is certainly true that advocates have made important gains, their successes may ultimately prove to be fragile. Even if genetic mutations continue to matter in a way that they did not in the 1960s and 1970s, we cannot be certain of the ends toward which they will be mobilized. The XYY-criminality nexus examined in chapter 3 should not be treated as just a historical oddity: the history of genetics and human difference is a varied and often disquieting story. Furthermore, this book has been almost entirely limited to highly developed, Western countries with their (at least partly) liberal political regimes. But genetic testing is starting to gain significant traction elsewhere, notably in China, where Sequenom immediately launched the first version of MaterniT21™.

Noninvasive prenatal genetic screening shows how the future for genomic designation will depend on developments in everything from the biotech industry to prevailing norms for managing abnormal populations. It could mean that many more young children who have these mutations will actually receive the relevant genetic diagnosis, dramatically increasing the number of patients and families in groups like the International 22q11.2 Foundation and the broader 22q movement. It could also mean that far fewer people with these mutations are born, thereby reducing the population prevalence of the genetic disorders that these patient groups and movements represent. Or, it could very well mean both. In other words, the burgeoning NIPT industry has the potential to dramatically increase ascertainment *and* lower the number of people born with these mutations. Furthermore, it may well change the socioeconomic, geographic, religious, and cultural makeup of the populations with genetic disorders like 22q11.2DS and XYY syndrome. A lot will depend on the capacity of experts and advocates to shape how noninvasive prenatal screening is used. The networks built up around mutations like the 22q11.2 microdeletion may be able to mitigate the potential loss of population and potentially even benefit from increased ascertainment and early engagement with the diagnosed and their families. At the same time, the explosion of noninvasive prenatal screening is yet another example of the way broader trends in genetics, medicine, and society will always shape the future for genomic designation.

Conclusion

Genomic designation has been a constant in human genetics for more than half a century now. Ever since genetic mutations became visible under the microscope, they have been used to recalibrate existing diagnoses, rework relations between disorders, and delineate entirely new conditions that could never have been discerned on the basis of what the populations in question are actually like. The turn to high-throughput sequencing and twenty-first-century clinical genomics has only pushed this trend forward. Whether it was seeing extra X or eighteenth chromosomes in 1959 or finding a point mutation in the *MTOR* gene just a couple of years ago, geneticists have been quick to think of newly observed mutations as novel clinical entities. In other cases, findings from genetic tests have served to reshape long-standing disease categories, be it XXY and Klinefelter syndrome in 1959 or the 7q11.2 microdeletion and Williams syndrome more recently. As we saw, research on the 22q11.2 microdeletion actually led to the "lumping" together of several older syndromes and the creation of a completely new, bewilderingly variable medical condition. In short, finding a new mutation can reshape medical classification in many different ways.

This much is clear: genetic mutations have come to mean far more than the "gene-for" model can accommodate. They have become the basis for a new form of human classification. Knowledge about a genetic mutation can be even more powerful when it does *not* line up with existing disease categories. Even when a mutation does not cause a phenotype that is consistent or specific enough for clinical diagnosis, people may still come to see it as a new disease entity.

Today, knowing that someone has a 22q11.2 microdeletion, a CGG repeat expansion on his *FMR1* gene, or an extra Y chromosome can reshape the way we understand and approach that person, sometimes quite radically. They have given rise to support groups, foundations, specialist clinics and literatures, and a series of alliances spanning experts from a wide array of biomedical fields, caregivers, various stakeholders, advocates, and, last but not least, patients and their families.

And yet, we saw that it was several decades before significant numbers of these other actors joined medical geneticists in thinking about mutations as the best way to carve up illness and difference. The mutations at the core of this book have come a long way as facts over the last few decades. They had to be mobilized in order to create what Ian Hacking would call new kinds of people.

Our story began in 1959, when genomic designation emerged quite rapidly in the new field of cytogenetics. However, back then, there was just not all that much one could do with these mutations and the categories of people they indexed. They were facts in the domain of human genetics, but they were not really medical facts, psychological facts, or social facts.

Fast forwarding a few decades, our journey culminated with a discussion of the way these mutations have come to really matter to growing numbers of people. Actors have worked to forge the networks of research, collaboration, and collective action that can turn a genetic mutation like the 22q11.2 microdeletion into an object of knowledge that can truly reshape people's lives. Some of those same mutations are being leveraged as biological models for common conditions with which they overlap, like obesity, autism, schizophrenia, and ADHD. Knowing about these mutations can now profoundly impact the way parents, doctors, and patients think about and treat illness, and even reshape the boundaries between the normal and the pathological.

Drawing on the framework of "reiterated fact-making," we saw how some mutations have been transformed from obscure objects of esoteric genetics research into powerful markers of human difference. A huge part of this story concerns a series of broader developments: deinstitutionalization and the emergence of contemporary patient advocacy created the historical conditions and repertoires of collective action that have served conditions like 22q11.2DS so well; the looping processes at work in conditions like autism created new opportunities for genetic disorders like Fragile X; advances in genetic testing and communications technologies have made it far easier to detect genetic mutations and to build new communities around them; changes in related fields like genetic counseling and clinical psychology, along with a broader turn to "personalized medicine," have allowed the knowledge that a person has a particular genetic mutation to shape practice in fields that have been historically disinterested or even hostile toward genetics; the way the public imagination has fastened onto the genome as perhaps *the* site for understanding human disease and difference. All these and more clearly shape the way people respond to a diagnosis that ties a patient's fate to a genetic mutation.

But creating robust new kinds of people out of syndromes like XXX or 5p– also took concerted work by experts and advocates laboring under the banner of a particular mutation and the population that has it. They had to creatively adapt existing repertoires of patient advocacy. They had to forge productive points of interface with clinical medicine and leverage the genetic specificity of their condition to attract biomedical research. In sum, they have to work within vast fields like pediatric medicine, psychiatry, and special education, even as they strive to redirect resources and reshape practice in the name of a genomically designated condition and its patients. Theirs is in many ways a perfect example of the "duality" of structure and agency (Sewell 1992): when advocates are most successful at mobilizing mutations, it is because they have found ways to reroute existing resources and rework prevailing conceptual schemas for dealing with human difference. In sum, we have seen how new combinations of actors, repertoires of mobilization, and conditions of possibility can make and remake genetic mutations as powerful facts. Through these hybrid forms of research and collective action, the categories born of genomic designation are becoming what Ian Hacking might call a new kind of human kind.

Finally, genomic designation seems poised to become a much more widespread, salient feature of contemporary medicine. Researchers are identifying new mutations all the time as genetic testing becomes more affordable, available, and accurate. As a result, new genomically designated conditions are being reported week in and week out. When a clinical genetics team finds a mutation in a patient, they now have publicly available databases to help them figure out if it is pathogenic, if there are other affected patients out there, and if it means they have an established genetic disorder. Meanwhile, parents can draw upon established repertoires of patient advocacy and use social media to connect with other families and kick-start the laborious process of mobilizing a rare mutation. New conditions like *NGLY1* and *ADCY5* have made progress in just the last few years that once would have taken decades.

At the same time, the new noninvasive prenatal landscape may shift the ground beneath advocates' feet. The mutations discussed in this book are increasingly likely to be discovered just a couple of months into pregnancy, leaving would-be parents with deeply vexed decisions to make. Even generally mild disorders like the XXX and XYY syndromes, as well as uncertain ones like 22q11.2DS, were quickly added to these new prenatal screens. For the companies making and marketing these tests, the goals is clear: offer as many mutations as possible early in pregnancy while still ensuring accuracy and affordability. We may soon have noninvasive prenatal genetic screens that cover hundreds or even thousands of mutations. Part of the rationale for offering these tests is preparation and early intervention. But the bigger, if largely unspoken rationale is the identification and selective termination of fetuses with genetic disorders. What will happen if genomically designated conditions are widely seen as both avoidable and worth avoiding? The rapid uptake of NIPT has profound implications for genomically designated conditions like 22q11.2DS: ascertainment may skyrocket, swelling the ranks of advocacy organizations, even as their populations decrease and undergo demographic change.

Clearly then, the fate of these genomically designated conditions is profoundly uncertain. It depends on forces beyond the control of geneticists and patient advocates alike. Much will depend on who has access to genetic testing, not to mention the sorts of resources it takes to truly enact a diagnosis like Fragile X or 22q11.2DS. That, in turn, means genomic designation will remain beholden to our strained and inequitable educational, research, and health care systems.

Open Futures for Genomic Designation

This book has offered a sociological account of the way mutations can accrue clinical and social power, not an evaluation of the risks and rewards, harms and benefits, that come with genomic designation. Indeed, the contrast between XYY as the "criminal chromosome" from the 1960s and 1970s and its newfound status as a mild developmental disorder today makes it plain to see that the implications of genomic designation can vary wildly, even when it comes to the same mutation. The pertinent questions for policy and medical ethics are therefore not centrally about genomic designation per se, but about what is done with it. That is no simple question. Far more research is needed before we can even begin to thoroughly answer such questions.

Perhaps the most crucial issue, which I have only just begun to address, is the potential for iatrogenic harm, self-fulfilling prophecies, and many other possible pitfalls that genomic designation may create for patients. That is quite intentional. Unfortunately, there is just not enough evidence to make such an evaluation. We lack the kind of rigorous, unbiased knowledge about most genetic disorders that would allow us to get a sense of the range and complexity of their phenotypes, never mind the sort of evidence that would allow us to assess the effects of receiving the relevant genetic diagnosis on people's health care and well-being. It is easy to imagine some of the items that might appear on either side of the ledger. On the one hand, we might be rightly wary of the way genomic designation can bias expectations and create self-fulfilling prophecies, lead to overtreatment and anxiety, or represent a new back door to eugenics. On the other, we might look forward to the day when genetic specificity leads to truly targeted drugs and treatment regimes, more accurate prospect horizons, and empowered communities united by genetic kinship. The only certainty is that we need much more research on the many different ways in which knowledge about mutations is actually being used.

At the same time, genomic designation could exacerbate existing inequalities. It takes resources just to get access to genetic testing, never mind tap into the myriad services that are recommended for many genetic disorders. We even saw how a mutation can recast a child as developmentally impaired in some way, even when that impairment falls well below our usual thresholds of clinical significance. Will parents with a mean IQ of 115 argue that their child's score of 85 is the symptom of a genetic disorder? What steps might they be willing to take? Will accommodations be made on that basis? Middle- and upper-class parents have long sought, understandably, to give their children every possible advantage in life. Genetics may be poised to give parents whose kids seem fine, but not where they *should* be, a sort of biomedical ammunition to make claims on strained early intervention, special education, and other sorts of services. More generally, people with access to genetic testing and sufficient economic, social, and cultural capital may end up garnering educational and medical resources that would not otherwise be made available for their children. Finally, as prenatal testing continues its uneven expansion, we face the disquieting prospect of a rising correlation between socioeconomic disadvantage and a host of genetic disorders.

The proliferation of genetic testing is not a worldwide phenomenon. Hence this book focused on the United States, with the occasional foray into Canada and Western Europe. But mutations like the ones discussed in this book are increasingly being tested for and acted upon in China, India, and many other non-Western countries. We need to pay close attention to the way mutations are mobilized over the coming years in many different places, not least the world's most populous regions. Genomic designation will inevitably be shaped by historical context, local health care systems, ideas about genetics and disability, and many other factors besides. Countries like China and Singapore, for example, which have neither our liberal ideology nor our disastrous experience with early twentieth-century eugenics, are investing huge amounts of resources in genomics research. There is a lot of work left to do—be it among underserved populations in the United States or people in the Global South—before we can understand genomic designation's true impact moving forward.

This book also focused largely on the genomic designation of childhood developmental difference. However, conditions like *ADCY5*, XYY, Prader-Willi syndrome, 22q11.2DS, and Williams syndrome show how genomic designation has the capacity to inform understanding of and treatment in areas ranging from cardiology and endocrinology to obesity studies and muscle disorders. Meanwhile, there is reason to believe that the genomic designation of tumors and metabolic disorders will yield direct therapeutic benefits much sooner than it will for developmental disorders. If we want to understand how genetics can reshape medical classification more broadly, we will need to look at these and many other sorts of maladies.

Things are moving quickly for genetic medicine in general and genomic designation in particular. We cannot therefore assume that all of the important issues have already come into view. Nor should we assume that the models of collaborative research and advocacy that I have paid so much attention to are the final chapter in the history of mobilizing mutations. The dynamics of "biocapital" (Rose 2007a; Sunder Rajan, 2006) should not be underestimated. There is an enormous amount of money to be made in genomic testing, pharmaceutical development, and other industries with a vested interest in the idea that mutations are an essential part of understanding what makes us sick or different.

Indeed, there is no reason why genomic designation must remain limited to medicalized populations (see Shostak, Conrad, and Horwitz 2008 on the path-dependent relationship between genetics and medicalization). We just saw how knowledge about a mutation like the 16p11.2 and 22q11.2 microdeletions or the Fragile X premutation can turn subclinical traits into features of a genetic condition, remaking the boundary between the normal and the pathological in the process. Meanwhile, the popularity of direct-to-consumer genetic testing is suggestive of the potential for genomic designation to give rise to new categories of identity formation and self-practice that are only indirectly connected to issues of medicine and developmental disability (Nelson 2008; Abu El-Haj 2007). Indeed, this has already started to happen in genetic ancestry testing with the designation of various haplogroups and "subclades" (haplotype subgroups), like the various R1b groups,[1] and the emergence of various Yahoo! groups and discussion boards where lay experts seek to make sense of their ancestral genomic inheritance.[2] Of course, these sorts of groups are less reliant on credentialed scientific experts, peer review, and other checks on scientific credibility. The same could have been said for direct-to-consumer genetic testing for health risks before the FDA stepped in to regulate it in 2014—regulations that have already been watered down in the shift from President Obama's FDA to President Trump's (see US Food and Drug Administration 2017).

It is impossible to say where all this will lead. But if people can find meaning in the alignment of the planets at the moment they were born, who can say what others might find when they begin to interpret their genomes? In other words, if astrology has convinced millions of people that they are a certain type of person, who is to say that poorly understood changes in what many a scientist has called the "book of life" could not do the same? With money to be made from genomic testing and social media platforms there to help us to connect with other people who bear a particular mutation or variant, genomic designation could be turned toward all sorts of newfangled group building and identity formation.

Finally, genomic designation could very well remain confined to a fairly small corner of medicine, or perhaps even fade back into irrelevance. Either way, it will be worth tracing what Alondra Nelson (2016) might call, via Arjun Appadurai (1988), the "social lives" of the DNA mutations discussed in this book.

Parting Thoughts

It is time to start taking genomic designation seriously. The ever-growing capacity to identify mutations and our tendency to treat knowledge about the genome as indicating something essential to the self makes this plain to see. Ian Hacking has pointed out that, despite both humanist and scientific arguments to the contrary, "People can hardly avoid thinking of their genetic inheritance as part of what constitutes them, as part of who they are, as their essence" (2006a:92). As he put it (88), "Knowledge of genetic 'identities' will forge social ones, creating new communities of shared recognition based on partial science. That is not intrinsically bad, but it is still a phenomenon that can be grossly abused." Such a warning takes on even greater significance with genomic designation, especially as the number and range of human kinds tied to genetic mutations continues to grow. We need to start paying attention to the way that people mobilize mutations, not just as proxies or genes for other things, but as essential referents of new categories of human difference.

Hacking was right to point out that "biologizing" a human kind changes it in important ways. What he and other scholars of science and medicine have failed to account for, however, is the way that findings from genetics can do far more than just change the way we think about established categories. Genomic designation does not just recast or reduce human traits and maladies, nor does it merely essentialize, stigmatize, or destigmatize abnormal persons. Rather than simply shaping our understanding of existing categories of human difference along genetic lines, genomic designation actually produces new categories of persons.

That does not, however, mean that geneticists and allied biomedical experts attain unquestioned authority over the way we understand difference and abnormality. On the contrary, what it means to have a genomically designated condition—both in terms of its clinical profile and the forms of practice it gives rise to—is decisively shaped by the work of many different sorts of credentialed and lay experts. It takes a village to turn a genetic mutation into a rich category of human difference. Given the right alliances and the right forms of mobilization, mutations can give rise to new and dynamic categories that profoundly shape the experience of illness and difference. By tracing these shifting alliances, we have seen how mutations can be used to create new kinds of people in the full sense of the term.

To that end, I hope others will devote more sustained attention to the perspectives of people with these genetic mutations themselves. My greatest regret about this book is the relative absence of patient voices or accounts of their day-in-day-out experiences. For practical and IRB-related reasons, I was not able to conduct detailed ethnographic work with patients in specialist clinics, psychologists' offices, schools, summer camps, homes, or any of the other sites where knowledge about mutations is brought to bear. This leaves an opening for a micro-sociological study of the way conditions like Fragile X, 22q11.2DS, and XYY syndrome are looping and shaping people's lives.

Affixing kinds of people to genetic mutations forecloses certain processes of looping, but it also enables others. It is quite clear who can be diagnosed with a genomically designated condition, yet anything but clear who will be tested and what will be done with the knowledge that they have a particular genetic mutation. Thinking through reiterated fact-making, we have seen how the very same object of knowledge—a genetic mutation—can take many different forms: an esoteric finding in a human genetics journal, a "syndrome" in the literature, or a robust kind of person underwritten by an extensive network of research and practice.

After decades of building up knowledge, resources, and alliances, groups dedicated to people with genomically designated conditions have made enormous inroads. However, we also saw that they did so under conditions not of their own choosing or their own making. The power of conditions like Fragile X and 22q11.2 Deletion Syndrome will always depend on much broader technoscientific trends and social forces. Whatever the future holds, we should pay close attention to the myriad ways in which knowledge about genetic mutations can reshape what it means to be ill, different, and ultimately, human.

Notes

INTRODUCTION

1. A host of work in the social studies of science has convincingly argued that the "social" is not a distinct or coherent dimension of reality, and one cannot provide a "social explanation" of science or anything else (see esp. Latour 1993, 1999, 2007; Callon 1995). All a sociologist can do, from this perspective, is trace more or less stable sets of relations among many different sorts of objects.

2. Haydu (1998) explains, "There must be *some* correspondence between the observer's conception of a recurring problem and the social actors' experiences of confronting common obstacles and devising ways to surmount them" (355). Consider Haydu's casing of US industrial-relations regimes: "Making 1900 the cutoff thus provides for more 'controlled' comparisons between periods and trains attention on what both observers today and social actors in 1900 would recognize as common dilemmas of management" (361). This encapsulates why reiterated problem-solving needs to be amended for our purposes.

3. After all, we do not want to treat the work of advocates and genetic counselors as "exogenous," as Haydu frames state intervention in the formulation of a new regime of labor relations in the 1930s (1998:364).

4. Fleck briefly discusses "'mutations' in thought style" (1981:26), even citing the shift to relativity theory in modern physics (one of Kuhn's "revolutions"). Hence, he recognized that "the modern concept of disease entity, for example, is an outcome of [a historical development] and by no means the only logical possibility" (21) decades before

Foucault's groundbreaking articulation of much the same point (1973; see chap. 1).

5. In a narrow sense, genomic designation upends the sequence of delineating a disease entity—after all, it often begins with the isolation of a medical condition according to a biomarker. However, we will see how genomically designated conditions also require long processes of cooperative research spanning lay and expert knowledge before they can function as powerful categories of difference.

6. To make this point, Fleck describes a bacteriological examination (1981:113–15). He contrasts the lab expert's technical report—itself an idealization—with the simplified report on the microscopically visible rods indicating "diphtheria bacilli" that would be given to a general practitioner. As Fleck puts it, "This finding is specially written to suit the general practitioner, but it does not represent the knowledge of the expert. It is vivid, simplified, and apodictic." Eventually, the fact becomes even more solidified as we move to the sphere of the "generally educated," such that the "mother of the child whose throat swab had been examined is simply informed: 'Your child has diphtheria.'" The mother's understanding of diphtheria, he insisted, also affects the bacteriologist's expertise: popular knowledge stabilizes a fact and "reacts in turn upon the expert" (113).

7. Reiterated fact-making therefore provides for a *comparative* study of, as Callon put it (1995:54), the way an actant's "identity depends on the state of the network and the translations under way, that is, on the history in which they are participating."

8. For example, Keith Wailoo adopts something like a reiterated fact-making approach in his brilliant book on sickle-cell disease (2001), especially in his analysis of the clinical and social conditions of the sickle-cell's visibility and the way it has been shaped and reshaped by American culture and politics over several decades. Charles Rosenberg's work (1966, 2009) on successive cholera epidemics in the United States is another outstanding example.

9. Granted, there may have been fewer, since medical advances have, for example, allowed a significant number of 22q11.2DS patients with infant heart malformations to survive. Meanwhile, an increase in average parental age will have increased genomically designated populations, and the development of prenatal genetic testing will have had the opposite effect.

10. Hacking abandoned the term *human kind* on the basis of "a simple deduction: there is no such thing as a natural kind [the concept had become untenable in analytic philosophy] . . . a fortiori, there is no such thing as a human kind" (Hacking 2007:n17). Hence the turn to the less metaphysically loaded "kind of person."

11. With this in mind, let's sidestep Latour's objection that it is invalid to say that a person, like Ramses II, suffered from a condition, like tuberculosis, in an era prior to development of the sociotechnical capacity to diagnose

it. Latour (2000:250; see also 1999) was adamant when it came to things like Koch's bacillus (the bacteria that causes tuberculosis) or, by extension, genetic mutations: "Those types of facts cannot escape their network of production." There have undoubtedly been millions of people over the course of human history who would have been diagnosable with conditions like 22q11.2DS or XYY syndrome were they alive today. If we found a preserved person or tissue sample, we could even "extend the network" by testing them for various mutations. Hence, we could at least say that a person did have a 22q11.2 microdeletion or an extra Y chromosome. (Whether Latour is right that they had the 22q11.2 microdeletion *all along*, but only *after*" [2000:266; emphasis in original] we tested their long-deceased corpse is above my pay grade.)

12. This might seem like a surprising claim, but advances in medical care can significantly increase the size of a population (e.g., with 22q11.2DS, given the high frequency of infant heart malformations), while national and institutional variation in prenatal testing and selective termination rates for genetic disorders ensure that the incidence of certain genetic mutations varies considerably according to time and place.

CHAPTER ONE

1. By *genomic* I do not mean observations particular to new genomics technologies, such as high-throughput sequencing, but observations of the genetic material contained overwhelmingly in our chromosomes that constitutes the human genome. Genomic designation could and did occur through karyotype analysis (below).

2. For example, Miller et al. (2005) found that the identification of single-gene mutations associated with Huntington's disease, cystic fibrosis, and tuberous sclerosis had very different nosological implications in each case, sometimes being used to "rule in" or "rule out" borderline cases of a diagnosis and sometimes being subordinated to clinical judgment. More recently, Timmermans and Buchbinder (2010, 2012) found that newborn testing for rare genetic disorders produced a class of "patients in waiting" who had the marker but not the characteristic symptoms. As a result, experts were compelled to engage in ontological "bridging work" in order to reconcile this unexpected lack of alignment between biomarker and the symptomatology of the medical condition it was supposed to indicate. Bourret, Keating, and Cambrosio (2011) have examined how knowledge about genomic markers is produced through "clinical collectives" and can impact classification and judgment in oncology. Finally, as I discuss in in chapter 7, Rabeharisoa and Bourret (2009) discuss the "bioclinical collectives" that "simultaneously produc[e] the clinical relevance *and* the biological significance of mutations" (693) for each patient at each local site.

3. Earlier descriptions of what was probably the same phenotype were made by Jean Etienne-Dominique Esquirol in 1838 and Edouard Séguin in 1846 (see Roubertoux and Kerdelhué 2006), but these lacked the diagnostic specificity, influence, and longevity of Down's work.

4. However, researchers immediately began to search for other aberrations related to chromosome 21 (e.g., partial duplication or translocation) that could account for the phenotype. Separate studies were conducted on patients with classic mongolism and older mothers vs. those with a somewhat different profile and young mothers, showing that these corresponded to full chromosome 21 trisomy and chromosome 21 translocations, respectively (see Harper 2006:68).

5. While it has been claimed that trisomy 13 is coextensive with a clinical phenotype first described by Danish physician Thomas Bartholin in 1657 (see Warburg and Mikkelsen 1963 for what I believe is the first claim to this effect) and described clinically by Warburg (1960), it is quite clear that Patau et al.'s discovery did lead to the delineation of a new medical condition.

6. While the deletion can range from 185,000 to 9 million base pairs, there is little observed correlation between the deletion size and the severity of the phenotype as long the *SHANK3* gene is missing (Phelan and McDermid 2012).

7. See "Phelan-McDermid Syndrome Foundation History," at https://web .archive.org/web/20130515171149/http://22q13.org/j15/index.php?option= com_content&view=article&id=97&Itemid=113.

8. See "What Is Phelan-McDermid Syndrome?," at https://www.pmsf.org/ about_pms/.

9. Assendelft 2017. See also Agency for Persons with Disabilities, "Offering Waiver Enrollment to People with Phelan-McDermid Syndrome," at http://apd.myflorida.com/docs/PhelanFlyer2016.pdf.

10. Some of these sources are no longer available from PMSF. However, their website contains a wealth of updated material on the features and medical issues associated with PMS. See, for example, https://www.pmsf.org/about _pms/, https://www.pmsf.org/about_pms/medical-issues/, and https://www .pmsf.org/about_pms/features-of-pms_gb/.

11. This has in fact been an issue since the outset of the mongolism/trisomy 21 association. While Lejeune, Gautier, and Turpin published the first paper on the association in 1959, we will see in chapter 2 that several other teams were on the verge of reporting the same finding. A much larger study in Edinburgh by Jacobs, Court Brown, et al.(1959) examined the chromosomes of around forty patients diagnosed with mongolism, but found six who had the normal chromosome complement of forty-six. Jacobs claimed (more than forty years later) that when they had the leading British expert on mongolism, Lionel Penrose, come up from London, he rediagnosed the patients in precise accordance with the trisomy theory of

Down syndrome without prior knowledge of their karyotypes. Similarly, Warkany (1960:415) showed how it was almost immediately employed in research environments to help adjudicate clinically contested cases. Nevertheless, especially in postnatal cases, the observation of trisomy or translocation 21 is often used to *confirm* a clinical diagnosis that can be made on the basis of phenotypic criteria (e.g., Devlin and Morrison 2004).

12. This does not mean that every patient has an *identical* genetic mutation. For example, chromosomal deletions and duplications can vary in size, and single-gene variants can disrupt the production of a particular protein even if the precise site or mechanism of mutation is different. The point is that they are considered to be the same mutation, and that continuity is calibrated and maintained across different genetic testing platforms. Crucially, this means that "people with mutation x" picks out a consistent population.

13. See *OMIM: Online Mendelian Inheritance in Man*, "Smith-Kingsmore Syndrome," at https://www.omim.org/entry/616638; see also Lee et al. 2012.

14. Surprisingly, an award-winning 2007 *New York Times* article used 16p11.2 as its headline case of "genetic kinship," even though 22q13 was also discussed in the article (Harmon 2007a).

15. The deletion is usually around three million base pairs long, and, although deletion size can vary considerably, existing studies have found no meaningful correlation between deletion size or break points and phenotypic severity or range (Philip and Bassett 2011; McDonald-McGinn et al. 2001). There is some debate about the status of mutations on the key gene TBX1.

16. Although one single-paragraph report in the supplemental pages of the *American Journal of Human Genetics* (Goldberg et al. 1985:A54) noted clinical overlap between VCFS and DiGeorge syndrome, it had no impact on the field (see Navon and Shwed 2012).

17. See http://www.22q.org/index.php/what-is-22q/same-name-campaign.

18. Of course, this is very different from the boundary work that divides science and nonscience (Gieryn 1983).

19. Lippman's seminal discussion of geneticization (1991a) was actually about far more than the identification of genomically specific etiologies, focusing more on the reduction of human difference and the foreclosing of possibilities for development on the basis of a presumed genetic basis for disease. Indeed, it did not necessarily require an actual etiological finding (see chapter 4 for a case in point).

20. See also Featherstone and Atkinson's (2011) excellent analysis of the way that Rett syndrome's association with mutations in the *MECP2* gene led to various nosological conundrums, new avenues of research, a new basis for hope and mobilization, and different enactments across diverse settings. For our purposes, their analysis of Rett syndrome demonstrates that actors at some sites can embrace this kind of genomically designated recalibration with respect to a particular condition, even while others do not.

21. See "Diagnosing Williams Syndrome," https://web.archive.org/web/
20140718075150/http://www.williams-syndrome.org:80/diagnosing
-williams-syndrome/diagnosing-williams-syndrome.

CHAPTER TWO

1. Lejeune et al. 1960 was written before the Denver system for numbering
chromosomes became available. At that stage, only different-sized groups
could be confidently distinguished. Indeed, the autosomal chromosomes
are numbered according to size with the exception of chromosomes 21
and 22, which are reversed, because the label "21 trisomy" was considered
too entrenched to be revised by the time their true size was determined
(Harper 2006:146).

2. Furthermore, reports in the *Lancet* the following year demonstrated that a
variant of Down syndrome could be caused by a chromosomal translocation inherited from asymptomatic parents (Carter et al. 1960; Penrose,
Ellis, and Delhanty 1960; Polani et al. 1960), spurring interest in prenatal
diagnosis (see Harper 2006:68–69).

3. These two findings—monosomy X in Turner syndrome and XXY in
Klinefelter syndrome—were also decisive in establishing the idea that the
Y chromosome was "sex determining" for males.

4. Each chromosome was divided into short (*p* for *petit*) and long (*q*, which
simply follows *p*) arms and then labeled by region (first digit) and band
(second digit), later followed by decimal points. Thus, 22q13 refers to the
twenty-second chromosome's long arm, region 1, band 3.

5. Fleck's distinction between journal and vademecum science offers an
important rejoinder to Daston and Galison's recent work on objectivity
in modern Western science, which used such atlases as their main source
material (Daston and Galison 2010). As Fleck points out, esoteric journal
articles tend to be far more hesitant and circumspect, embracing the fal-
libility of the authors pending validation by the scientific collective. If
"objectivity is the suppression of some aspect of the self, the countering of
subjectivity" (Daston and Galison 2010:36), then much of the published
work in contemporary medical genetics is far less objective than Daston
and Galison would have us believe. Written some seventy-five years earlier, Fleck's account of modern science allows us to say that, by working
with atlases, Daston and Galison were effectively selecting on their dependent variable: atlases belong to the realm of vademecum science, and
their very purpose is to present an objective, disembodied, and purified
account of the more fluid, guarded, and circumspect knowledge developed in esoteric or journal science. In genetics at least, science is often less
"objective" than they imply.

6. Even though Triple X syndrome often causes no phenotypic symptoms
(though it is associated with increased height and risk of developmental

abnormalities), its observation through prenatal testing regimes has led to a significant number of terminated pregnancies, as I discuss later.

7. See Finucane, Haas-Givler, and Simon (2003) on the challenge the association with eugenics posed to genetic counseling's adoption in schools.

8. However, the authors also noted, "Each of his [two] wives gave birth to at least one abnormal child," and each had one miscarriage: one eighteen-year-old daughter found to have no breast development or, following an operation, internal sexual organs, though she had a normal XX sex chromosome complement; further, a twenty-two-month-old daughter from the second marriage was a "typical 47-chromosome mongoloid." Five other biological children were "apparently living or well," though because they were adopted, it was not possible to study their chromosomes (Sandberg et al. 1961:489).

9. The *Lancet* had *not* reported an association between said trait and XYY. Nevertheless, a letter in response later that year (Collier 1966) stated, "The condition of hypertrichosis pinnae auris (H.P.A.), the Y-linkage of which is still debated, has also been reported in Italians, Israelis, and Singhalese; I report here its occurrence in a native of the British Isles who attended this hospital; . . . the Y chromosome was at the upper limit of normal, being always larger than the no. 21 and in one case equal to the no. 17" (1036).

10. A letter published in the *Lancet* by a pathologist in response to this point (Park 1966:1468) noted that this is "a matter clearly relevant to current events and, as you suggested, one of much psychiatric and medicolegal significance: for example, is a YY psychopathic criminal (to be) regarded in law differently from an XY psychopathic criminal? . . . Should the chances [of rehabilitation] be slender or nil, much of the time directed towards rehabilitation is in effect time wasted, and this, if true, would be a pity, for a great deal of sympathetic thought and care are devoted to these and other delinquent persons; psychiatrists, prison staffs, and others may be blaming themselves unnecessarily for failure to achieve better results than they do." He concluded with the hope that UK government officials were taking research on XYY and criminality very seriously.

11. Today, *infertility* is more likely to be investigated in XYY syndrome (Kim et al. 2013).

12. This did not stop Alan Dershowitz, some thirty years later, from warning of the risks of using XYY "in the service of crime prevention or criminal responsibility" (2007:274), while at the same time railing against the dangers of scientific censorship born of fear of finding that there really is a link between chromosomal abnormalities and violence. (Passages in the chapter suggest it was written much earlier.)

13. Papers with XYY in the title were published at a rate of around 28.5 per year between 1966 and 1981 (457 total over sixteen years), with a peak of 54 and 53 in 1969 and 1970 respectively. By contrast, a mean of only around 7.5 per year were published between 1982 and 2017 (275 total over

thirty-six years). The actual search string used in ISI's Web of Science was "TI=(XYY* OR "YY SYNDROME" OR "DOUBLE Y CHROMOSOM*" OR "Jacob's syndrome")" (24 papers using the other two terms, almost all of them in the late 1960s).

14. See the websites of those two organizations: https://fivepminus.org/ and http://www.chromosome18.org/.

15. See the organization's website: http://www.trisomy18.org/.

16. See "Letter from Victoria Miller," at https://web.archive.org/web/201311 05165752/http:/www.trisomy18.org/site/PageServer?pagename=aboutus _founders_welcome.

17. See "Federal Research Funding," at https://web.archive.org/web/ 20130919034920/http://www.trisomy18.org/site/PageServer?pagename= involved_advocacy_funding.

18. See the organization's website: https://genetic.org/.

19. For Mayo Clinic, see https://www.mayoclinic.org/diseases-conditions/ triple-x-syndrome/symptoms-causes/syc-20350977. For WebMD, see https://web.archive.org/web/20110417114459/http://children.webmd.com: 80/triplo-x-syndrome. For Healthline, see https://www.healthline.com/ health/triple-x-syndrome.

20. See "Educational and Informational Brochures," https://web.archive.org/ web/20150129003641/http://www.genetic.org/Knowledge/Brochures.aspx. The AXYS website (https://genetic.org/) now contains updated brochures on all of the major sex chromosome aneuploidies.

21. This is not to say that we are now immune to programs of research that seek the cause of violence and crime in the human genome. As the next chapter shows, one extremely rare genomically designated syndrome gave rise to the much-hyped notion of a common "warrior gene." The NIH ran into considerable opposition and had to halt plans to hold a conference entitled "Genetic Factors in Crime: Findings, Uses and Implications" in 1992 (Hilts 1992). Finally, plans to sequence the genome of the Newtown, CT, killer, Adam Lanza, eerily recall the association between XYY and infamous serial killer Richard Speck forty years ago, though it also imme- diately elicited scientific skepticism (Kolata 2012a).

22. As any good consumer of the British press would surely agree, few newspa- pers would be more likely to latch on to the idea of genetically determined criminals than the *Daily Mail*.

23. For research results and study/trial announcements publicized by AXYS, see "47,XYY," at https://genetic.org/category/47xyy/; and "Research Oppor- tunities for Families," at https://genetic.org/about/research/opportunities -for-families/.

24. For a public-facing example, see the entry for XYY syndrome in the National Organization for Rare Disorders (NORD) Rare Disease Database: https://rarediseases.org/rare-diseases/xyy-syndrome/.

CHAPTER THREE

1. Rabinow's seminal statement on the emergence of "biosociality," for example, noted that, "given the way genes are currently located on chromosomes, i.e., linkage maps, the easiest genome to map and sequence would necessarily be composed of the largest number of abnormal genes. In other words, the pathological would be the path to the norm" (1996:97). Similarly, Cambrosio and his colleagues (Cambrosio et al. 2009) discussed the "bio-clinical hybrids," like mice models and biomarkers, that increasingly circulate between the biologist's lab and the clinic, blurring the line between the normal and the pathological in fields like cancer genetics (see also Keating and Cambrosio 2006). Perhaps the most direct engagement is found in the recent discussion of the dynamic of "singularization-generalization" (Rabeharisoa et al. 2014), which describes hybrid communities of families, clinicians, and researchers who make reflexive decisions about framing their rare disease as singular or unique vs. a focus on the commonalities shared with other conditions. The authors even note the dilemma faced by organizations when researchers seek to use their rare condition as a model or "guinea pig" for more prevalent forms of disease (207–8). However, none of these studies examines leveraging in any detail.

2. This works both through the breeding of particular variants, and the molecular "knock-out" of genes and genomic regions, or inducement of other sorts of mutations. By comparing "wild types" (normal), heterozygous mutants (one mutation), and homozygous mutants (mutations on both chromosomes pairs), connections between genes, physiology, and function can be inferred. Such a strategy plays a major role in a number of biomedical fields.

3. See "Diagnosing Williams Syndrome," https://web.archive.org/web/2014 0718075150/http://www.williams-syndrome.org:80/diagnosing-williams -syndrome/diagnosing-williams-syndrome.

4. A transcript of the program is available at https://web.archive.org/web/ 20111126163945/http://www.pbs.org/saf/1205/resources/transcript.htm.

5. Lenhoff (1997:73) recounts an episode when John Burn noted in the *Journal of Medical Genetics* that he could not comment on whether Williams syndrome children had elfin facies, because he had "never seen an elf." A few years later, in 1990, the former president of the Williams Syndrome Association delivered a pithy retort at their annual meeting: "Of course Dr. Burn has seen elves before, because he has seen our Williams syndrome children."

6. See "WSA Mission," at http://www.williams-syndrome.org/content/wsa -mission.

7. See "Current Studies" in the "Researchers" section: https://williams -syndrome.org/researcher/current-studies; for the registry, see https:// williams-syndrome.org/registry-families.

8. See "Williams Syndrome and Research," at http://www.williams-syndrome
.org/media/williams-syndrome-and-research.

9. Caspi et al. defined antisocial behavior as (1) adolescent conduct disorder
according to *DSM-IV* criteria; (2) convictions for violent crimes; (3) "a personality disposition toward violence" in a psychological examination at
age twenty-six; or (4) symptoms of "antisocial personality disorder" at age
twenty-six by people nominated by the subject as "someone who knows
you well" (2002:852).

10. There are also less common 3.5R and 5R alleles whose impact on function
are more ambiguous.

11. Roettger et al. (2016) subsequently found an independent effect of the
MAOA 2R allele on "delinquency"—operationalized as a composite of
eight actions (e.g., property damage, theft, selling drugs, getting in a fight,
threatening to use or using a weapon) among an expanded Add Health
sample of 6,001 males, 76 of whom had the 2R allele.

12. Excerpt from Walter Ward, "The Thug Gene?," posted by WhiteRights on
https://www.stormfront.org/forum/t1167567/, July 13, 2016. Ward's article
originally appeared in *Taki's Magazine* on March 7, 2011.

13. See "The Warrior Gene," at http://www.thewarriorgene.com/.

14. See "Born to Rage?," at http://www.drphil.com/slideshows/slideshow/
6293/?id=6293&slide=0&showID=1626&preview=&versionID=, three
pages.

15. In contrast to our contemporary understanding of Fragile X's complex
phenotype, Martin and Bell were clear in their assessment that "physically
the affected males are not abnormal. They are in general of sturdy build,
but they do not show any distinctiveness in shape or head or face. . . .
Their sexual development appears to be normal" (1943:155).

16. A 2001 review put it, somewhat anachronistically, like this: "The cytogenetic test employed by [studies in the 1980s] has since been shown to
be inaccurate, generating both false negative and positive results." They
also note that the new tests reduced Fragile X's prevalence by at least half
(Crawford, Acuña, and Sherman 2001:360).

17. In 1992, a new fragile site dubbed "FRAXE" was discovered in the q27–28
region of the X chromosome (Sutherland and Baker 1992). FRAXE was
quickly shown to be caused by a GCC repeat expansion (Knight et al.
1993) that was soon associated with a novel gene: Fragile X mental retardation 2 or *FMR2* (Gu et al. 1996). An early study of FRAXE, based entirely
on patients who were referred for Fragile X testing, explained, "Although
FRAXA [an alternate term for Fragile X] and FRAXE are indistinguishable
by use of conventional cytogenetic means, they can be delineated at the
molecular level, and this provides the basis for differential diagnosis"
(Knight et al. 1996:910). While FRAXE tends to be milder than post-1991
Fragile X, the differences are not nearly clear enough to strongly guide
diagnosis.

18. See UC Davis Health 2016. The story also reports that "Leonard Abbeduto, director of the UC Davis MIND Institute and co-leader of the research at UC Davis, said it will not only help participating families, but also change how the field conducts clinical trials of new drugs for people with intellectual and developmental disabilities."

19. NIH Reporter (https://projectreporter.nih.gov/reporter.cfm), active projects' total funding for Fragile X, Williams syndrome, and *MAOA*.

20. The NIH is the only major agency to fund Williams syndrome and *MAOA* research at significant levels, while Fragile X receives funding from several others (including the Department of Defense).

CHAPTER FOUR

1. That said, long-term increases in average parental age, leading to more de novo mutations, may have played a small but significant role (Liu, King, and Bearman 2010).

2. Hence Rimland repeatedly endorsed the psychogenic explanation's main piece of evidence: autism parents were cold, highly intellectual, prone to abstract occupations, and lacking an interest in people (Rimland 1964:160).

3. While the introduction of larger sample sizes and more sophisticated heritability estimation techniques in recent years has led to the publication of considerably lower heritability estimates (Liu, King, and Bearman 2010; Colvert et al. 2015), there is intriguing evidence that these more sophisticated estimates have also increased alongside autism's rise in prevalence (Liu King, and Bearman 2010). Regardless, the unfolding of this third loop of autism heritability was estimated only through small-n twin studies.

4. Much of this increase came during a period of expanding total NIH budgets. However, the steep rise in NIH spending on autism research has continued even amid the stagnating overall NIH budgets of recent years. For data on NIH annual budgets, see "Spending History by Institute/Center, Mechanism, etc. (1983 to present)," at http://officeofbudget.od.nih.gov/spending_hist.html.

5. Of course, other related factors were important as well: autism heritability findings supported the focus on genetics; genetics research more generally was growing quickly, with technological innovation serving as an important driver (Ledbetter 2008); and epidemiological evidence that autism prevalence was growing, and the rhetoric of "epidemic," also provided a powerful rationale for conducting research on the genetics of autism.

6. Even before *DSM-III* came out in 1980, some researchers claimed that children with autism were comorbid for mental retardation in up to 94% of cases (e.g., DeMyer et al. 1974; see also Feinstein 2010:145–46).

7. Rimland had argued forcefully against autism/mental retardation comorbidity decades earlier (1964:10–11, 139, 160), but he ended up embracing idea that there were high rates of autism in Fragile X *mental retardation* (as it was still called). His influential outlet, the *Autism Research Review International*, even reported Fragile X–related findings enthusiastically to its readership of autism parents and allied researchers (1987, 1989, 1991).

8. Some doubted the validity of IQ tests in autism patients altogether (Kraijer 1997:23, 37–42; Wing 1973). In a sense, this line of reasoning was as old as autism itself: even Kanner (1949, 11, 27–28) referred to autism's "apparent feeblemindedness."

9. It was precisely such variegated diagnostic criteria, formally incorporated into *DSM-III-R* (1987; see also Reiss and Freund 1990 and 1992 on *DSM-III-R* autism diagnosis and FXS) and *DSM-IV* (1994), that allowed researchers and clinicians to see FXS and autism as both tightly intertwined and importantly distinct. Indeed, the current studies demonstrating much higher rates of autism or ASD in FXS take this inclusive approach even further.

10. Elsewhere, Rutter and Bailey called the strength of the autism–Fragile X correlation into question on the grounds that they were distinct "behavioural phenotypes" (Bailey et al. 1993:676) and that stricter diagnostic criteria for autism (682), as well as more stringent cytogenetic techniques (683), weakened the association considerably; they even excluded from their follow-up study an MZ twin pair who had been part of Folstein and Rutter's sample on the grounds that they had since been diagnosed with Fragile X (Bailey et al. 1995:67).

11. See the National Fragile X Foundation's page "FXS and Autism: Similar but Different" for a similar account: https://web.archive.org/web/20170112031659/https://fragilex.org/fragile-x/fragile-x-syndrome/autism-and-fragile-x-syndrome/fxs-and-autism-similar-but-different/.

12. A small number of reviews began discussing associations between autism and a handful of chromosomal abnormalities in the mid-1980s, but with the exception of Fragile X, they remained limited to summarizing isolated case reports (see Reiss, Feinstein, and Rosenbaum 1986 for the most thorough example). By the late 1990s and early 2000s, by contrast, there were many more review papers discussing the relationship between autism and a range of long-standing genetic disorders in much greater detail (e.g., Gillberg 1998; Bespalova and Buxbaum 2003; Cohen et al. 2005; Folstein and Rosen-Sheidley 2001).

13. For a more detailed version of this analysis, see Navon and Eyal 2014.

14. See "Genetics and Genomics," at https://web.archive.org/web/20161219001732/https://www.autismspeaks.org/science/initiatives/autism-genome-project.

15. See note 14 above. See also the MSSNG website: https://www.mss.ng/.

16. Geschwind won awards from those groups, served on their advisory boards, and worked as a founding member and chief scientific advisor for the Autism Genetic Resource Exchange; see Autism Speaks 2008.

17. See also Geschwind's recent piece in *Nature Medicine* (Torre-Ubieta et al. 2016).

18. Indeed, a paper entitled "Convergence of Genes and Cellular Pathways Dysregulated in Autism Spectrum Disorders" (Pinto et al. 2014), featuring 112 authors from around the world, including Geschwind and many other leading lights in autism genetics, recently appeared in the *American Journal of Human Genetics*.

19. When Miller declined (he is already working with several other similar foundations, including the 22q11.2DS foundation), the PMSF hired him to oversee the hiring process instead.

20. See Nelson 2018 for a superb account of animal models in psychiatric research.

21. See "PMSF Research," at https://www.pmsf.org/research/; for the registry, see https://pmsiregistry.patientcrossroads.org/.

22. ADHD's prevalence has also grown by orders of magnitude, and it is increasingly characterized by high heritability estimates and genetic heterogeneity (e.g., Lo-Castro, D'Agati, and Curatolo 2011; Schachar 2014). It is hardly surprising then that Fragile X and other genetic disorders have already been leveraged as models for attention disorder.

CHAPTER FIVE

1. In 2010 they met in the British city of Coventry; in 2014 they met in Mallorca, Spain; in 2016 they met on Lake Garda in Sirmione, Italy; and in 2018 they met in Whistler, Canada.

2. To be sure, genomic designation still functions within much larger discursive and institutional systems—clinical medicine, liberal governance, modern biopower, and biopolitics, just to take a few dealt with by Foucault himself (2009, 1973, 2010).

3. I am drawing on the distinction in science studies between translation and simple diffusion here (see esp. Latour 1988:132–44).

4. Callon and Rabeharisoa in particular have shown how patients and their advocates have become important actors in biomedical research as part of "hybrid collectives" (2003, 2004, 2008; Rabeharisoa and Callon 2002; Rabeharisoa et al. 2012). More generally STS scholars have turned their attention to the way that biomedical knowledge is "coproduced" (Jasanoff 2013) by scientific researchers and the social organizations formed around disease categories. Scholars like Steven Epstein have also shown how the distinction between researcher and activist has been broken down by the emergence of lay experts (Epstein 1996; see also Eyal et al. 2010), and Panofsky has shown how advocacy groups for genetic disorders have

worked to foster social ties with biomedical experts that will impact their research agendas moving forward (2011).

5. See the organization's website: http://www.geneticalliance.org/.

6. See "Fragile X Clinics," at https://fragilex.org/treatment-intervention/fragile-x-clinics/.

7. See "Press Archives," January 2015, at http://www.22q.org/awareness-events/press-archives/.

8. See "Media Information," at https://web.archive.org/web/20160315191000/http://www.genetic.org/About/Media.aspx.

9. For a current list of countries, see the "International Contacts" page of the foundation's website: http://www.22q.org/resources-for-22q/for-families/family-support-network/international-contacts/.

10. A study published in *Clinical Genetics* in 2008 identified an infant that had inherited a 22q11.2 duplication from a seemingly normal mother. The family turned out to have eight 22q11.2 duplication bearers across three generations. The abstract explained, "Phenotypic variation include[d] heart defect (1 in 8 individuals, 1/8), submucous cleft palate (2/8), intellectual disability (2/8), speech delay (2/8), behaviour problems (3/8) and brachydactyly (3/8)" (Yu et al. 2008).

11. See "22q11.2 Duplication," at http://www.22q.org/about-22q/new-diagnosed/22q11-2-duplication-2/.

12. The same breakpoints that predispose the loss of chromosomal material during meiosis can lead to the mirror-opposite gain, or three copies instead of the usual two. Hence we have not only 17p11.2 deletion and duplication syndromes (Smith-Magenis and Potocki-Lupski syndromes, respectively), but also a 7q11.23 duplication syndrome as the reciprocal of Williams syndrome. As with other mutations, many of these CNVs have been reported in the medical genetics literature; some have been genomically designated as novel medical conditions in that literature, and a small handful have taken on considerable social and clinical meaning.

13. See "About 22q," at http://www.22q.org/about-22q/.

14. See stephiemoo121212's YouTube channel, at https://www.youtube.com/channel/UCp55aQnIKDavtCQ98oEpY5g. See also Wright 2016 for an example of interest from the autism community, and below on ADHD and schizophrenia.

15. See "Prevalence of 22q11.2 Deletion and Duplication Syndromes, July 2015" on the foundation's "News" page, at http://www.22q.org/awareness-events/news/; from the website of the UK charity Max Appeal, "What Is the Prevalence of 22q Deletion in the Population?," at http://www.maxappeal.org.uk/news/content.asp?ni=240; and from the website of the 22q11.2 Society, "Higher Prevalence Than Previously Estimated," at http://22qsociety.org/news/content.asp?ni=232&pv=1. The International 22q11.2 Foundation's "22q11.2 Deletion" page states (under "The Syndrome"), "Present in 1 out of every 1,000 live pregnancies, in 1 in 68 children with

congenital heart disease, and in 5 to 8 percent of children born with cleft palate, the 22q11.2 deletion is almost as common as Down syndrome"; see http://www.22q.org/about-22q/new-diagnosed/deletion/.

16. Furthermore, at least in 22q11.2DS, the fact that it is the facial phenotype that often leads to testing results in decreased ascertainment of non-Caucasian patients, as their craniofacial features are less distinct (or so say the mostly white doctors who fail to recognize them).

17. I do not want to advance the comparison too forcefully—many factors make XYY syndrome in the 1970s and 22q11.2DS today *dis*analogous, not least the frequency and severity of serious medical complications and the wildly divergent social circuits within which they are mobilized. Nevertheless, the lead researcher on the Harvard XYY screening study, Stanley Walzer, was an ardent proponent of early diagnosis and intervention— perhaps *the* watchwords of contemporary advocacy for genetic and developmental disorders. However, he was ahead of his time in the sense that screening programs for XYY circa 1974 would probably have been absorbed into oppressive networks dedicated to crime and male degeneracy rather than collaborative research and patient advocacy.

18. See "Annual 22q at the Zoo," at http://www.22q.org/awareness-events/awareness/annual-22q-at-the-zoo/.

19. See "Resources" > "Clinics" > "International," at http://www.22q.org/resources-for-22q/clinics/international/.

20. See "Resources for 22q," at http://www.22q.org/resources-for-22q/.

21. See the 2015 conference brochure at http://media.chop.edu/data/files/pdfs/cme-22q-ibbc-2015.pdf.

22. See IBBC's "Project Overview" page, at http://22q11-ibbc.org/about/.

23. The drug, NFC-1, is a nonstimulant neuromodulator designed to treat patients with "mGluR+ ADHD." The mGluR pathway has been implicated in a host of neurodevelopmental disorders like ADHD, sleep disturbances, and autism spectrum disorders, attracting widespread scientific attention in the process (Osherovich 2012; Wenger, Kao, et al. 2016). It is also the pathway that is being targeted in most of the trials for Fragile X and autism discussed in previous chapters. Around 85% of 22q11.2DS patients are missing a gene that is involved in the mGluR pathway, *RANBP1*, making 22q11.2 microdeletions a potential model for the treatment of neurodevelopmental disorders.

24. See "New Finding Regarding Potential Treatment of ADHD and Anxiety and Its Implications for the 22q Community, September 2015" on the foundation's "News" page, at http://www.22q.org/awareness-events/news/; and http://www.22q.org/awareness-events/news/new-finding-regarding -potential-treatment-of-adhd-and-anxiety-and-its-implications-for-the -22q-community/.

25. See the International 22q11.2 Foundation's "Dragonfly Summer Camp," at http://www.22q.org/awareness-events/dragonfly-summer-camp/.

CHAPTER SIX

1. In 2017 GlaxoSmithKline began offering a gene therapy to treat and perhaps even cure the extremely rare condition, severe combined immune deficiency (often called "bubble boy" disease)—a development that has given researchers, advocates, and pharmaceutical companies added hope as they seek to develop targeted treatments for hundreds of single-gene disorders (Mullin 2017; Regalado 2016).

2. See the brochure "47,XYY Syndrome," at https://genetic.org/wp-content/uploads/2016/09/AXYS-XYY-Brochure-updated-12-10-16.pdf.

3. See the VCFSEF Twitter page at https://twitter.com/vcfsefoundation (my emphasis).

4. See "Same Name Campaign," at http://www.22q.org/awareness-events/awareness/same-name-campaign/.

5. As Armstrong (2011) has shown, even the dominant *International Classification of Diseases* (*ICD*) system still faces acute obstacles and resistances in general practitioners' mostly symptoms-oriented practice. It is hardly surprising, then, that actors working with genomically designated conditions often encounter recalcitrance and find themselves having to work with other modes of medical classification.

6. See "About" > "22q" > "Newly Diagnosed" > "Healthcare Guidelines," at http://www.22q.org/about-22q/new-diagnosed/healthcare-guidelines-2/.

7. For example, studying genomically designated syndromes supports Rabeharisoa and Bourret's argument (2009:697) that "contrary to the discourse on the 'geneticization' of diseases, . . . the introduction of genetics into oncology and into psychiatry does not by any means amount to reductionism"; rather, "genetics reinforces the complexity of pathological categories." I also found that conditions like 22q11.2DS compel researchers, clinicians, and advocates to work to "invent or reinvent a clinic capable of working on these multiple and complex pathological entities."

8. Indeed, precisely the same kind of genetic mutations that Rabeharisoa and Bourret discuss have started to powerfully shape clinical practice. Rabeharisoa and Bourret cite a presentation in which "a child psychiatrist reviewed his collaboration with the pediatric geneticists, and reported on 26 'diagnoses.' . . . Apart from 11 diagnoses of Fragile X and some isolated diagnoses of rare syndromes, the 'diagnoses' mentioned locations of chromosomal abnormalities" (707). At most, this group discussed these chromosomal abnormalities as potential "binding objects" between pathological categories, rather than diagnostic categories in their own right. In other settings, disease categories named after chromosomal locations *have* achieved the status of a diagnosis (sans quotation marks). Under the right circumstances, our knowledge about them can inform practice and take on profound meaning for the patients and families to whom they are delivered.

CHAPTER SEVEN

1. Until recent revisions, Wechsler IQ tests generated scores for two subscales along with a full-scale IQ: verbal IQ (measuring abilities like comprehension and working memory) and performance (measuring visuospatial organization and processing speed).
2. See "Resources" > "Growth Charts," at http://www.22q.org/resources-for -22q/growth-charts-2/.
3. Unfortunately, my IRB protocol at the time did not allow me to formally interview these patients.
4. Other incidental findings that support the idea of substantially higher prevalence include identical twins with very different phenotypes and several pairs of cousins with independent de novo cases of 22q.
5. It is thought that around 90% of 22q11.2DS cases are the result of de novo mutations. However, parents with 22q have a 50% chance of passing it on to their child, so it is a heritable condition, even though it is not usually actually inherited from a parent.
6. See, e.g., Ambry Genetics, "Fragile X-Associated Disorders," at http:// www.ambrygen.com/tests/fragile-x-associated-disorders; and Myriad Women's Health (formerly Counsyl), "Fragile X Syndrome," at https:// myriadwomenshealth.com/diseases/fragile-x-syndrome/.
7. See "The Three Fragile X-Associated Disorders," at https://fragilex.org/ fragile-x/.
8. A 2016 paper examined nonclinically referred adults who did not have either FXTAS or a child with Fragile X in order to control for ascertainment bias and confounding variables. They found significantly higher rates of "broad autism spectrum" symptoms among premutation males and obsessive-compulsive symptoms among females (Schneider et al. 2016).
9. While a couple of previous social scientific studies have addressed the Fragile X premutation, none have grappled with its transformation from a carrier gene into a disease variant of its own. Dorothy Nelkin (1996) used the case of Fragile X testing in special education classes in Colorado to explore "the growing practice of genetic testing in American society" (537). While the paper is very insightful, Nelkin does not distinguish between mildly affected girls with Fragile X and Fragile X premutation carriers. More recent work by Raspberry and Skinner (2011b, 2011a) has examined the way a positive test for the Fragile X premutation brings with it an expanded notion of "genetic responsibility." Without question, the inheritance pattern of Fragile X is an essential part of the way families think about and deal with the disorder, and it also plays a key role in the patient movement. However, Raspberry and Skinner do not address the fact that the Fragile X premutation is now thought to have its own phenotype.
10. See "Fragile X-Associated Tremor/Ataxia Syndrome | FXTAS," at https:// fragilex.org/fragile-x/fxtas/; "Fragile X-Associated Primary Ovarian

Insufficiency | FXPOI," at https://fragilex.org/fragile-x/fxpoi/; and "Premutation Carriers," at https://fragilex.org/fragile-x/carriers/.

CHAPTER EIGHT

1. I mean this in the actor-network theoretical sense of an actor who translates without reshaping the knowledge or object in question. Below, I outline how genetic counselors have become *mediators* who do transform the meaning of mutations (Latour 1999:307).
2. See "Genetic Services," at https://www.elwyn.org/services/adults-21/health -services/genetic-services/.
3. See "Genetic Evaluations," at https://web.archive.org/web/20160316035112/ http://www.elwyngenetics.org./GeneticsEvals.html.
4. Arc of the United States, previously the Association for Retarded Citizens, is the major support and lobbying organization for people with intellectual and developmental disabilities in the United States.
5. See the brochure "22q11.2 Deletion Syndrome: Consultative Services for Schools," at https://web.archive.org/web/20160316035226/http://www .elwyngenetics.org./Elwyn%2022q%20brochure2013pub.pdf.
6. See ICD-11 (https://icd.who.int/), especially the many entries in the subsections to "20 Developmental Anomalies" (December 2018): https://icd .who.int/browse11/l-m/en#/http%3a%2f%2fid.who.int%2ficd%2fentity %2f223744320.
7. See the Human Disease Genes website: http://www.ppm1dgene.com/.
8. In 2010, a "consensus statement" by the International Standard Cytogenetic Array Consortium was published in the *American Journal of Human Genetics*. They advocated the use of a nontargeted, higher-yield chromosomal microarray as a "first-tier clinical diagnostic test," in place of karyotyping, "for patients with unexplained DD/ID, ASD, or MCA [multiple congenital anomalies]" (Miller et al. 2010:757).
9. See "Seasoned ADCY5.org Team" on the ADCY5.org home page, at http:// www.adcy5.org/home.html.
10. See the ADNPKids website: https://www.adnpkids.com/.
11. There has been extensive coverage of the problems associated with false positives, including cases where terminations were carried out without invasive diagnostic testing (NIPT is just a screen, after all). There has been speculative discussion about the prospect of "designer babies" and concerns that NIPT would be used for sex selections. Finally, our old friend geneticization has been invoked, and appropriately so, given that prenatal genetic testing was the empirical backdrop for Abby Lippman's seminal discussion of the way our conception of human difference was being reduced to genetics.
12. There are scattered studies that report rates of testing and aneuploidy findings in particular locales but do not present data on resulting ter-

minations (e.g., Hook and Schreinemachers 1983; Naber, Huether, and Goodwin 1987). The highest rates of prenatal genetic testing in these first decades appear to come from Denmark, where by 1979–80 Mikkelsen et al. (1983) could note that the Down syndrome births stood at 0.86 per 1,000 compared to 1.17 when prenatally diagnosed cases were included.

13. Shaffer, Caughey, and Norton (2006) report that termination rates for SCAs were higher following CVS rather than amniocentesis testing (but not for the more severe autosomal trisomies)—"77% vs 55%, p = 0.015" (669). They plausibly ascribe this result, as Verp et al. (1988) did nearly twenty years earlier, to the fact that CVS tends to be performed between the tenth and twelfth weeks of pregnancy vs. the fifteenth and twentieth weeks in the case of amniocentesis, as well as to the decreased tolerance for genetic abnormality of women opting for CVS testing.

14. Small amounts of cell-free DNA (cfDNA) from the fetus circulate in its mother's blood. By screening both fetal and maternal cfDNA, NIPT kits are able to distinguish between them and then identify genomic anomalies in the fetal genome.

15. In 2014 Sequenom, Inc. reported, "Approximately 148,500 MaterniT21 PLUS test commercial samples were accessioned in 2013, 143% more than in 2012; 93% of accessions were from U.S. patients; international test volumes and revenues continue to show strong growth" (Sequenom 2014). Early sales surpassed even their own expectations, and led their total revenues for diagnostic services to go from $8.3 million in 2011 to $119.6 million in 2013—a shift their annual report ascribes to MaterniT21™. For the 2012 report (which also contains the 2011 figures), see http://www.sequenom.com/press/sequenom-inc-reports-financial-results-fourth-quarter-and-full-year-2012 (accessed March 12, 2014). See also Heger 2013.

16. The National Down Syndrome Society has not taken a position on prenatal testing or termination per se. Instead, they focus on facilitating access to genetic counselors and other genetic experts for parents who have received a prenatal diagnosis and legally mandating the provision of accurate information about Down syndrome by advocating for the Accurate Education for Prenatal Screenings Act (HR 3441) (see "Noninvasive Prenatal Tests (NIPTs)," at https://www.ndss.org/advocate/ndss-legislative-agenda/healthcare-research/noninvasive-prenatal-tests-nipts). To this end, they have drafted model legislation, which passed in Massachusetts in June 2012. As a 2012 press release from the Massachusetts Down Syndrome Congress explained, the legislation ensures that "medical professionals are required to give parents who receive a prenatal or postnatal diagnosis 'up-to-date, evidence-based, written information about Down syndrome that has been reviewed by medical experts and national Down syndrome organizations'" and that parents are "given contact information for the MDSC's Parent's First Call Program and support services,"

as well as other Down syndrome advocacy resources. The press release explicitly noted the significance of the new wave of noninvasive prenatal genetic test kits, which, they explained, "signaled a not-far-off future in which expectant parents will routinely receive an accurate prenatal diagnosis for Down syndrome and other chromosomal conditions early in their pregnancy" (see the MDSC's "Legislative Update," at http://archive.constantcontact.com/fs037/1102107208525/archive/1110304047480.html).

17. See Virginia Isaacs's letter at https://genetic.org/wp-content/uploads/2016/08/AXYS-Letter-to-parents-with-a-prenatal-dx.pdf.

18. In late 2012, Verinata reported findings at the American Society of Human Genetics that suggest noninvasive prenatal testing for chromosomal abnormalities smaller than full aneuploidy were on their way. This led their CEO to say, "Looking beyond our current product offering . . . clearly demonstrates the power and potential of massively parallel sequencing to detect alterations within individual chromosomes, similar to chromosomal microarrays" (Verinata Health 2012a).

19. See the brochure at https://www.sequenom.com/uploads/collateral/MaterniT-GENOME-provider-brochure_Rep-1037-v1-0217.pdf.

20. The US assistant secretary for Health, Education and Welfare put it like this in 1975: "One of the main points of emphasis in the Department of HEW is prevention of disability. By focusing on prevention we increase the resources available for other programs. Few advances compare with amniocentesis in their capability for prevention of disability" (cited in Paul 1995:132).

21. A large meta-analysis covering five countries found that ~92% of 5,035 cases were aborted (Mansfield, Hopfer, and Marteau 1999), although a more recent study suggested that rates in the United States are somewhat lower and highly variable across sites (Natoli et al. 2012). In many countries, increased average maternal age and relatively low prenatal testing rates ensure that a small increase in prevalence is still observed. In other places, it is very much the opposite. For example, in Paris and Taiwan it is estimated that 85% and 80% respectively of Down syndrome fetuses are aborted due to much higher prenatal testing uptake and similarly high rates of termination upon receiving a Down syndrome diagnosis (Leroi 2006).

CONCLUSION

1. See, for example, Family Tree DNA's page for the haplogroup R1b paternal lineage: https://www.familytreedna.com/groups/r-1b/about.

2. To take the same R1b haplogroup: https://groups.yahoo.com/neo/groups/R1b-YDNA/info.

References

Abbott, Andrew. 1988. *System of Professions: Essay on the Division of Expert Labor.* University of Chicago Press.

Abrahams, Brett S., and Daniel H. Geschwind. 2008. "Advances in Autism Genetics: On the Threshold of a New Neurobiology." *Nature Reviews Genetics* 9(5):341–55.

Abrams, N., and E. Pergament. 1971. "Childhood Psychosis Combined with XYY Abnormalities." *Journal of Genetic Psychology* 118(1):13–16.

Abu El-Haj, Nadia. 2007. "The Genetic Reinscription of Race." *Annual Review of Anthropology* 36(1):283–300.

ACMG Board of Directors. 2012. "Points to Consider in the Clinical Application of Genomic Sequencing." *Genetics in Medicine* 14(8):759–61.

Adams, Virginia. 1977. "Causes of Crime, Maybe." *New York Times,* December 18, 188.

Agarwal, Ashwin, Lauren C. Sayres, Mildred K. Cho, Robert Cook-Deegan, and Subhashini Chandrasekharan. 2013. "Commercial Landscape of Noninvasive Prenatal Testing in the United States." *Prenatal Diagnosis* 33(6):521–31.

Aglan, M. S., A. K. Kamel, and N. A. Helmy. 2008. "Partial Trisomy of the Distal Part of 10q: A Report of Two Egyptian Cases." *Genetic Counseling* (Geneva, Switzerland) 19(2):199–209.

Alfi, O., G. N. Donnell, B. F. Crandall, A. Derencsenyi, and R. Menon. 1973. "Deletion of the Short Arm of Chromosome No. 9 (46,9p-): A New Deletion Syndrome." *Annales de Génétique* 16(1):17–22.

Allan, W., C. N. Herndon, F. C. Dudley, et al. 1944. "Some Examples of the Inheritance of Mental Deficiency: Apparently Sex-Linked Idiocy and Microcephaly." *American Journal of Mental Deficiency* 48:325–34.

Allderdice, P. W., et al. 1969. "The 13q-Deletion Syndrome." *American Journal of Human Genetics* 21(5):499–512.

Allen, John, Dr. Marian K. DeMyer, James A. Norton, William Pontius, and Ellen Yang. 1971. "Intellectuality in Parents of Psychotic, Subnormal, and Normal Children." *Journal of Autism and Childhood Schizophrenia* 1(3):311–26.

Alpman, Asude, et al. 2005. "Ring Chromosome 20 Syndrome with Intractable Epilepsy." *Developmental Medicine and Child Neurology* 47(5):343–46.

American College of Medical Genetics and Genomics. 2016. "Updated Position Statement on Noninvasive Prenatal Screening for Detection of Fetal Aneuploidy." ScienceDaily, July 28. https://www.sciencedaily.com/releases/2016/07/160728125016.htm.

American Psychiatric Association. 1980. *Diagnostic and Statistical Manual of Mental Disorders: DSM-III.* American Psychiatric Association.

———. 1987. *Diagnostic and Statistical Manual of Mental Disorders: DSM-III-R.* Rev. ed. American Psychiatric Association.

———. 1994. *Diagnostic and Statistical Manual of Mental Disorders: DSM-IV.* American Psychiatric Association.

———. 2013. *Diagnostic and Statistical Manual of Mental Disorders: DSM-V.* American Psychiatric Association.

Appadurai, Arjun. 1988. *The Social Life of Things: Commodities in Cultural Perspective.* Cambridge University Press.

Archambault, Louise, dir. 2013. *Gabrielle.* Seville Pictures (Canada).

Armstrong, David. 1995. "The Rise of Surveillance Medicine." *Sociology of Health & Illness* 17(3):393–404.

———. 2011. "Diagnosis and Nosology in Primary Care." *Social Science & Medicine* 73(6):801–7.

Aronowitz, Robert A. 1999. *Making Sense of Illness: Science, Society and Disease.* Cambridge University Press.

Assendelft, Nick. 2012. "Conference Wrap Up." Phelan-McDermid Syndrome Foundation, September 12. https://web.archive.org/web/20130515191414/http://22q13.org/j15/index.php?option=com_content&view=article&id=242&Itemid=213.

———. 2017. "Transition Will Position PMS Foundation for the Future." Phelan-McDermid Syndrome Foundation blog, February 25. http://www.pmsf.org/transition-will-position-pms-foundation-for-the-future/.

Autism Research Review International. 1987. "Autism, Fragile X Connection Investigated." *Autism Research Review International* 1(1):6–7.

———. 1989. "Link between Autism, Genes Is Explored." *Autism Research Review International* 3(2):1–2, 6.

———. 1991. "Fragile X Gene Discovery Announced." *Autism Research Review International* 5(2):1–2.

Autism Speaks. 2008. "2008 Annual Volunteer Conference Awards." Autism Speaks, March 13. https://web.archive.org/web/20170921171529/https://

www.autismspeaks.org/news/news-item/2008-annual-volunteer-conference
-awards.

Bailey, A., et al. 1993. "Prevalence of the Fragile X Anomaly amongst Autistic Twins and Singletons." *Journal of Child Psychology and Psychiatry* 34(5):673–88.

———. 1995. "Autism as a Strongly Genetic Disorder: Evidence from a British Twin Study." *Psychological Medicine* 25(01):63–77.

Bailey, Donald B., Melissa Raspa, Murrey Olmsted, and David B. Holiday. 2008. "Co-occurring Conditions Associated with *FMR1* Gene Variations: Findings from a National Parent Survey." *American Journal of Medical Genetics, Part A* 146A(16):2060–69.

Bailey, Donald B., Debra Skinner, Arlene M. Davis, Ian Whitmarsh, and Cynthia Powell. 2008. "Ethical, Legal, and Social Concerns about Expanded Newborn Screening: Fragile X Syndrome as a Prototype for Emerging Issues." *Pediatrics* 121(3):e693–e704.

Baily, Mary Ann, and Thomas H. Murray. 2008. "Ethics, Evidence, and Cost in Newborn Screening." *Hastings Center Report* 38(3):23–31.

Baio, Jon. 2018. "Prevalence of Autism Spectrum Disorder among Children Aged 8 Years—Autism and Developmental Disabilities Monitoring Network, 11 Sites, United States, 2014." *Morbidity and Mortality Weekly Report Surveillance Summaries* 67(6).

Bales, Abigail M., Christina A. Zaleski, and Elizabeth W. McPherson. 2010. "Newborn Screening Programs: Should 22q11 Deletion Syndrome Be Added?" *Genetics in Medicine* 12(3):135–44.

Ballif, Blake C., et al. 2007. "Discovery of a Previously Unrecognized Microdeletion Syndrome of 16p11.2–p12.2." *Nature Genetics* 39(9):1071–73.

Barbaro, Michela, et al. 2009. "Characterization of Deletions at 9p Affecting the Candidate Regions for Sex Reversal and Deletion 9p Syndrome by MLPA." *European Journal of Human Genetics* 17(11):1439–47.

Barry, Jessica C., et al. 2017. "Identification of 22q11.2 Deletion Syndrome via Newborn Screening for Severe Combined Immunodeficiency." *Journal of Clinical Immunology* 37(5):476–85.

Bassett, Anne S., et al. 2011. "Practical Guidelines for Managing Patients with 22q11.2 Deletion Syndrome." *Journal of Pediatrics* 159(2):332–39.e1.

Bastarache, Lisa, et al. 2018. "Phenotype Risk Scores Identify Patients with Unrecognized Mendelian Disease Patterns." *Science* 359(6381):1233–39.

Baty, Bonnie J., Brent L. Blackburn, and John C. Carey. 2005. "Natural History of Trisomy 18 and Trisomy 13: I. Growth, Physical Assessment, Medical Histories, Survival, and Recurrence Risk." *American Journal of Medical Genetics* 49(2):175–88.

Bauer, Diane. 1972. "Maryland Tests for Criminal Potential." In *Experimentation with Human Beings: The Authority of the Investigator, Subject, Professions, and State in the Human Experimentation Process*, edited by J. Katz. Russell Sage Foundation.

———, et al. 1980. "Special Supplement: The XYY Controversy: Researching Violence and Genetics." *Hastings Center Report* 10(4):1–31.

Baumgardner, Thomas L., Kathleen E. Green, and Allan Reiss. 1994. "A Behavioral Neurogenetics Approach to Developmental Disabilities: Gene-Brain-Behavior Associations." *Current Opinion in Neurology* 7(2):172–78.

Beaver, Kevin M., J. C. Barnes, and Brian B. Boutwell. 2014. "The 2-Repeat Allele of the *MAOA* Gene Confers an Increased Risk for Shooting and Stabbing Behaviors." *Psychiatric Quarterly* 85(3):257–65.

Beaver, Kevin M., Matt DeLisi, Michael G. Vaughn, and J. C. Barnes. 2010. "Monoamine Oxidase A Genotype Is Associated with Gang Membership and Weapon Use." *Comprehensive Psychiatry* 51:130–34.

Beaver, Kevin M., et al. 2013. "Exploring the Association between the 2-Repeat Allele of the *MAOA* Gene Promoter Polymorphism and Psychopathic Personality Traits, Arrests, Incarceration, and Lifetime Antisocial Behavior." *Personality and Individual Differences* 54(2):164–68.

Beck, Melinda. 2012. "Progress in Identifying the Genetic Roots of Autism." *Wall Street Journal*, September 24.

Becker, Howard Saul. 1963. *Outsiders: Studies in the Sociology of Deviance*. Free Press of Glencoe.

Beckwith, Jonathan. 1975. "Harvard XYY Study." *Science* 187(4174):298–99.

———. 2002. *Making Genes, Making Waves: A Social Activist in Science*. Harvard University Press.

Beckwith, Jonathan, and Jonathan King. 1974. "The XYY Syndrome: A Dangerous Myth." *New Scientist* 64(923):474–76.

Belluck, Pam. 2014. "New DNA Test Better at Predicting Some Disorders in Babies, Study Finds." *New York Times*, February 26.

Belluck, Pam, and Benedict Carey. 2013. "Psychiatry's New Guide Falls Short, Experts Say." *New York Times*, May 6.

Berg, Jonathan S., Lorraine Potocki, and Carlos A. Bacino. 2010. "Common Recurrent Microduplication Syndromes: Diagnosis and Management in Clinical Practice." *American Journal of Medical Genetics, Part A* 152A(5):1066–78.

Berry-Kravis, Elizabeth, et al. 2003. "Tremor and Ataxia in Fragile X Premutation Carriers: Blinded Videotape Study." *Annals of Neurology* 53(5):616–23.

Bespalova, I. N., and J. D. Buxbaum. 2003. "Disease Susceptibility Genes for Autism." *Annals of Medicine* 35(4):274–81.

Best, Rachel Kahn. 2012. "Disease Politics and Medical Research Funding: Three Ways Advocacy Shapes Policy." *American Sociological Review* 77(5):780–803.

Betancur, Catalina. 2011. "Etiological Heterogeneity in Autism Spectrum Disorders: More Than 100 Genetic and Genomic Disorders and Still Counting." *Brain Research* 1380:42–77.

Bettelheim, Bruno. 1967. *Empty Fortress*. Simon and Schuster.

Beuren, A. J., J. Apitz, and D. Harmjanz. 1962. "Supravalvular Aortic Stenosis in Association with Mental Retardation and a Certain Facial Appearance." *Circulation* 26:1235–40.

Bianchi, Diana W., et al. 2014. "DNA Sequencing versus Standard Prenatal Aneuploidy Screening." *New England Journal of Medicine* 370(9): 799–808.

Bill, Brent R., and Daniel H. Geschwind. 2009. "Genetic Advances in Autism: Heterogeneity and Convergence on Shared Pathways." *Current Opinion in Genetics & Development* 19(3):271–78.

Bishop, Dorothy V. M. 2010. "Which Neurodevelopmental Disorders Get Researched and Why?" *PLOS One* 5(11).

Bishop, Dorothy V. M., et al. 2011. "Autism, Language and Communication in Children with Sex Chromosome Trisomies." *Archives of Disease in Childhood* 96(10):954–59.

Black, Herbert. 1968. "1 Man in 300 May Inherit 'Violent' Gene." *Boston Globe*, August 7.

Bliss, Geraldine. 2011. "The Phelan-McDermid Syndrome Foundation." *Autism Speaks Official Blog*, January 11. https://autismspeaksblog.wordpress.com/tag/the-phelan-mcdermid-syndrome-foundation/.

———. 2012. "2012 Symposium Rationale." Phelan-McDermid Syndrome Foundation. (Document available from Daniel Navon.)

Boghosiansell, L., et al. 1994. "Molecular Mapping of the Edwards-Syndrome Phenotype to 2 Noncontiguous Regions on Chromosome-18." *American Journal of Human Genetics* 55(3):476–83.

Böök, Jan A. 1964. "Some Mechanisms of Chromosome Variations and Their Relation to Human Malformations." *Eugenics Review* 56(3):151–57.

Borg, I., J. D. Delhanty, and M. Baraitser. 1995. "Detection of Hemizygosity at the Elastin Locus by FISH Analysis as a Diagnostic Test in Both Classical and Atypical Cases of Williams Syndrome." *Journal of Medical Genetics* 32(9):692–96.

Borgaonkar, Digamber S. 1972. "Chromosome Survey of Maryland Boys." *American Journal of Human Genetics* 24(6):13a.

———. 1975. *Chromosomal Variation in Man: A Catalog of Chromosomal Variants and Anomalies*. Johns Hopkins University Press.

Bosk, Charles L. 1992. *All God's Mistakes: Genetic Counseling in a Pediatric Hospital*. 1st ed. University of Chicago Press.

Boucher, Geoff. 1994. "A Williams Child Parent's Educated Guess on Origin of Fairy and Elf Folk Tales." *Los Angeles Times*, August 21.

Bourgeois, James A., et al. 2011. "Lifetime Prevalence of Mood and Anxiety Disorders in Fragile X Premutation Carriers." *Journal of Clinical Psychiatry* 72(2):175–82.

Bourret, Pascale, Peter Keating, and Alberto Cambrosio. 2011. "Regulating Diagnosis in Post-genomic Medicine: Re-aligning Clinical Judgment?" *Social Science & Medicine* 73(6):816–24.

Bowker, Geoffrey C., and Susan Leigh Star. 2000. *Sorting Things Out: Classification and Its Consequences*. MIT Press.

Bozdagi, Ozlem, Teresa Tavassoli, and Joseph D. Buxbaum. 2013. "Insulin-like Growth Factor-1 Rescues Synaptic and Motor Deficits in a Mouse Model of Autism and Developmental Delay." *Molecular Autism* 4:9.

Brandler, William M., and Jonathan Sebat. 2015. "From De Novo Mutations to Personalized Therapeutic Interventions in Autism." *Annual Review of Medicine* 66(1):487–507.

Bretelle, Florence, et al. 2010. "Prenatal and Postnatal Diagnosis of 22q11.2 Deletion Syndrome." *European Journal of Medical Genetics* 53(6):367–70.

Brkanac, Zoran, Wendy H. Raskind, and Bryan H. King. 2008. "Pharmacology and Genetics of Autism: Implications for Diagnosis and Treatment." *Personalized Medicine* 5(6):599–607.

Brody, Jane E. 1968. "Rate of Crime-Linked Genetic Flaw Is Revised; Abnormality Found in Men Shows Evidence of Having Much Higher Incidence." *New York Times*, August 7, 34.

———. 1974a. "Harvard Backs Genetic Study." *New York Times*, December 14, 20.

———. 1974b. "Scientists' Group Terms Boston Study of Children with Extra Sex Chromosome Unethical and Harmful; Wider Fears Cited." *New York Times*, November 15.

———. 1975. "Babies' Screening Is Ended in Boston; Extra Chromosome Study Stirred Controversy on Its Ethics and Value." *New York Times*, June 20, 6.

Brooks-Crozier, Jennifer Melien. 2011. "The Nature and Nurture of Violence: Early Intervention Services for the Families of *MAOA*-Low Children as a Means to Reduce Violent Crime and the Costs of Violent Crime." *Connecticut Law Review* 44(2):531–73.

Brown, A., et al. 1996. "Two Patients with Duplication of 17p11.2: The Reciprocal of the Smith-Magenis Syndrome Deletion?" *American Journal of Medical Genetics* 63(2):373–77.

Brown, S., J. Russo, D. Chitayat, and D. Warburton. 1995. "The 13q– Syndrome: The Molecular Definition of a Critical Deletion Region in Band 13q32." *American Journal of Human Genetics* 57(4):859–66.

Brown, W. Ted, et al. 1982. "Autism Is Associated with the Fragile-X Syndrome." *Journal of Autism and Developmental Disorders* 12(3):303–8.

———. 1986. "Fragile X and Autism: A Multicenter Survey." *American Journal of Medical Genetics* 23(1–2):341–52.

Brunner, Han G. 1996. "MAOA Deficiency and Abnormal Behavior: Perspectives on an Association." In *Genetics of Criminal and Antisocial Behaviour*, edited by G. R. Bock and J. A. Goode, 155–67. Wiley.

Brunner, Han G., M. R. Nelen, X. Breakefield, H. Ropers, and B. van Oost. 1993. "Abnormal Behavior Associated with a Point Mutation in the Structural Gene for Monoamine Oxidase A." *Science* 262(5133):578–80.

Brunner, Han G., M. R. Nelen, P. van Zandvoort, et al. 1993. "X-Linked Borderline Mental Retardation with Prominent Behavioral Disturbance:

Phenotype, Genetic Localization, and Evidence for Disturbed Monoamine Metabolism." *American Journal of Human Genetics* 52(6):1032–39.

Buiting, K., et al. 1992. "A Putative Gene Family in 15q11–13 and 16p11.2: Possible Implications for Prader-Willi and Angelman Syndromes." *Proceedings of the National Academy of Sciences* 89(12):5457–61.

Bumiller, Kristin. 2009. "The Geneticization of Autism: From New Reproductive Technologies to the Conception of Genetic Normalcy." *Signs* 34(4):875–99.

Burn, J. 1999. "Closing Time for CATCH22." *Journal of Medical Genetics* 36(10):737–38.

Callon, Michel. 1986. "Some Elements of a Sociology of Translation: Domestication of the Scallops and the Fishermen of St Brieuc Bay." *Power Action and Belief a New Sociology of Knowledge* 32(4):196–223.

———. 1995. "Four Models for the Dynamics of Science." In *Handbook of Science and Technology Studies*, edited by S. Jasanoff, G. E. Markle, J. C. Peterson, and T. J. Pinch, 29–63. Sage.

Callon, Michel, and Vololona Rabeharisoa. 2003. "Research 'in the Wild' and the Shaping of New Social Identities." *Technology in Society* 25(2):193–204.

———. 2004. "Gino's Lesson on Humanity: Genetics, Mutual Entanglements and the Sociologist's Role." *Economy and Society* 33(1):1.

———. 2008. "The Growing Engagement of Emergent Concerned Groups in Political and Economic Life: Lessons from the French Association of Neuromuscular Disease Patients." *Science, Technology & Human Values* 33(2):230–61.

Cambrosio, Alberto, Peter Keating, Pascale Bourret, Philippe Mustar, and Susan Rogers. 2009. "Genomic Platforms and Hybrid Formations." In *Handbook of Genetics and Society: Mapping the New Genomic Era*, edited by P. Atkinson, P. E. Glasner, and M. Lock, 502–20. Routledge.

Campbell, Linda E., et al. 2009. "A Comparative Study of Cognition and Brain Anatomy between Two Neurodevelopmental Disorders: 22q11.2 Deletion Syndrome and Williams Syndrome." *Neuropsychologia* 47(4):1034–44.

Canguilhem, Georges. (1965) 2008. *Knowledge of Life*. 3rd ed. Fordham University Press.

———. (1943) 1991. *The Normal and the Pathological*. Zone Books.

Carlson, Tucker. 2012. "Eugenics, American Style." *Slate*, February 21.

Carolina, I., N. Geddes, J. Sibbald, S. A. Larkins, and E. V. Davison. 2005. "The Emerging 22q11 Duplication Syndrome: Two Familial Cases." *Journal of Medical Genetics* 42:S87.

Carter, C. O., J. L. Hamerton, P. E. Polani, A. Gunalp, and S. D. Weller. 1960. "Chromosome Translocation as a Cause of Familial Mongolism." *Lancet* 2(7152):678–80.

Caspi, Avshalom, et al. 2002. "Role of Genotype in the Cycle of Violence in Maltreated Children." *Science* 297(5582):851–54.

Check Hayden, Erika. 2008. "Biological Tools Revamp Disease Classification." *Nature* 453(7196):709.

———. 2012. "Fetal Tests Spur Legal Battle." *Nature* 486(7404):454.

———. 2013a. "Data Barriers Limit Genetic Diagnosis: Tools for Data-Sharing Promise to Improve Chances of Connecting Mutations with Symptoms of Rare Diseases." *Nature* 494(7436):156–58.

———. 2013b. "Geneticists Push for Global Data-Sharing: International Organization Aims to Promote Exchange and Linking of DNA Sequences and Clinical Information." *Nature* 498(7452):16–18.

———. 2014. "Prenatal-Screening Companies Expand Scope of DNA Tests." *Nature* 507(7490):19.

Chedd, Graham. 2001. "Growing Up Different." *Scientific American Frontiers*. PBS television series.

Chen, Dong-Hui, et al. 2015. "*ADCY5*-Related Dyskinesia Broader Spectrum and Genotype–Phenotype Correlations." *Neurology* 85(23):2026–35.

Chen, Ying-Zhang, et al. 2012. "Autosomal Dominant Familial Dyskinesia and Facial Myokymia: Single Exome Sequencing Identifies a Mutation in Adenylyl Cyclase 5." *Archives of Neurology* 69(5):630–35.

———. 2014. "Gain-of-Function *ADCY5* Mutations in Familial Dyskinesia with Facial Myokymia." *Annals of Neurology* 75(4):542–49.

Chiurazzi, Pietro, Charles E. Schwartz, Jozef Gecz, and Giovanni Neri. 2008. "XLMR Genes: Update 2007." *European Journal of Human Genetics* 16(4):422–34.

"Chromosome Precedent in Trials Is Disputed." 1969. *Washington Post*, February 3, A10.

Clarke, Adele E., Janet K. Shim, Laura Mamo, Jennifer Ruth Fosket, and Jennifer R. Fishman. 2003. "Biomedicalization: Technoscientific Transformations of Health, Illness, and U.S. Biomedicine." *American Sociological Review* 68(2):161–94.

Clifford, Sally, et al. 2007. "Autism Spectrum Phenotype in Males and Females with Fragile X Full Mutation and Premutation." *Journal of Autism and Developmental Disorders* 37(4):738–47.

Cody, Jannine. 2009. "Reply to Letter from Drs. Ledbetter, Saul, and Moeschler." *Genetics in Medicine* 11(9):682–83.

Cohen, David, et al. 2005. "Specific Genetic Disorders and Autism: Clinical Contribution towards Their Identification." *Journal of Autism and Developmental Disorders* 35(1):103–16.

Cohen, I. L., et al. 1991. "Why Are Autism and the Fragile-X Syndrome Associated? Conceptual and Methodological Issues." *American Journal of Human Genetics* 48(2):195–202.

Cohn, Victor. 1968. "A Criminal by Heredity? Testing for 'Criminal Heredity' Urged by Three Geneticists." *Washington Post, Times Herald*, August 7, A1.

Collier, J. G. 1966. "The YY Syndrome." *Lancet* 287(7445):1036.

Collins, Francis S., Eric D. Green, Alan E. Guttmacher, and Mark S. Guyer. 2003. "A Vision for the Future of Genomics Research." *Nature* 422(6934):835–47.

Colvert, Emma, Beata Tick, Fiona McEwan, Catherine Stewart, et al. 2015. "Heritability of Autism Spectrum Disorder in a UK Population-Based Twin Sample." *JAMA Psychiatry.*

Colvin, Arlie. 2014. *Jack and His Extra Y.* Amazon CreateSpace.

Comfort, Nathaniel. 2013. "Is Individuality the Savior of Eugenics?" Guest blog, *Scientific American,* August 23. http://blogs.scientificamerican.com/guest-blog/2013/08/23/is-individuality-the-savior-of-eugenics/.

———. 2014. *The Science of Human Perfection: How Genes Became the Heart of American Medicine.* Reprint ed. Yale University Press.

Condit, Celeste M. 2010. "Public Attitudes and Beliefs about Genetics." *Annual Review of Genomics and Human Genetics* 11:339–59.

"Congenital Criminals?" 1970. *Newsweek,* May 18, 98–99.

Conley, Dalton, and Emily Rauscher. 2013. "Genetic Interactions with Prenatal Social Environment: Effects on Academic and Behavioral Outcomes." *Journal of Health and Social Behavior* 54(1):109–27.

Conrad, Peter. 1975. "The Discovery of Hyperkinesis: Notes on the Medicalization of Deviant Behavior." *Social Problems* 23(1):12–21.

———. 1992. "Medicalization and Social Control." *Annual Review of Sociology* 18:209–32.

———. 2007. *The Medicalization of Society: On the Transformation of Human Conditions into Treatable Disorders.* Johns Hopkins University Press.

Conway, Gerard S., Shyamani Hettiarachchi, Anna Murray, and Patricia A. Jacobs. 1995. "Fragile X Premutations in Familial Premature Ovarian Failure." *Lancet* 346(8970):309–10.

Cordeiro, Lisa, Nicole Tartaglia, David Roeltgen, and Judith Ross. 2012. "Social Deficits in Male Children and Adolescents with Sex Chromosome Aneuploidy: A Comparison of XXY, XYY, and XXYY Syndromes." *Research in Developmental Disabilities* 33(4):1254–63.

Costain, G., E., W. C. Chow, P. N. Ray, and A. S. Bassett. 2012. "Caregiver and Adult Patient Perspectives on the Importance of a Diagnosis of 22q11.2 Deletion Syndrome." *Journal of Intellectual Disability Research* 56(6):641–51.

Costales, Jesse L., and Alexander Kolevzon. 2015. "Phelan–McDermid Syndrome and *SHANK3*: Implications for Treatment." *Neurotherapeutics* 12(3):620–30.

Court Brown, W. M. 1968. "Males with an XYY Sex Chromosome Complement." *Journal of Medical Genetics* 5(4):341–59.

Court Brown, W. M., W. H. Price, and P. A. Jacobs. 1968. "The XYY Male." *British Medical Journal* 4(5629):513.

Court Brown, W. M., et al. 1964. *Abnormalities of the Sex Chromosome Complement in Man : Privy Council Medical Research Council Special Report Series No. 305.* Her Majesty's Stationery Office.

Courtens, Winnie, Inge Schramme, and Annick Laridon. 2008. "Microduplication 22q11.2: A Benign Polymorphism or a Syndrome with a Very Large

Clinical Variability and Reduced Penetrance?—Report of Two Families." *American Journal of Medical Genetics, Part A* 146A(6):758–63.

Crampton, Peter, and Chris Parkin. 2007. "Warrior Genes and Risk-Taking Science." *New Zealand Medical Journal* 120(1250):U2439.

Crane, Diana. 1969. "Social Structure in a Group of Scientists: A Test of the 'Invisible College' Hypothesis." *American Sociological Review* 34(3):335–52.

Crawford, Dana C., Juan M. Acuña, and Stephanie L. Sherman. 2001. "*FMR1* and the Fragile X Syndrome: Human Genome Epidemiology Review." *Genetics in Medicine* 3(5):359–71.

"Criminal Law: Question of Y." 1968. *Time*, October 25, 76.

Culliton, Barbara J. 1975. "XYY: Harvard Researcher under Fire Stops Newborn Screening." *Science* 188(4195):1284–85.

D'Angelo, Carla S., et al. 2010. "Extending the Phenotype of Monosomy 1p36 Syndrome and Mapping of a Critical Region for Obesity and Hyperphagia." *American Journal of Medical Genetics, Part A* 152A(1):102–10.

Daston, Lorraine J., and Peter Galison. 2010. *Objectivity*. Zone Books.

Davies, Gail. 2010. "Captivating Behaviour: Mouse Models, Experimental Genetics and Reductionist Returns in the Neurosciences." *Sociological Review* 58(s1):53–72.

Davies, J., A. Jaffé, and A. Bush. 1998. "Distal 10q Trisomy Syndrome with Unusual Cardiac and Pulmonary Abnormalities." *Journal of Medical Genetics* 35(1):72–74.

Day, Philip, dir. 2010. "Born to Rage?" *National Geographic Explorer*, season 25, episode 4.

De Caro, John J., Celia Dominguez, and Stephanie L. Sherman. 2008. "Reproductive Health of Adolescent Girls Who Carry the *FMR1* Premutation." *Annals of the New York Academy of Sciences* 1135(1):99–111.

de Grouchy, J., J. Bonnette, and C. Salmon. 1966. "[Deletion of the Short Arm of Chromosome 18]." *Annales de Génétique* 9(1):19–26.

de Grouchy, J., M. Lamy, S. Thieffry, M. Arthuis, and C. H. Salmon. 1963. "Dysmorphie complexe avec oligophrénie: Délétion des bras courts d'un chromosome 17–18." *Comptes rendus de l'Académie des Sciences* (Paris) 258:1028–29.

de Grouchy, J., A. Rossier, and N. Joab. 1967. "Une nouvelle observation d'abberation chromosome 18p–" [A New Observation of Chromosome Aberrations 18p]. *Annales de Génétique* 10(4):221–23.

de Grouchy, J., and Catherine Turleau. 1977. *Clinical Atlas of Human Chromosomes*. Wiley.

de la Chapelle, A., R. Herva, M. Koivisto, and P. Aula. 1981. "A Deletion in Chromosome 22 Can Cause DiGeorge Syndrome." *Human Genetics* 57(3):253–56.

Della Cava, Marco R. 2010. "Henry Rollins, 'Born to Rage' Hunt Anger's Genetic Roots." *USA Today*, December 13. Available at http://www.usatoday.com/life/television/news/2010-12-14-ragetv14_ST_N.htm.

Delude, Cathryn M. 2015. "Deep Phenotyping: The Details of Disease." *Nature* 527(7576):S14–15.

DeMyer, Dr. Marian K., et al. 1974. "The Measured Intelligence of Autistic Children." *Journal of Autism and Childhood Schizophrenia* 4(1):42–60.

Dershowitz, Alan M. 2007. *Preemption: A Knife That Cuts Both Ways.* W. W. Norton.

de Saussure, Ferdinand. 2011. *Course in General Linguistics.* Columbia University Press.

Devlin, L., and P. J. Morrison. 2004. "Accuracy of the Clinical Diagnosis of Down Syndrome." *Ulster Medical Journal* 73(1):4–12.

Dhar, S. U., et al. 2010. "22q13.3 Deletion Syndrome: Clinical and Molecular Analysis Using Array CGH." *American Journal of Medical Genetics, Part A* 152A(3):573–81.

DiGeorge, A. M. 1968. "Congenital Absence of the Thymus and Its Immunologic Consequences: Concurrence with Congenital Hypoparathyroidism." *Birth Defects* 4(1):116–21.

Dixon, Darrin P. 2008. "Informed Consent or Institutionalized Eugenics? How the Medical Profession Encourages Abortion of Fetuses with Down Syndrome." *Issues in Law & Medicine* 24(1):3–59.

Dobbs, David. 2007. "The Gregarious Brain." *New York Times*, July 8. Available at http://www.nytimes.com/2007/07/08/magazine/08sociability-t.html?_r=2&pagewanted=all.

Dolan, Michelle, et al. 2010. "A Novel Microdeletion/Microduplication Syndrome of 19p13.13." *Genetics in Medicine* 12(8):503–11.

Donnai, D., and A. Karmiloff-Smith. 2000. "Williams Syndrome: From Genotype through to the Cognitive Phenotype." *American Journal of Medical Genetics* 97(2):164–71.

Down, John Langdon. 1866. "Observations on an Ethnic Classification of Idiots." *London Hospital Reports* 3:259–62.

Drew, Liam J., et al. 2011. "The 22q11.2 Microdeletion: Fifteen Years of Insights into the Genetic and Neural Complexity of Psychiatric Disorders." *International Journal of Developmental Neuroscience* 29(3):259–81.

Driscoll, Deborah A., et al. 1992. "Deletions and Microdeletions of 22q11.2 in Velo-Cardio-Facial Syndrome." *American Journal of Medical Genetics* 44(2):261–68.

Dumars, K. W., C. Gaskill, and N. Kitzmiller. 1964. "Le Cri du Chat (Crying Cat) Syndrome." *American Journal of Diseases of Children* 108:533–37.

Dupont, Céline, et al. 2015. "Prenatal Diagnosis of 24 Cases of Microduplication 22q11.2: An Investigation of Phenotype-Genotype Correlations." *Prenatal Diagnosis* 35(1):35–43.

Durkheim, Émile. (1912) 2001. *The Elementary Forms of Religious Life.* Oxford University Press.

Duster, Troy. (1990) 2003. *Backdoor to Eugenics.* 2nd ed. Routledge.

Edelmann, L., et al. 1999. "A Common Molecular Basis for Rearrangement Disorders on Chromosome 22q11." *Human Molecular Genetics* 8(7):1157–67.

Edwards, Jim. 2011. "Death of an Insider: R&D Chief Passes Before She Can Testify in Stock Fraud Case." CBS News, March 25. http://www.cbsnews.com/8301-505123_162-42847754/death-of-an-insider-rd-chief-passes-before-she-can-testify-in-stock-fraud-case/.

Edwards, Jim, D. G. Harnden, A. H. Cameron, V. M. Crosse, and O. H. Wolff. 1960. "A New Trisomic Syndrome." *Lancet* 1(7128):787–90.

Einfeld, Stewart, Helen Molony, and Wayne Hall. 1989. "Autism Is Not Associated with the Fragile X Syndrome." *American Journal of Medical Genetics* 34(2):187–93.

Einfeld, Stewart, Bruce J. Tonge, and Vaughan W. Rees. 2001. "Longitudinal Course of Behavioral and Emotional Problems in Williams Syndrome." *American Journal on Mental Retardation* 106(1):73–81.

Elghezal, Hatem, et al. 2007. "Ring Chromosome 20 Syndrome without Deletions of the Subtelomeric and CHRNA4–KCNQ2 Genes Loci." *European Journal of Medical Genetics* 50(6):441–45.

Ellis, J. R., O. J. Miller, L. S. Penrose, and G. E. B. Scott. 1961. "A Male with XXYY Chromosomes." *Annals of Human Genetics* 25(2):145–51.

Enns, Gregory M., et al. 2014. "Mutations in *NGLY1* Cause an Inherited Disorder of the Endoplasmic Reticulum-Associated Degradation Pathway." *Genetics in Medicine* 16(10):751–58.

Ensenauer, Regina E., et al. 2003. "Microduplication 22q11.2, an Emerging Syndrome: Clinical, Cytogenetic, and Molecular Analysis of Thirteen Patients." *American Journal of Human Genetics* 73(5):1027–40.

Entine, Jon. 2013. "DNA Screening Is Part of the New Eugenics—and That's Okay." *Genetic Literacy Project*, July 8. http://www.geneticliteracyproject.org/2013/07/08/dna-screening-is-part-of-the-new-eugenics-and-thats-okay/#.UyDTSFFdUdD.

Epstein, Charles J. 2002. "From Down Syndrome to the 'Human' in 'Human Genetics.'" *American Journal of Human Genetics* 70(2):300–313.

Epstein, Steven. 1995. "The Construction of Lay Expertise: AIDS Activism and the Forging of Credibility in the Reform of Clinical Trials." *Science, Technology & Human Values* 20(4):408–37.

———. 1996. *Impure Science: AIDS, Activism, and the Politics of Knowledge*. University of California Press.

———. 2007a. *Inclusion: The Politics of Difference in Medical Research*. University of Chicago Press.

———. 2007b. "Patient Groups and Health Movements." In *The Handbook of Science and Technology Studies*, edited by E. J. Hackett, O. Amsterdamska, M. E. Lynch, and J. Wajcman, 499–539. MIT Press.

———. 2016. "The Politics of Health Mobilization in the United States: The Promise and Pitfalls of 'Disease Constituencies.'" *Social Science & Medicine* 165:246–54.

Eyal, Gil. 2013. "For a Sociology of Expertise: The Social Origins of the Autism Epidemic." *American Journal of Sociology* 118(4):863–907.

Eyal, Gil, B. Hart, E. Onculer, N. Oren, and N. Rossi. 2010. *The Autism Matrix*. Polity.

Family Tree DNA. 2010. "The Warrior Gene." http://thewarriorgene.com/The WarriorGene.html.

Fan, H. Christina, and Stephen R. Quake. 2010. "Noninvasive Diagnosis of Fetal Aneuploidy by Sequencing." US Patent no. 20100138165.

Fan, H. Christina, et al. 2012. "Non-invasive Prenatal Measurement of the Fetal Genome." *Nature* 487(7407):320–24.

Fang, J. S., et al. 2008. "Cytogenetic and Molecular Characterization of a Three-Generation Family with Chromosome 5p Terminal Deletion." *Clinical Genetics* 73(6):585–90.

Featherstone, Katie, and Paul Atkinson. 2011. *Creating Conditions: The Making and Remaking of a Genetic Syndrome*. Routledge.

Feenstra, Ilse, et al. 2007. "Genotype-Phenotype Mapping of Chromosome 18q Deletions by High-Resolution Array CGH: An Update of the Phenotypic Map." *American Journal of Medical Genetics, Part A* 143A(16):1858–67.

Feinstein, Adam. 2010. *A History of Autism: Conversations with the Pioneers*. John Wiley & Sons.

Feinstein, Carl. 2009. "Stranded, Part II." *Journal of the American Academy of Child and Adolescent Psychiatry* 48(11):1049–50.

Fernandez, Magali, et al. 2001. "Familial Dyskinesia and Facial Myokymia (FDFM): A Novel Movement Disorder." *Annals of Neurology* 49(4):486–92.

Ferreira, Carlos R., Clara D. M. van Karnebeek, Jerry Vockley, and Nenad Blau. 2018. "A Proposed Nosology of Inborn Errors of Metabolism." *Genetics in Medicine*. https://doi.org/10.1038/s41436-018-0022-8.

Fincher, David, dir. 1992. *Alien 3*. Twentieth Century Fox.

Finucane, Brenda, Thomas D. Challman, Christa Lese Martin, and David H. Ledbetter. 2016. "Shift Happens: Family Background Influences Clinical Variability in Genetic Neurodevelopmental Disorders." *Genetics in Medicine* 18(4):302–4.

Finucane, Brenda, Barbara Haas-Givler, and Elliott W. Simon. 2003. "Genetics, Mental Retardation, and the Forging of New Alliances." *American Journal of Medical Genetics, Part C* 117C(1):66–72.

Finucane, Brenda, Deborah Konar, Barbara Haas-Givler, Michael B. Kurtt, and Charles I. Scott Jr. 1994. "The Spasmodic Upper-body Squeeze: A Characteristic Behavior in Smith-Magenis Syndrome." *Developmental Medicine and Child Neurology* 36(1):78–83.

Firth, Helen V. 2013. "22q11.2 Duplication." In *GeneReviews*. University of Washington, Seattle.

Fischbach, Gerald. 2007. "Summary of Simons Foundation Autism Research Initiative." Presented at the US Department of Health and Human Services Interagency Autism Coordinating Committee, full committee meeting, November 30, Washington, DC.

Fleck, Ludwik. (1935) 1981. *Genesis and Development of a Scientific Fact.* University of Chicago Press.

Folstein, Susan. 1996. "Twin and Adoption Studies in Child and Adolescent Psychiatric Disorders." *Current Opinion in Pediatrics* 8(4):339–47.

Folstein, Susan, and Beth Rosen-Sheidley. 2001. "Genetics of Autism: Complex Aetiology for a Heterogeneous Disorder." *Nature Reviews Genetics* 2(12):943–55.

Folstein, Susan, and Michael Rutter. 1977a. "Genetic Influences and Infantile Autism." *Nature* 265(5596):726–28.

———. 1977b. "Infantile Autism: A Genetic Study of 21 Twin Pairs." *Journal of Child Psychology and Psychiatry* 18(4):297–321.

Ford, C. E., K. W. Jones, P. E. Polani, J. C. De Almeida, and J. H. Briggs. 1959. "A Sex-Chromosome Anomaly in a Case of Gonadal Dysgenesis (Turner's Syndrome)." *Lancet* 273(7075):711–13.

Foucault, Michel. 1973. *The Birth of the Clinic: An Archaeology of Medical Perception.* Pantheon Books.

———. 1977. "The Confession of the Flesh." In *Power/Knowledge: Selected Interviews and Other Writings, 1972–1977*, edited by C. Gordon, 194–228. Pantheon Books.

———. 1990a. *Politics, Philosophy, Culture: Interviews and Other Writings, 1977–1984.* Psychology Press.

———. 1990b. *The History of Sexuality.* Vol. 1. *An Introduction.* Vintage.

———. 2002. *Archaeology of Knowledge.* Routledge.

———. 2003. *"Society Must Be Defended": Lectures at the Collège de France, 1975–1976.* Reprint. Picador.

———. 2009. *Security, Territory, Population: Lectures at the Collège de France 1977–1978.* Edited by M. Senellart. Picador.

———. 2010. *The Birth of Biopolitics: Lectures at the Collège de France, 1978–1979.* Reprint. Picador.

Fox, Richard G. 1969. "XYY Chromosomes and Crime." *Australian & New Zealand Journal of Criminology* 2(1):5–19.

Franzke, A. W. 1975. "Letter: Telling Parents about XYY Sons." *New England Journal of Medicine* 293(2):100–101.

Freese, Jeremy, and Sara Shostak. 2009. "Genetics and Social Inquiry." *Annual Review of Sociology* 35(1):107–28.

Frith, Uta. 2003. *Autism: Explaining the Enigma.* Wiley-Blackwell.

Fujimura, Joan H., Troy Duster, and Ramya Rajagopalan. 2008. "Introduction: Race, Genetics, and Disease Questions of Evidence, Matters of Consequence." *Social Studies of Science* 38(5):643–56.

Fullwiley, Duana. 2011. *The Encultured Gene: Sickle Cell Health Politics and Biological Difference in West Africa.* Princeton University Press.

Gajecka, Marzena, Katherine L. Mackay, and Lisa G. Shaffer. 2007. "Monosomy 1p36 Deletion Syndrome." *American Journal of Medical Genetics, Part C* 145C(4):346–56.

Galasso, Cinzia, et al. 2008. "Deletion 2q37: An Identifiable Clinical Syndrome with Mental Retardation and Autism." *Journal of Child Neurology* 23(7):802–6.

Galison, Peter. 1997. *Image and Logic: A Material Culture of Microphysics*. University of Chicago Press.

Garrison, Lloyd. 1968. "French Murder Jury Rejects Chromosome Defect as Defense." *New York Times*, October 15.

Gawde, H., et al. 2006. "Chromosome 22 Microdeletion by F.I.S.H. in Isolated Congenital Heart Disease." *Indian Journal of Pediatrics* 73(10):885–88.

Geerts, M., J. Steyaert, and J. P. Fryns. 2003. "The XYY Syndrome: A Follow-up Study on 38 Boys." *Genetic Counseling* 14(3):267–79.

"Genetics: Of Chromosomes & Crime." 1968. *Time*, May 3.

Geschwind, Daniel H. 2008. "Autism: Many Genes, Common Pathways?" *Cell* 135(3):391–95.

Gibbons, Ann. 2004. "Tracking the Evolutionary History of a 'Warrior' Gene." *Science* 304(5672):818.

Gieryn, Thomas F. 1983. "Boundary-Work and the Demarcation of Science from Non-Science: Strains and Interests in Professional Ideologies of Scientists." *American Sociological Review* 48(6):781–95.

Giles, Annabel. 2008. "The XYY Factor: How a Rare Chromosome Disorder Brought My Son a World of Pain." *Daily Mail*, November 1.

Gillberg, Christopher. 1983. "Identical Triplets with Infantile-Autism and the Fragile-X Syndrome." *British Journal of Psychiatry* 143(September):256–60.

———. 1998. "Chromosomal Disorders and Autism." *Journal of Autism and Developmental Disorders* 28(5):415–25.

Gillberg, Christopher, Inger Winnergard, and Jan Wahlström. 1984. "The Sex Chromosomes: One Key to Autism? An XYY Case of Infantile Autism." *Applied Research in Mental Retardation* 5(3):353–60.

Glass, B. 1971. "Science: Endless Horizons or Golden Age?" *Science* 171(3966):23–29.

Goh, Kwang-Il, et al. 2007. "The Human Disease Network." *Proceedings of the National Academy of Sciences* 104(21):8685–90.

Goizet, C., et al. 2000. "Case with Autistic Syndrome and Chromosome 22q13.3 Deletion Detected by FISH." *American Journal of Medical Genetics* 96(6):839–44.

Goldberg, R., R. Marion, M. Borderon, A. Wiznia, and R. J. Shprintzen. 1985. "Phenotypic Overlap between Velo-Cardio-Facial Syndrome and DiGeorge Sequence." *American Journal of Human Genetics* 37(supp.):A54.

Goldsmith, Jonathan C., et al. 2012. "Framing the Research Agenda for Sickle Cell Trait: Building on the Current Understanding of Clinical Events and Their Potential Implications." *American Journal of Hematology* 87(3):340–46.

Goodrich-Hunsaker, Naomi J., et al. 2011. "Young Adult Female Fragile X Premutation Carriers Show Age- and Genetically-Modulated Cognitive Impairments." *Brain and Cognition* 75(3):255–60.

Gottesman, Irving I., and Todd D. Gould. 2003. "The Endophenotype Concept in Psychiatry: Etymology and Strategic Intentions." *American Journal of Psychiatry* 160(4):636–45.

Gottesman, Irving I., and James Shields. 1972. *Schizophrenia and Genetics: A Twin Study Vantage Point*. Academic Press.

Gould, Stephen Jay. 1996. *The Mismeasure of Man*. W. W. Norton.

Gozes, Illana, et al. 2015. "The Compassionate Side of Neuroscience: Tony Sermone's Undiagnosed Genetic Journey—ADNP Mutation." *Journal of Molecular Neuroscience* 56(4):751–57.

Grati, Francesca Romana, et al. 2015. "Prevalence of Recurrent Pathogenic Microdeletions and Microduplications in over 9500 Pregnancies." *Prenatal Diagnosis* 35(8):801–9.

Green, Robert C., et al. 2013. "ACMG Recommendations for Reporting of Incidental Findings in Clinical Exome and Genome Sequencing." *Genetics in Medicine* 15(7):565–74.

Greenberg, F., et al. 1984. "Familial DiGeorge Syndrome and Associated Partial Monosomy of Chromosome 22." *Human Genetics* 65(4):317–19.

Gregg, Anthony R., et al. 2016. "Noninvasive Prenatal Screening for Fetal Aneuploidy, 2016 Update: A Position Statement of the American College of Medical Genetics and Genomics." *Genetics in Medicine* 18(10):1056–65.

Griffiths, Dorothy, and Robert King. 2004. *Demystifying Syndromes: Clinical and Educational Implications of Common Syndromes Associated with Persons with Intellectual Disabilities*. National Association for the Dually Diagnosed.

Grinker, Roy Richard. 2008. *Unstrange Minds: Remapping the World of Autism*. Basic Books.

Grisart, B., et al. 2009. "17q21.31 Microduplication Patients Are Characterised by Behavioural Problems and Poor Social Interaction." *Journal of Medical Genetics* 46(8):524–30.

Gropman, Andrea L., Wallace C. Duncan, and Ann C. M. Smith. 2006. "Neurologic and Developmental Features of the Smith-Magenis Syndrome (Del 17p11.2)." *Pediatric Neurology* 34(5):337–50.

Gu, Yanghong, Ying Shen, Richard A. Gibbs, and David L. Nelson. 1996. "Identification of *FMR2*, a Novel Gene Associated with the *FRAXE* CCG Repeat and CpG Island." *Nature Genetics* 13(1):109–13.

Guo, Guang, Xiao-Ming Ou, Michael Roettger, and Jean C. Shih. 2008. "The VNTR 2 Repeat in *MAOA* and Delinquent Behavior in Adolescence and Young Adulthood: Associations and *MAOA* Promoter Activity." *European Journal of Human Genetics* 16(5):626–34.

Gustavson, K. H., W. Arancibia, U. Eriksson, and L. Svennerholm. 1986. "Deleted Ring Chromosome 22 in a Mentally Retarded Boy." *Clinical Genetics* 29(4):337–41.

Guzman, Maria Luisa, et al. 2012. "Growth in Chilean Infants with Chromosome 22q11 Microdeletion Syndrome." *American Journal of Medical Genetics, Part A* 158A(11):2682–86.

Habel, Alex, Michael-John McGinn, Elaine H. Zackai, Nancy Unanue, and Donna M. McDonald-McGinn. 2012. "Syndrome-Specific Growth Charts for 22q11.2 Deletion Syndrome in Caucasian Children." *American Journal of Medical Genetics, Part A* 158A(11):2665–71.

Haberstick, Brett C. et al. 2014. "*MAOA* Genotype, Childhood Maltreatment, and Their Interaction in the Etiology of Adult Antisocial Behaviors." *Biological Psychiatry* 75(1):25–30.

Hacking, Ian. 1995. "The Looping Effects of Human Kinds." In *Causal Cognition: A Multidisciplinary Debate*, Symposia of the Fyssen Foundation, edited by D. Sperber, D. Premack, and A. J. Premack, 351–94. Oxford University Press.

———. 1998a. *Mad Travelers: Reflections on the Reality of Transient Mental Illnesses*. University of Virginia Press.

———. (1995) 1998b. *Rewriting the Soul*. Princeton University Press.

———. 2006a. "Genetics, Biosocial Groups and the Future of Identity." *Daedalus* 135(4):81–95.

———. 2006b. "What Is Tom Saying to Maureen?" *London Review of Books*, May 11, 3–7.

———. 2007. "Kinds of People: Moving Targets." *Proceedings of the British Academy* 51:285–318.

Hagerman, Paul J., and Randi J. Hagerman. 2004. "Fragile X–Associated Tremor/Ataxia Syndrome (FXTAS)." *Mental Retardation and Developmental Disabilities Research Reviews* 10(1):25–30.

Hagerman, Randi Jenssen. 1999. *Neurodevelopmental Disorders: Diagnosis and Treatment*. Oxford University Press.

Hagerman, Randi Jenssen, and A. W. Jackson. 1985. "Autism or Fragile-X Syndrome." *Journal of the American Academy of Child and Adolescent Psychiatry* 24(2):239–40.

Hagerman, Randi Jenssen, et al. 1986. "An Analysis of Autism in Fifty Males with the Fragile X Syndrome." *American Journal of Medical Genetics* 23(1–2):359–74.

———. 2001. "Intention Tremor, Parkinsonism, and Generalized Brain Atrophy in Male Carriers of Fragile X." *Neurology* 57(1):127–30.

Halder, Ashutosh, Manish Jain, Isha Chaudhary, and Madhulika Kabra. 2010. "Prevalence of 22q11.2 Microdeletion in 146 Patients with Cardiac Malformation in a Referral Hospital of North India." *BioMedCentral Medical Genetics* 11:101.

Hall, J. G. 1993. "CATCH 22." *Journal of Medical Genetics* 30(10):801–2.

Hamamy, Hanan A., and Sophie Dahoun. 2004. "Parental Decisions Following the Prenatal Diagnosis of Sex Chromosome Abnormalities." *European Journal of Obstetrics & Gynecology and Reproductive Biology* 116(1):58–62.

Hamerton, John L. 1963. *Chromosomes in Medicine*. Medical Advisory Committee of the National Spastics Society, in Association with Wm. Heinemann (Medical Books).

———. 1971. *Human Cytogenetics: Clinical Cytogenetics*. Academic Press.

———. 1976. "Human Population Cytogenetics: Dilemmas and Problems." *American Journal of Human Genetics* 28(2):107–22.

Hammond, Peter. 2007. "The Use of 3D Face Shape Modelling in Dysmorphology." *Archives of Disease in Childhood* 92(12):1120–26.

Hansen, Bent Sigurd. 2005. "Something Rotten in the State of Denmark: Eugenics and the Ascent of the Welfare State." In *Eugenics and the Welfare State: Sterilization Policy in Demark, Sweden, Norway, and Finland*, edited by G. Broberg and N. Roll-Hansen, 9–76. Michigan State University Press.

Harel, T., and J. R. Lupski. 2018. "Genomic Disorders 20 Years on— Mechanisms for Clinical Manifestations." *Clinical Genetics* 93(3):439–49.

Harmon, Amy. 2007a. "After DNA Diagnosis: 'Hello, 16p11.2. Are You Just Like Me?'" *New York Times*, December 28.

———. 2007b. "Prenatal Test Puts Down Syndrome in Hard Focus." *New York Times*, May 9.

Harper, Peter. 2006. *First Years of Human Chromosomes: The Beginnings of Human Cytogenetics*. Scion.

Harris, James C. 2017. "Understanding Psychiatric Disorders in People with 22q11.2 Deletion and Duplication." *JAMA Psychiatry* 74(3):290–92.

Hassed, S. J., D. Hopcus-Niccum, L. Zhang, S. Li, and J. J. Mulvihill. 2004. "A New Genomic Duplication Syndrome Complementary to the Velocardio-facial (22q11 Deletion) Syndrome." *Clinical Genetics* 65(5):400–404.

Hauge, Xueya, et al. 2008. "Detailed Characterization of, and Clinical Correlations in, 10 Patients with Distal Deletions of Chromosome 9p." *Genetics in Medicine* 10(8):599–611.

Hauschka, T. S., A. A. Sandberg, M. N. Goldstein, J. E. Hasson, and G. F. Koepf. 1962. "An XYY Man with Progeny Indicating Familial Tendency to Non-Disjunction." *American Journal of Human Genetics* 14(1):22–30.

Haydu, Jeffrey. 1998. "Making Use of the Past: Time Periods as Cases to Compare and as Sequences of Problem Solving." *American Journal of Sociology* 104(2):339–71.

Heath, Deborah, Rayna Rapp, and Karen-Sue Taussig. 2004. "Genetic Citizenship." In *A Companion to the Anthropology of Politics*, edited by D. Nugent and J. Vincent, 152–67. Blackwell.

Hedgecoe, Adam M. 1998. "Geneticization, Medicalisation and Polemics." *Medicine, Health Care and Philosophy* 1(3):235–43.

———. 2000. "The Popularization of Genetics as Geneticization." *Public Understanding of Science* 9(2):183.

———. 2001. "Schizophrenia and the Narrative of Enlightened Geneticization." *Social Studies of Science* 31(6):875–911.

———. 2003. "Expansion and Uncertainty: Cystic Fibrosis, Classification and Genetics." *Sociology of Health & Illness* 25(1):50–70.

Heger, Monica. 2013. "Facing Increased Competition, Sequenom Sees Continued Growth of MaterniT21 Test in Q4 2012." GenomeWeb, March 13.

http://www.genomeweb.com/sequencing/facing-increased-competition -sequenom-sees-continued-growth-maternit21-test-q4-2.

———. 2014. "Sequenom Eyes Low-Risk NIPT Market; Inks Contract with Aetna." GenomeWeb, March 5. http://www.genomeweb.com/sequencing/ sequenom-eyes-low-risk-nipt-market-inks-contract-aetna.

———. 2017. "Natera Moves beyond Chromosomal Aneuploidy to Screen Non-invasively for De Novo Single Gene Mutations." GenomeWeb, May 10. https://www.genomeweb.com/molecular-diagnostics/natera-moves -beyond-chromosomal-aneuploidy-screen-noninvasively-de-novo-single.

Helsmoortel, Céline, et al. 2014. "A SWI/SNF-Related Autism Syndrome Caused by *De Novo* Mutations in *ADNP.*" *Nature Genetics* 46(4):380–84.

Henderson, Lindsay B., et al. 2014. "The Impact of Chromosomal Microarray on Clinical Management: A Retrospective Analysis." *Genetics in Medicine* 16(9):657–64.

Herva, R., I. Saarinen, and L. Leikkonen. 1977. "The r(20) Syndrome." *Journal of Medical Genetics* 14(4):281–83.

Hilts, Philip J. 1992. "U.S. Puts a Halt to Talks Tying Genes to Crime." *New York Times*, September 5.

Hinkel, G. K., et al. 1997. "Overgrowth and Retarded Development Associated with Chromosome 22q13 Deletion." *Monatsschrift Kinderheilkunde* 145(9):892–96.

Hogan, Andrew J. 2016. *Life Histories of Genetic Disease: Patterns and Prevention in Postwar Medical Genetics*. Johns Hopkins University Press.

Hogart, A., et al. 2009. "Chromosome 15q11–13 Duplication Syndrome: Brain Reveals Epigenetic Alterations in Gene Expression Not Predicted from Copy Number." *Journal of Medical Genetics* 46(2):86–93.

Hollmer, Mark. 2014. "Sequenom Counts on Prenatal Test Growth to Reverse Its Fortunes." FierceDiagnostics, March 3. https://web.archive.org/web/ 20150314204217/http://www.fiercediagnostics.com/story/sequenom -counts-prenatal-test-growth-reverse-its-fortunes/2014-03-03.

Hook, E. B., and D. M. Schreinemachers. 1983. "Trends in Utilization of Prenatal Cytogenetic Diagnosis by New York State Residents in 1979 and 1980." *American Journal of Public Health* 73(2):198–202.

Horgan, John. 2011. "Born Outlaws? A Criminally Feeble Proposition." *Chronicle of Higher Education*, July 17.

Horwitz, Allan V. 2002. *Creating Mental Illness*. University of Chicago Press.

Hsu, T. C. 1979. *Human and Mammalian Cytogenetics: An Historical Perspective*. Springer Science & Business Media.

Hughes, Susan Starling, Stephanie Fiedler, Lei Zhang, and Alison Kaye. 2016. "22Q11.2 Duplication Syndrome: Guiding Medical Management." *Cleft Palate-Craniofacial Journal* 53(4):E126.

Huynh, Minh-Tuan, et al. 2018. "A Heterozygous Microdeletion of 20q13.13 Encompassing *ADNP* Gene in a Child with Helsmoortel–van Der Aa Syndrome." *European Journal of Human Genetics* 26(10):1497–1501.

Illumina. 2017. "Illumina Introduces the NovaSeq Series." Press release, January 9. https://www.illumina.com/company/news-center/press-releases/press-release-details.html?newsid=2236383.

Insel, Thomas. 2013. "Transforming Diagnosis." *NIMH Director's Blog*, April 29. http://www.nimh.nih.gov/about/director/2013/transforming-diagnosis.shtml.

Insel, Thomas, and Bruce N. Cuthbert. 2009. "Endophenotypes: Bridging Genomic Complexity and Disorder Heterogeneity." *Biological Psychiatry* 66(11):988–89.

Jacob, François. (1973) 1993. *The Logic of Life*. New edition. Princeton University Press.

Jacobs, Patricia A. 1982. "The William Allan Memorial Award Address: Human Population Cytogenetics: The First Twenty-Five Years." *American Journal of Human Genetics* 34(5):689–98.

Jacobs, Patricia A., A. G. Baikie, et al. 1959. "Evidence for the Existence of the Human 'Super Female.'" *Lancet* 274(7100):423–25.

Jacobs, Patricia A., Muriel Brunton, Marie M. Melville, R. P. Brittain, and W. F. McClemont. 1965. "Aggressive Behaviour, Mental Sub-normality and the XYY Male." *Nature* 208(5017):1351–52.

Jacobs, Patricia A., W. M. Court Brown, A. G. Baikie, and J. A. Strong. 1959. "The Somatic Chromosomes in Mongolism." *Lancet* 273(7075):710.

Jacobs, Patricia A., W. H. Price, W. M. Court Brown, R. P. Brittain, and P. B. Whatmore. 1968. "Chromosome Studies on Men in a Maximum Security Hospital." *Annals of Human Genetics* 31(4):339–58.

Jacobs, Patricia A., and J. A. Strong. 1959. "A Case of Human Intersexuality Having a Possible XXY Sex-Determining Mechanism." *Nature* 183(4657):302–3.

Jacobson, C., et al. 2010. "Core Neuropsychological Characteristics of Children and Adolescents with 22q11.2 Deletion." *Journal of Intellectual Disability Research* 54(8):701–13.

Jansen, Sandra, et al. 2017. "De Novo Truncating Mutations in the Last and Penultimate Exons of *PPM1D* Cause an Intellectual Disability Syndrome." *American Journal of Human Genetics* 100(4):650–58.

Jarvik, Lissy F., Victor Klodin, and Steven S. Matsuyama. 1973. "Human Aggression and the Extra Y Chromosome: Fact or Fantasy?" *American Psychologist* 28(8):674–82.

Järvinen-Pasley, Anna, et al. 2008. "Defining the Social Phenotype in Williams Syndrome: A Model for Linking Gene, the Brain, and Behavior." *Development and Psychopathology* 20(1):1–35.

Jasanoff, Sheila. 2013. *States of Knowledge: The Co-Production of Science and the Social Order*. Taylor & Francis.

Javitt, D. C., et al. 2011. "Translating Glutamate: From Pathophysiology to Treatment." *Science Translational Medicine* 3(102/102mr2).

Jeon, Kwon Chan, Lei-Shih Chen, and Patricia Goodson. 2012. "Decision to Abort After a Prenatal Diagnosis of Sex Chromosome Abnormality: A Systematic Review of the Literature." *Genetics in Medicine* 14(1):27–38.

Johnston, A. W., M. A. Ferguson-Smith, S. D. Handmaker, Howard W. Jones, and Georgeanna S. Jones. 1961. "The Triple-X Syndrome." *British Medical Journal* 2(5259):1046–52.

Jones, Wendy, et al. 2000. "II. Hypersociability in Williams Syndrome." *Journal of Cognitive Neuroscience* 12(supp. 1):30–46.

Jorde, Lynn B. 2012. "2011 Presidential Address: From Classroom to Courtroom to Clinic—Closing the Gaps in Human Genetics Education." *American Journal of Human Genetics* 90(3):387–89.

Jorge, Rita, Carmen Silva, Sofia Águeda, Sofia Dória, and Miguel Leão. 2015. "Intellectual Disability and Overgrowth—A New Case of 19p13.13 Microdeletion Syndrome with Digital Abnormalities." *American Journal of Medical Genetics, Part A* 167(11):2839–43.

Kanner, Leo. 1943. "Autistic Disturbances of Affective Contact." *Acta Paedopsychiatrica* 35(4):100–136.

———. 1949. *Feeblemindedness: Absolute, Relative and Apparent.* Child Care Monographs. Child Care Publications.

Kaplan, Paige, Paul P. Wang, and Uta Francke. 2001. "Williams (Williams-Beuren) Syndrome: A Distinct Neurobehavioral Disorder." *Journal of Child Neurology* 16(3):177–90.

Karayiorgou, Maria, Tony J. Simon, and Joseph A. Gogos. 2010. "22q11.2 Microdeletions: Linking DNA Structural Variation to Brain Dysfunction and Schizophrenia." *Nature Reviews Neuroscience* 11(6):402–16.

Kay, Lily E. 1996. *The Molecular Vision of Life: Caltech, the Rockefeller Foundation, and the Rise of the New Biology.* Oxford University Press.

Keating, Peter, and Alberto Cambrosio. 2006. *Biomedical Platforms: Realigning the Normal and the Pathological in Late-Twentieth-Century Medicine.* MIT Press.

Keller, Evelyn Fox. 2002. *The Century of the Gene.* Harvard University Press.

Kenna, Heather A., et al. 2013. "High Rates of Comorbid Depressive and Anxiety Disorders among Women with Premutation of the *FMR1* Gene." *American Journal of Medical Genetics, Part B* 162B(8):872–78.

Kent, Jon, dir. 2011. *Embraceable.* Documentary film.

Kerr, Anne. 2000. "(Re)Constructing Genetic Disease." *Social Studies of Science* 30(6):847–94.

———. 2004. "Giving Up on Geneticization: A Comment on Hedgecoe's 'Expansion and Uncertainty: Cystic Fibrosis, Classification and Genetics.'" *Sociology of Health & Illness* 26(1):102–6.

Kerr, Anne, Sarah Cunningham-Burley, and Amanda Amos. 1998. "Eugenics and the New Genetics in Britain: Examining Contemporary Professionals' Accounts." *Science, Technology & Human Values* 23(2):175–98.

Kevles, Daniel J. 1985. *In the Name of Eugenics: Genetics and the Uses of Human Heredity.* University of California Press.

Kim, Ina W., Arjun C. Khadilkar, Edmund Y. Ko, and Edmund S. Sabanegh. 2013. "47,XYY Syndrome and Male Infertility." *Reviews in Urology* 15(4):188–96.

King, Marissa D. 2008. "Diagnosis, Substitution, and Diffusion in the Autism Epidemic." PhD diss. Columbia University, Department of Sociology.

King, Marissa D., and Peter Bearman. 2009. "Diagnostic Change and the Increased Prevalence of Autism." *International Journal of Epidemiology* 38(5):1224–34.

Kingsbury, Kathleen. 2009. "Which Kids Join Gangs? A Genetic Explanation." *Time*, June 10. Available at http://www.time.com/time/health/article/0,8599,1903703,00.html.

Kirk, E. P., et al. 2009. "The Clinical Variability of the *MECP2* Duplication Syndrome: Description of Two Families with Duplications Excluding L1CAM and FLNA." *Clinical Genetics* 75(3):301–3.

Kitzman, Jacob O., et al. 2012. "Noninvasive Whole-Genome Sequencing of a Human Fetus." *Science Translational Medicine* 4(137/137ra76).

Klaassen, Petra, et al. 2016. "Explaining the Variable Penetrance of CNVs: Parental Intelligence Modulates Expression of Intellectual Impairment Caused by the 22q11.2 Deletion." *American Journal of Medical Genetics, Part B* 171(6):790–96.

Klein-Tasman, Bonita P., Kristin D. Phillips, Catherine E. Lord, Carolyn B. Mervis, and Frank Gallo. 2009. "Overlap with the Autism Spectrum in Young Children with Williams Syndrome." *Journal of Developmental and Behavioral Pediatrics* 30(4):289–99.

Kline, A. D., et al. 1993. "Molecular Analysis of the 18q– Syndrome—and Correlation with Phenotype." *American Journal of Human Genetics* 52(5):895–906.

Knight, S. J., et al. 1993. "Trinucleotide Repeat Amplification and Hypermethylation of a CpG Island in *FRAXE* Mental Retardation." *Cell* 74(1):127–34.

———. 1996. "A Study of FRAXE in Mentally Retarded Individuals Referred for Fragile X Syndrome (FRAXA) Testing in the United Kingdom." *American Journal of Human Genetics* 58(5):906–13.

Knox, Richard. 1974. "Scientists Oppose Survey of Chromosome Disorder." *Boston Globe*, November 16, 3.

Kogan, Michael D., Stephen J. Blumberg, Laura A. Schieve, Coleen A. Boyle, James M. Perrin, et al. 2009. "Prevalence of Parent-Reported Diagnosis of Autism Spectrum Disorder among Children in the US, 2007." *Pediatrics* 124(5):1395–1403.

Kohane, I. S., D. R. Masys, and R. B. Altman. 2006. "The Incidentalome: A Threat to Genomic Medicine." *Journal of the American Medical Association* 296(2):212–15.

Kolata, Gina. 2012a. "Scientists to Seek Clues to Violence in Genome of Gunman in Newtown, Conn." *New York Times*, December 24.

———. 2012b. "Study Says DNA's Power to Predict Illness Is Limited." *New York Times*, April 2.

Kolevzon, Alexander. 2012. "Clinical Trial in 22q13 Deletion Syndrome (Phelan-McDermid Syndrome)." Available at https://clinicaltrials.gov/ct2/show/NCT01525901.

Kolevzon, Alexander, et al. 2014. "A Pilot Controlled Trial of Insulin-like Growth Factor-1 in Children with Phelan-McDermid Syndrome." *Molecular Autism* 5(1):54.

Koolen, David A., et al. 2006. "A New Chromosome 17q21.31 Microdeletion Syndrome Associated with a Common Inversion Polymorphism." *Nature Genetics* 38(9):999–1001.

———. 2008. "Clinical and Molecular Delineation of the 17q21.31 Microdeletion Syndrome." *Journal of Medical Genetics* 45(11):710–20.

Koroshetz, Walter. 2007. "Summary of Autism Spectrum Disorder (ASD) Related Activities National Institute of Neurological Disorders and Stroke." Presented at the US Department of Health and Human Services Interagency Autism Coordinating Committee, full committee meeting, November 30, Washington, DC.

Kosmicki, Jack A., et al. 2017. "Refining the Role of *De Novo* Protein-Truncating Variants in Neurodevelopmental Disorders by Using Population Reference Samples." *Nature Genetics* 49(4):504–10.

Kouser, Mehreen. 2011. "Shank Synaptic Genes in Autism: Human Genetics to Mouse Models and Therapeutics." *Autism Speaks Official Blog*, May 24. https://autismspeaksblog.wordpress.com/2011/05/24/shan/.

Kraijer, Dirk W. 1997. *Autism and Autistic-like Conditions in Mental Retardation.* Swets & Zeitlinger.

Kremer, E. J., et al. 1991. "Mapping of DNA Instability at the Fragile X to a Trinucleotide Repeat Sequence p(CCG)N." *Science* 252(5013):1711–14.

Kripke, Saul A. 1980. *Naming and Necessity.* Wiley.

Krueger, Dilja D., and Mark F. Bear. 2011. "Toward Fulfilling the Promise of Molecular Medicine in Fragile X Syndrome." *Annual Review of Medicine* 62(1):411–29.

Kruszka, Paul, et al. 2017. "22q11.2 Deletion Syndrome in Diverse Populations." *American Journal of Medical Genetics, Part A* 173(4):879–88.

Kuhl, Stefan. 2002. *The Nazi Connection: Eugenics, American Racism, and German National Socialism.* Rev. ed. Oxford University Press.

Küry, Sébastien, et al. 2017. "De Novo Disruption of the Proteasome Regulatory Subunit *PSMD12* Causes a Syndromic Neurodevelopmental Disorder." *American Journal of Human Genetics* 100(4):689.

Lacassie, Y., and M. I. Arriaza. 1996. "Opitz GBBB Syndrome and the 22q11.2 Deletion." *American Journal of Medical Genetics* 62(3):318.

Lam, Christina, et al. 2017. "Prospective Phenotyping of *NGLY1-CDDG*, the First Congenital Disorder of Deglycosylation." *Genetics in Medicine* 19(2):160–68.

Lamy, Maurice, and Jean de Grouchy. 1967. *L' homme et l'hérédité.* Hachette.

Lappé, Martine, and Hannah Landecker. 2015. "Sociology in an Age of Genomic Instability: Copy Number Variation, Somatic Mosaicism, and the Fallen Genome." In *Genetics, Health and Society.* Vol. 16, *Advances in Medical Sociology,* 157–86. Emerald Group.

Larson, R. S., and M. G. Butler. 1995. "Use of Fluorescence in Situ Hybridization (FISH) in the Diagnosis of DiGeorge Sequence and Related Diseases." *Diagnostic Molecular Pathology: The American Journal of Surgical Pathology, Part B* 4(4):274–78.

Latimer, Joanna, et al. 2006. "Rebirthing the Clinic." *Science, Technology & Human Values* 31(5):599–630.

Latour, Bruno. 1988. *Science in Action: How to Follow Scientists and Engineers Through Society*. Harvard University Press.

———. 1993. *The Pasteurization of France*. Harvard University Press.

———. 1999. *Pandora's Hope: Essays on the Reality of Science Studies*. Harvard University Press.

———. 2000. "On the Partial Existence of Existing and Nonexisting Objects." In *Biographies of Scientific Objects*, edited by L. Daston, 247–69. University of Chicago Press.

———. 2007. *Reassembling the Social: An Introduction to Actor-Network-Theory*. Oxford University Press.

Law, John. 1992. "Notes on the Theory of the Actor-Network: Ordering, Strategy, and Heterogeneity." *Systemic Practice and Action Research* 5(4):379–93.

Laws, Glynis, and Dorothy V. M. Bishop. 2004. "Pragmatic Language Impairment and Social Deficits in Williams Syndrome: A Comparison with Down's Syndrome and Specific Language Impairment." *International Journal of Language & Communication Disorders* 39(1):45–64.

Lea, Rod, and Geoffrey Chambers. 2007. "Monoamine Oxidase, Addiction, and the 'Warrior' Gene Hypothesis." *Journal of the New Zealand Medical Association* 120(1250):U2441.

Lea, Rod, D. Hall, M. Green, and Geoffrey Chambers. 2005. "Tracking the Evolutionary History of the Warrior Gene in the South Pacific." Presented at the Molecular Biology and Evolution Conference in Auckland, June.

LeCouteur, A., et al. 1996. "A Broader Phenotype of Autism: The Clinical Spectrum in Twins RID A-9625-2011." *Journal of Child Psychology and Psychiatry and Allied Disciplines* 37(7):785–801.

Ledbetter, David H. 2008. "Cytogenetic Technology—Genotype and Phenotype." *New England Journal of Medicine* 359(16):1728–30.

———. 2009a. "'New Microdeletion Syndromes: Complex, but No New Paradigms.'" *Journal of Medical Genetics* 46(8):576.

———. 2009b. "Response to Saul and Moeschler 'How Best to Use CGH Arrays in the Clinical Setting.'" *Genetics in Medicine* 11(5):371–72.

Lederberg, Joshua. 1968. "'Criminal Genetic Types' Pose a Research Dilemma." *Washington Post*, October 19, A15.

Lee, Jeong Ho, et al. 2012. "*De Novo* Somatic Mutations in Components of the PI3K-AKT3-mTOR Pathway Cause Hemimegalencephaly." *Nature Genetics* 44(8):941–45.

Leggett, Victoria, Patricia Jacobs, Kate Nation, Gaia Scerif, and Dorothy V. M. Bishop. 2010. "Neurocognitive Outcomes of Individuals with a Sex Chromosome Trisomy: XXX, XYY, or XXY: A Systematic Review." *Developmental Medicine and Child Neurology* 52(2):119–29.

Lejeune, Jérôme, et al. 1960. "A Proposed Standard System of Nomenclature of Human Mitotic Chromosomes." *Lancet* 275(7133):1063–65.

———. 1963. "[3 Cases of Partial Deletion of the Short Arm of a 5 Chromosome]." *Comptes rendus hebdomadaires des séances de l'Académie des Sciences* 257:3098–3102.

Lejeune, Jérôme, M. Gautier, and R. Turpin. 1959. "Etude des chromosomes somatiques de neuf enfants mongoliens" [Study of Somatic Chromosomes from 9 Mongoloid Children]. *Comptes rendus hebdomadaires des séances de l'Académie des Sciences* 248(11):1721–22.

Lejeune, Jérôme, and Raymond Turpin. 1961. "Chromosomal Aberrations in Man." *American Journal of Human Genetics* 13(1, pt. 2):175–84.

Lenhoff, Howard M. 1999. "A Real-World Source for the 'Little People': A Comparison of Fairies to Individuals with Williams Syndrome." In *Nursery Realms: Children in the Worlds of Science Fiction, Fantasy, and Horror*, edited by G. Westfahl and G. E. Slusser, 150–60. University of Georgia Press.

Lenhoff, Howard M., Paul P. Wang, Frank Greenberg, and Ursula Bellugi. 1997. "Williams Syndrome and the Brain." *Scientific American* 277(6):68–73.

Leroi, Armand Marie. 2006. "The Future of Neo-Eugenics. Now That Many People Approve the Elimination of Certain Genetically Defective Fetuses, Is Society Closer to Screening All Fetuses for All Known Mutations?" *EMBO Reports* 7(12):1184–87.

Lindee, M. Susan. 2005. *Moments of Truth in Genetic Medicine*. Johns Hopkins University Press.

Lippman, Abby. 1991a. "Prenatal Genetic Testing and Screening: Constructing Needs and Reinforcing Inequities." *American Journal of Law & Medicine* 17:15–50.

———. 1991b. "The Geneticization of Health and Illness: Implications for Social Practice." *Endocrinologie* 29(1–2):85–90.

———. 1994. "The Genetic Construction of Prenatal Testing: Choice, Consent, or Conformity for Women?" In *Women and Prenatal Testing: Facing the Challenges of Genetic Technology*, edited by K. H. Rothenberg and E. J. Thomson, 9–34. Ohio State University Press.

———. 1998. "The Politics of Health: Geneticization versus Health Promotion." In *The Politics of Women's Health: Exploring Agency and Autonomy*, edited by S. Sherwin, 64–82. Temple University Press.

Lipson, A., B. Emanuel, P. Colley, K. Fagan, and D. A. Driscoll. 1994. "'CATCH 22' sans Cardiac Anomaly, Thymic Hypoplasia, Cleft-Palate, and Hypocalcemia: cAtch 22. A Common Result of 22q11 Deficiency?" *Journal of Medical Genetics* 31(9):741.

Liu, Ka-Yuet, Marissa King, and Peter S. Bearman. 2010. "Social Influence and the Autism Epidemic." *American Journal of Sociology* 115(5):1387–1434.

Lo, Y. M., et al. 1997. "Presence of Fetal DNA in Maternal Plasma and Serum." *Lancet* 350(9076):485–87.

Lo-Castro, Adriana, Elisa D'Agati, and Paolo Curatolo. 2011. "ADHD and Genetic Syndromes." *Brain and Development* 33(6):456–61.

Lock, Margaret. 2005. "Eclipse of the Gene and the Return of Divination." *Current Anthropology* 46(S5):S47–70.

Loscalzo, Joseph, Isaac Kohane, and Albert-Laszlo Barabasi. 2007. "Human Disease Classification in the Postgenomic Era: A Complex Systems Approach to Human Pathobiology." *Molecular Systems Biology* 3(124). https://doi.org/10.1038/msb4100163.

Losowsky, M. S. 1961. "Hereditary Mental Defect Showing the Pattern of Sex Influence." *Journal of Mental Deficiency Research* 5(1):60–62.

Lovett, Edward. 2012. "Williams Syndrome Grows in Awareness, Research." ABC News, March 16. http://abcnews.go.com/blogs/health/2012/03/16/williams-syndrome-grows-in-awareness-research/.

Lowery, M. C., et al. 1995. "Strong Correlation of Elastin Deletions, Detected by FISH, with Williams-Syndrome—Evaluation of 235 Patients." *American Journal of Human Genetics* 57(1):49–53.

Löwy, Ilana. 2014. "How Genetics Came to the Unborn: 1960–2000." *Studies in History and Philosophy of Science, Part C: Studies in History and Philosophy of Biological and Biomedical Sciences* 47, part A:154–62.

Lubs, H. A. 1969. "A Marker X Chromosome." *American Journal of Human Genetics* 21(3):231–44.

Lynch, D. R., et al. 1995. "Cerebellar Atrophy in a Patient with Velocardiofacial Syndrome." *Journal of Medical Genetics* 32(7):561–63.

Lyons, Richard D. 1968a. "Genetic Abnormality Is Linked to Crime; Genetics Linked to Violent Crimes." *New York Times*, April 21, 1.

———. 1968b. "Ultimate Speck Appeal May Cite a Genetic Defect." *New York Times*, April 22.

MacMillan, Donald L., Melvyn I. Semmel, and Michael M. Gerber. 1994. "The Social Context of Dunn Then and Now." *Journal of Special Education* 27(4):466–80.

Manning, M. A., et al. 2004. "Terminal 22q Deletion Syndrome: A Newly Recognized Cause of Speech and Language Disability in the Autism Spectrum." *Pediatrics* 114(2):451–57.

Manolio, Teri A., et al. 2013. "Implementing Genomic Medicine in the Clinic: The Future Is Here." *Genetics in Medicine* 15(4):258–67.

Mansfield, Caroline, Suellen Hopfer, and Theresa M. Marteau. 1999. "Termination Rates after Prenatal Diagnosis of Down Syndrome, Spina Bifida, Anencephaly, and Turner and Klinefelter Syndromes: A Systematic Literature Review." *Prenatal Diagnosis* 19(9):808–12.

Mardis, Elaine R. 2006. "Anticipating the $1,000 Genome." *Genome Biology* 7(7):112.

Marketwired. 2016. "Medgenics Reports First Quarter 2016 Financial Results and NFC-1 Program Update." Yahoo! Finance, May 10. http://

finance.yahoo.com/news/medgenics-reports-first-quarter-2016-120000994
.html.

Martin, Aryn. 2004. "Can't Any Body Count? Counting as an Epistemic Theme in the History of Human Chromosomes." *Social Studies of Science* 34(6): 923–48.

Martin, J. Purdon, and Julia Bell. 1943. "A Pedigree of Mental Defect Showing Sex-Linkage." *Journal of Neurology and Psychiatry* 6(3–4):154–57.

McCabe, Linda L., and Edward R. B. McCabe. 2011. "Down Syndrome: Coercion and Eugenics." *Genetics in Medicine* 13(8):708–10.

McDermott, Rose, Dustin Tingley, Jonathan Cowden, Giovanni Frazzetto, and Dominic D. P. Johnson. 2009. "Monoamine Oxidase A Gene (*MAOA*) Predicts Behavioral Aggression Following Provocation." *Proceedings of the National Academy of Sciences* 106(7):2118–23.

McDonald-McGinn, Donna. 2018. "22q11.2 Deletion Syndrome: A Tiny Piece Leading to a Big Picture." *American Journal of Medical Genetics, Part A* 176(10):2055–57.

McDonald-McGinn, Donna, E. H. Zackai, and D. Low. 1997. "What's in a Name? The 22q11.2 Deletion." *American Journal of Medical Genetics* 72(2):247–49.

McDonald-McGinn, Donna, et al. 1995. "Autosomal Dominant 'Opitz' GBBB Syndrome Due to a 22q11.2 Deletion." *American Journal of Medical Genetics* 59(1):103–13.

———. 2001. "Phenotype of the 22q11.2 Deletion in Individuals Identified Through an Affected Relative: Cast a Wide FISHing Net!" *Genetics in Medicine* 3(1):23–29.

———. 2015. "22q11.2 Deletion Syndrome." *Nature Reviews Disease Primers* 1:article #15071.

McKusick, Victor A. 1966. *Mendelian Inheritance in Man: A Catalog of Autosomal Dominant, Autosomal Recessive, and X-Linked Phenotypes.* Johns Hopkins University Press.

———. 1993. "Medical Genetics." *Journal of the American Medical Association* 270(19):2351–56.

———. 1998. *Mendelian Inheritance in Man: A Catalog of Human Genes and Genetic Disorders.* 12th ed. Johns Hopkins University Press.

McLennan, Yingratana, Jonathan Polussa, Flora Tassone, and Randi Hagerman. 2011. "Fragile X Syndrome." *Current Genomics* 12(3):216–24.

Mefford, Heather C., et al. 2008. "Recurrent Rearrangements of Chromosome 1q21.1 and Variable Pediatric Phenotypes." *New England Journal of Medicine* 359(16):1685–99.

Mencacci, Niccolo E., et al. 2015. "*ADCY5* Mutations Are Another Cause of Benign Hereditary Chorea." *Neurology* 85(1):80–88.

Meyer, David S., and Nancy Whittier. 1994. "Social Movement Spillover." *Social Problems* 41(2):277–98.

Meyer-Lindenberg, Andreas, Carolyn B. Mervis, and Karen Faith Berman. 2006. "Neural Mechanisms in Williams Syndrome: A Unique Window to

Genetic Influences on Cognition and Behaviour." *Nature Reviews Neuroscience* 7(5):380–93.

Meyer-Lindenberg, Andreas, et al. 2006. "Neural Mechanisms of Genetic Risk for Impulsivity and Violence in Humans." *Proceedings of the National Academy of Sciences* 103(16):6269–74.

Might, Matt. 2012. "Hunting Down My Son's Killer." Gizmodo, May 31. http://gizmodo.com/5914305/hunting-down-my-sons-killer.

Mikkelsen, M., G. Fischer, J. Hansen, B. Pilgaard, and J. Nielsen. 1983. "The Impact of Legal Termination of Pregnancy and of Prenatal Diagnosis on the Birth Prevalence of Down Syndrome in Denmark." *Annals of Human Genetics* 47(2):123–31.

Miller, David T., et al. 2010. "Consensus Statement: Chromosomal Microarray Is a First-Tier Clinical Diagnostic Test for Individuals with Developmental Disabilities or Congenital Anomalies." *American Journal of Human Genetics* 86(5):749–64.

Miller, Fiona Alice, Catherine Ahern, Jacqueline Ogilvie, Mita Giacomini, and Lisa Schwartz. 2005. "Ruling In and Ruling Out: Implications of Molecular Genetic Diagnoses for Disease Classification." *Social Science & Medicine* 61(12):2536–45.

Miller, Fiona Alice, Megan E. Begbie, Mita Giacomini, Catherine Ahern, and Erin A. Harvey. 2006. "Redefining Disease? The Nosologic Implications of Molecular Genetic Knowledge." *Perspectives in Biology and Medicine* 49(1):99–114.

Miller, Kimberley A. 2008. "FISH Diagnosis of 22q11.2 Deletion Syndrome." *Newborn and Infant Nursing Reviews* 8(1):e11–e19.

Miller, Robert. 2013. "Report on the 1st International Conference on the FMR1 Premutation." National Fragile X Foundation, July 17. https://fragilex.org/2013/keeping-you-informed/report-on-the-1st-international-conference-on-the-fmr1-premutation/.

Mnookin, Seth. 2014. "One of a Kind." *New Yorker*, July 21.

Moeschler, John B., T. K. Mohandas, Arnold B. Hawk, and Walter W. Noll. 2002. "Estimate of Prevalence of Proximal 15q Duplication Syndrome." *American Journal of Medical Genetics* 111(4):440–42.

Mol, Annemarie. 2002. *The Body Multiple: Ontology in Medical Practice*. Duke University Press.

Money, John, Charles Annecillo, Barry Van Orman, and Digamber S. Borgaonkar. 1974. "Cytogenetics, Hormones and Behavior Disability: Comparison of XYY and XXY Syndromes." *Clinical Genetics* 6(5):370–82.

Money, John, A. Franzke, and D. S. Borgaonkar. 1975. "XYY Syndrome, Stigmatization, Social Class, and Aggression: Study of 15 Cases." *Southern Medical Journal* 68(12):1536–42.

"The Mongol Chromosome and Some Others." 1960. *Lancet* 276(7159):1068–69.

Moosa, Shahida, et al. 2016. "Smith–Kingsmore Syndrome: A Third Family with the *MTOR* Mutation C.5395G>A p.(Glu1799Lys) and Evidence for

Paternal Gonadal Mosaicism." *American Journal of Medical Genetics, Part A* 173(1):264–67.

Morelle, Rebecca. 2007. "3D Face Scans Spot Gene Syndromes." BBC News, September 9.

Moreno-De-Luca, Andres, D. W. Evans, K. B. Boomer, et al. 2015. "The Role of Parental Cognitive, Behavioral, and Motor Profiles in Clinical Variability in Individuals with Chromosome 16p11.2 Deletions." *JAMA Psychiatry* 72(2):119–26.

Moreno-De-Luca, Andres, et al. 2013. "Developmental Brain Dysfunction: Revival and Expansion of Old Concepts Based on New Genetic Evidence." *Lancet Neurology* 12(4):406–14.

Morgan, Thomas Hunt. 1915. *The Mechanism of Mendelian Heredity.* Holt.

Morton, J. E., et al. 1997. "Fragile X Syndrome Is Less Common Than Previously Estimated." *Journal of Medical Genetics* 34(1):1–5.

Mukaddes, Nahit Motavalli, and Sabri Herguner. 2007. "Autistic Disorder and 22q11.2 Duplication." *World Journal of Biological Psychiatry* 8(2):127–30.

Müller-Wille, Staffan, and Hans-Jörg Rheinberger. 2012. *A Cultural History of Heredity.* University of Chicago Press.

Mullin, Emily. 2017. "A Year After Approval, a Gene-Therapy Cure Gets Its First Customer." *MIT Technology Review*, May 3. https://www.technologyreview.com/s/604295/a-year-after-approval-gene-therapy-cure-gets-its-first-customer/.

Naber, John M., Carl A. Huether, and Beth A. Goodwin. 1987. "Temporal Changes in Ohio Amniocentesis Utilization during the First Twelve Years (1972–1983), and Frequency of Chromosome Abnormalities Observed." *Prenatal Diagnosis* 7(1):51–65.

Nadesan, Majia Holmer. 2005. *Constructing Autism: Unravelling the "Truth" and Understanding the Social.* Psychology Press.

National Fragile X Foundation. [2018]. "2017 Annual Impact Report." https://fragilex.org/wp-content/uploads/2018/10/NFXF-2017-Annual-Impact-Report.pdf.

National Human Genome Research Institute. 2016. "The Cost of Sequencing a Human Genome." July 6. https://www.genome.gov/27565109/the-cost-of-sequencing-a-human-genome/.

Natoli, Jaime L., Deborah L. Ackerman, Suzanne McDermott, and Janice G. Edwards. 2012. "Prenatal Diagnosis of Down Syndrome: A Systematic Review of Termination Rates (1995–2011)." *Prenatal Diagnosis* 32(2):142–53.

Navon, Daniel. 2011. "Genomic Designation: How Genetics Can Delineate New, Phenotypically Diffuse Medical Categories." *Social Studies of Science* 41(2):203–26.

Navon, Daniel, and Gil Eyal. 2014. "The Trading Zone of Autism Genetics: Examining the Intersection of Genomic and Psychiatric Classification." *BioSocieties* 9(3):329–52.

————. 2016. "Looping Genomes: Diagnostic Change and the Genetic Makeup of the Autism Population." *American Journal of Sociology* 121(5):1416–71.

Navon, Daniel, and Uri Shwed. 2012. "The Chromosome 22q11.2 Deletion: From the Unification of Biomedical Fields to a New Kind of Genetic Condition." *Social Science & Medicine* 75(9):1633–41.

Need, Anna C., et al. 2012. "Clinical Application of Exome Sequencing in Undiagnosed Genetic Conditions." *Journal of Medical Genetics* 49:353–61.

Nelkin, Dorothy. 1996. "The Social Dynamics of Genetic Testing: The Case of Fragile-X." *Medical Anthropology Quarterly* 10(4):537–50.

Nelkin, Dorothy, and M. Susan Lindee. 2004. *The DNA Mystique: The Gene as a Cultural Icon*. University of Michigan Press.

Nelson, Alondra. 2008. "Bio Science Genetic Genealogy Testing and the Pursuit of African Ancestry." *Social Studies of Science* 38(5):759–83.

————. 2016. *The Social Life of DNA: Race, Reparations, and Reconciliation After the Genome*. Beacon Press.

Nelson, Nicole C. 2018. *Model Behavior: Animal Experiments, Complexity, and the Genetics of Psychiatric Disorders*. University of Chicago Press.

Nelson, Nicole C., Peter Keating, and Alberto Cambrosio. 2013. "On Being 'Actionable': Clinical Sequencing and the Emerging Contours of a Regime of Genomic Medicine in Oncology." *New Genetics and Society* 32(4):405–28.

Neri, Giovanni, and John M. Opitz. 2009. "Down Syndrome: Comments and Reflections on the 50th Anniversary of Lejeune's Discovery." *American Journal of Medical Genetics, Part A* 149A(12):2647–54.

New York Times. 1968a. "Murder Suspect Pleads Imbalance of Chromosomes." October 18, 18.

————. 1968b. "Nature or Nurture?" April 23, 46.

————. 1969a. "Geneticist Testifies at Murder Trial." April 24, 53.

————. 1969b. "Killer Gets 25-Year Term after Citing Genetic Defect." July 11, 42.

New Zealand Herald. 2009. "Scientist Debunks 'Warrior Gene.'" September 12.

Nickerson, E., F. Greenberg, M. T. Keating, C. McCaskill, and L. G. Shaffer. 1995. "Deletions of the Elastin Gene at 7q11.23 Occur in Approximately 90% of Patients with Williams Syndrome." *American Journal of Human Genetics* 56(5):1156–61.

Nielsen, Johannes, Kirsten Riber Christensen, Ursula Friedrich, Eva Zeuthen, and Olaf Østergaard. 1973. "Childhood of Males with the XYY Syndrome." *Journal of Autism and Developmental Disorders* 3(1):5–26.

Nordenbæk, Claudia, Meta Jørgensen, Kirsten Ohm Kyvik, and Niels Bilenberg. 2013. "A Danish Population-Based Twin Study on Autism Spectrum Disorders." *European Child & Adolescent Psychiatry* 23(1):35–43.

Novas, Carlos. 2006. "The Political Economy of Hope: Patients' Organizations, Science and Biovalue." *BioSocieties* 1(03):289–305.

The 1000 Genomes Project Consortium. 2010. "A Map of Human Genome Variation from Population-Scale Sequencing." *Nature* 467(7319):1061–73.

Opitz, John M., Allan T. Segal, Hallgrim Klove, Charles Mathews, and Robert L. Lehrke. 1965. "X-Linked Mental Retardation: Study of a Large Kindred with 20 Affected Members." *Journal of Pediatrics* 67(4):713–14.

Osborne, L. R., et al. 1996. "Identification of Genes from a 500-Kb Region at 7q11. 23 That Is Commonly Deleted in Williams Syndrome Patients." *Genomics* 36(2):328–36.

Osherovich, Lev. 2012. "Fine-Tuning MGluRs." *SciBX: Science-Business EXchange* 5(1):1–2.

Otto, James H., and A. Towle. 1973. *Modern Biology: 1973*. Book World Promotions.

Overhauser, J., et al. 1994. "Molecular and Phenotypic Mapping of the Short Arm of Chromosome 5: Sublocalization of the Critical Region for the Cri-Du-Chat Syndrome." *Human Molecular Genetics* 3(2):247–52.

Owen, Michael J., and Joanne L. Doherty. 2016. "What Can We Learn from the High Rates of Schizophrenia in People with 22q11.2 Deletion Syndrome?" *World Psychiatry* 15(1):23–25.

Palomaki, Glenn E., Edward M. Kloza, Geralyn M. Lambert-Messerlian, James E. Haddow, Louis M. Neveux, Mathias Ehrich, Dirk van den Boom, et al. 2011. "DNA Sequencing of Maternal Plasma to Detect Down Syndrome: An International Clinical Validation Study." *Genetics in Medicine* 13(11):913–20.

Panofsky, Aaron. 2011. "Generating Sociability to Drive Science: Patient Advocacy Organizations and Genetics Research." *Social Studies of Science* 41(1):31–57.

Park, W. Wallace. 1966. "The YY Syndrome." *Lancet* 288(7479):1468.

Parker, Charles E., Jamshed Mavalwala, John Melnyk, and Charles H. Fish. 1970. "The 48, XXYY Syndrome." *American Journal of Medicine* 48(6):777–81.

Parsons, Talcott. 1991. *The Social System*. Routledge.

Partridge, Myra. 2007. "Raise the Bar on FXTAS: Recognize It." *Psychiatric Times*, April 1. http://www.psychiatrictimes.com/articles/raise-bar-fxtas -recognize-it.

Patau, Klaus, David W. Smith, Eeva Therman, Stanley L. Inhorn, and Hans P. Wagner. 1960. "Multiple Congenital Anomaly Caused by an Extra Autosome." *Lancet* 275(7128):790–93.

Paul, Diane B. 1995. *Controlling Human Heredity, 1865 to the Present*. Humanities Press.

Peca, Joao, et al. 2011. "*SHANK3* Mutant Mice Display Autistic-like Behaviours and Striatal Dysfunction." *Nature* 472(7344):437–42.

Penrose, L. S., J. R. Ellis, and J. D. Delhanty. 1960. "Chromosomal Translocations in Mongolism and in Normal Relatives." *Lancet* 2(7147):409–10.

Pettus, Ashley. 2008. "A Spectrum of Disorders: The Urgent Search to Understand the Biological Basis of Autism." *Harvard Magazine* 110 (Jan.–Feb.):3.

Phelan, Jo C. 2005. "Geneticization of Deviant Behavior and Consequences for Stigma: The Case of Mental Illness." *Journal of Health and Social Behavior* 46(4):307–22.

Phelan, Katy, and H. E. McDermid. 2012. "The 22q13.3 Deletion Syndrome (Phelan-McDermid Syndrome)." *Molecular Syndromology* 2(3–5):186–201.

Phelan, Mary C. 2003. "Deletion 22q13 Syndrome." *Orphanet Encyclopedia*, September. Available at https://web.archive.org/web/20050215214608/https://www.orpha.net/data/patho/GB/uk-22q13.pdf.

———. 2008. "Deletion 22q13.3 Syndrome." *Orphanet Journal of Rare Diseases* 3(1, art. 14). https://ojrd.biomedcentral.com/track/pdf/10.1186/1750-1172-3-14.

Phelan, Mary C., R. C. Rogers, and L. K. Byrd. 1993. "Albright Hereditary Osteodystrophy and Del(2)(q37) in 2 Unrelated Individuals." *American Journal of Human Genetics* 53(3):S484.

Phelan, Mary C., R. C. Rogers, and R. E. Stevenson. 1988. "A De Novo Terminal Deletion of 22q." *American Journal of Human Genetics* 43(supp.):A118.

Phelan, Mary C., et al. 1992. "Cytogenetic, Biochemical, and Molecular Analyses of a 22q13 Deletion." *American Journal of Medical Genetics* 43(5):872–76.

———. 1995. "Albright Hereditary Osteodystrophy and Del(2)(Q37.3) in Four Unrelated Individuals." *American Journal of Medical Genetics* 58(1):1–7.

———. 2001. "22q13 Deletion Syndrome." *American Journal of Medical Genetics* 101(2):91–99.

Phelan-McDermid Syndrome Foundation. 2013. *Phelan-McDermid Syndrome Foundation Research Update, February 2013*. Phelan-McDermid Syndrome Foundation.

Pinker, Steven. 2007. *The Language Instinct: How the Mind Creates Language*. Harper Perennial Modern Classics.

Pinto, Dalila, et al. 2014. "Convergence of Genes and Cellular Pathways Dysregulated in Autism Spectrum Disorders." *American Journal of Human Genetics* 94(5):677–94.

Piton, Amélie, Claire Redin, and Jean-Louis Mandel. 2013. "XLID-Causing Mutations and Associated Genes Challenged in Light of Data from Large-Scale Human Exome Sequencing." *American Journal of Human Genetics* 93(2):368–83.

Piven, J., P. Palmer, D. Jacobi, D. Childress, and S. Arndt. 1997. "Broader Autism Phenotype: Evidence from a Family History Study of Multiple-Incidence Autism Families." *American Journal of Psychiatry* 154(2):185–90.

Polani, P. E., J. H. Briggs, C. E. Ford, C. M. Clarke, and J. M. Berg. 1960. "A Mongol Girl with 46 Chromosomes." *Lancet* 1(7127):721–24.

Pollack, Andrew. 2011. "Sequenom's Test for Down Syndrome Raises Hopes and Questions." *New York Times*, October 17.

———. 2013. "An Experimental Drug's Bitter End." *New York Times*, June 6.

———. 2014. "Seeking Clues to Obesity in Rare Hunger Disorder." *New York Times*, January 14.

Pollack, Harold. 2012. "Santorum: He's Not Funny Any More." The Reality-Based Community, February 19. http://www.samefacts.com/2012/02/religion-and-politics/santorum-hes-not-funny-any-more/.

Porter, Theodore. 2018. *Genetics in the Madhouse: The Unknown History of Human Heredity.* Princeton University Press.

Portnoï, M. F. 2009. "Microduplication 22q11.2: A New Chromosomal Syndrome." *European Journal of Medical Genetics* 52(2–3):88–93.

Portnoï, M. F., et al. 2005. "22q11.2 Duplication Syndrome: Two New Familial Cases with Some Overlapping Features with DiGeorge/Velocardiofacial Syndromes." *American Journal of Medical Genetics, Part A* 137(1):47–51.

Potocki, Lorraine, Christine J. Shaw, Pawel Stankiewicz, and James R. Lupski. 2003. "Variability in Clinical Phenotype despite Common Chromosomal Deletion in Smith-Magenis Syndrome [Del(17)(P11.2p11.2)]." *Genetics in Medicine* 5(6):430–34.

Potocki, Lorraine, et al. 2000. "Molecular Mechanism for Duplication 17p11.2: The Homologous Recombination Reciprocal of the Smith-Magenis Microdeletion." *Nature Genetics* 24(1):84–87.

———. 2007. "Characterization of Potocki-Lupski Syndrome (Dup(17) (P11.2p11.2)) and Delineation of a Dosage-Sensitive Critical Interval That Can Convey an Autism Phenotype." *American Journal of Human Genetics* 80(4):633–49.

Price, W. H., J. A. Strong, P. B. Whatmore, and W. F. McClemont. 1966. "Criminal Patients with XYY Sex-Chromosome Complement." *Lancet* 1(7437):565–66.

Price, W. H., and P. B. Whatmore. 1967. "Criminal Behaviour and the XYY Male." *Nature* 213(5078):815.

Pyeritz, Reed, J. Beckwith, and L. Miller. 1975. "Letter: XYY Disclosure Condemned." *New England Journal of Medicine* 293(10):508.

Pyeritz, Reed, Herb Schreier, Chuck Madansky, Larry Miller, and Jon Beckwith. 1977. "The XYY Male: The Making of a Myth." In *Biology as a Social Weapon*, edited by the Ann Arbor Science for the People Editorial Collective, 86–100. Burgess.

Quelin, C., et al. 2009. "Twelve New Patients with 13q Deletion Syndrome: Genotype–Phenotype Analyses in Progress." *European Journal of Medical Genetics* 52(1):41–46.

Rabeharisoa, Vololona, and Pascale Bourret. 2009. "Staging and Weighting Evidence in Biomedicine: Comparing Clinical Practices in Cancer Genetics and Psychiatric Genetics." *Social Studies of Science* 39(5):691–715.

Rabeharisoa, Vololona, and Michel Callon. 2002. "The Involvement of Patients' Associations in Research." *International Social Science Journal* 54(171):57–63.

Rabeharisoa, Vololona, et al. 2012. "The Dynamics of Causes and Conditions: The Rareness of Diseases in French and Portuguese Patients' Organizations' Engagement in Research." Centre de Sociologie de l'Innovation, CSI Working Papers Series, no. 026.

———. 2014. "From 'Politics of Numbers' to 'Politics of Singularisation': Patients' Activism and Engagement in Research on Rare Diseases in France and Portugal." *BioSocieties* 9(2):194–217.

Rabinow, Paul. (1992) 1996. *Essays on the Anthropology of Reason.* Princeton University Press.

Rader, Karen. 2004. *Making Mice: Standardizing Animals for American Biomedical Research, 1900–1955.* Princeton University Press.

Radford, Tim. 2002. "Scientists Identify Gene That May Trigger Violence in Abused Children." *Guardian*, August 2. Available at http://www.guardian.co.uk/uk/2002/aug/02/childprotection.medicalscience.

Rafferty, Andrew, and Domenico Montanaro. 2012. "Fact Check: Santorum Says Obama Looks Down on Disabled, Encouraging More Abortions." NBC News, February 18. http://firstread.nbcnews.com/_news/2012/02/18/10444238-santorum-says-obama-looks-down-on-disabled-encouraging-more-abortions.

Ramocki, Melissa B., Y. Jane Tavyev, and Sarika U. Peters. 2010. "The *MECP2* Duplication Syndrome." *American Journal of Medical Genetics, Part A* 152A(5):1079–88.

Ramocki, Melissa B., et al. 2009. "Autism and Other Neuropsychiatric Symptoms Are Prevalent in Individuals with *MeCP2* Duplication Syndrome." *Annals of Neurology* 66(6):771–82.

Ramsden, Edmund. 2009. "Confronting the Stigma of Eugenics: Genetics, Demography and the Problems of Population." *Social Studies of Science* 39(6):853–84.

Rapp, Rayna. 2000. *Testing Women, Testing the Fetus: The Social Impact of Amniocentesis in America.* Routledge.

Rappoport, Stanley, and William D. Kaplan. 1961. "Chromosomal Aberrations in Man." *Journal of Pediatrics* 59(3):415–38.

Raspa, Melissa, Anne C. Wheeler, and Catharine Riley. 2017. "Public Health Literature Review of Fragile X Syndrome." *Pediatrics* 139(supp. 3):S153–71.

Raspberry, Kelly, and Debra Skinner. 2011a. "Enacting Genetic Responsibility: Experiences of Mothers Who Carry the Fragile X Gene." *Sociology of Health & Illness* 33(3):420–33.

———. 2011b. "Negotiating Desires and Options: How Mothers Who Carry the Fragile X Gene Experience Reproductive Decisions." *Social Science & Medicine* 72(6):992–98.

Ratcliffe, S. 1999. "Long Term Outcome in Children of Sex Chromosome Abnormalities." *Archives of Disease in Childhood* 80(2):192–95.

Rees, E., et al. 2014. "Evidence That Duplications of 22q11.2 Protect against Schizophrenia." *Molecular Psychiatry* 19(1):37–40.

Regalado, Antonio. 2016. "Gene Therapy's First Out-and-Out Cure Is Here." *MIT Technology Review*, May 6. https://www.technologyreview.com/s/601390/gene-therapys-first-out-and-out-cure-is-here/.

Regier, D. A., W. E. Narrow, E. A. Kuhl, and D. J. Kupfer. 2009. "The Conceptual Development of DSM-V." *American Journal of Psychiatry* 166(6):645–50.

Reilly, C. 2012. "Behavioural Phenotypes and Special Educational Needs: Is Aetiology Important in the Classroom?" *Journal of Intellectual Disability Research* 56(10):929–46.

Reinhold, Robert. 1968. "Abortions Linked to Genetic Defect; Fetal Tests Said to Be Used as Basis for Operations." *New York Times*, September 2, 19.

Reiss, Allan L., Carl Feinstein, and Kenneth N. Rosenbaum. 1986. "Autism and Genetic Disorders." *Schizophrenia Bulletin* 12(4):724–38.

Reiss, Allan L., and L. Freund. 1990. "Fragile X Syndrome, *DSM-III*, and Autism." *Journal of the American Academy of Child and Adolescent Psychiatry* 29(6):885–91.

———. 1992. "Behavioral Phenotype of Fragile X Syndrome: DSM-III-R Autistic Behavior in Male Children." *American Journal of Medical Genetics* 43(1–2):35–46.

Reiss, Allan L., et al. 2004. "An Experiment of Nature: Brain Anatomy Parallels Cognition and Behavior in Williams Syndrome." *Journal of Neuroscience* 24(21):5009–15.

Repetto, G. M., et al. 2009. "Clinical Features of Chromosome 22q11.2 Microdeletion Syndrome in 208 Chilean Patients." *Clinical Genetics* 76(5):465–70.

Reti, Irving M., et al. 2010. "Monoamine Oxidase A Regulates Antisocial Personality in Whites with No History of Physical Abuse." *Comprehensive Psychiatry* 52(2):188–94.

Reuters. 2013. "Illumina to Buy Verinata Health for $350 Mln plus Milestone Payments." Reuters, January 7.

Reynolds, Justin. 2016. "Gene May Be Important in Autism Disorders, Other Neuropsychiatric Syndromes." FierceBiotech, January 20. http://www.fiercebiotech.com/research/gene-may-be-important-autism-disorders-other-neuropsychiatric-syndromes.

Rheinberger, Hans-Jörg. 1997. *Toward a History of Epistemic Things: Synthesizing Proteins in the Test Tube*. Stanford University Press.

———. 2010. *An Epistemology of the Concrete: Twentieth-Century Histories of Life*. Duke University Press.

———. 2013. "Heredity in the Twentieth Century: Some Epistemological Considerations." *Public Culture* 25(371):477–93.

Ricci, N., and P. Malacarne. 1964. "An XYY Human Male." *Lancet* 283(7335):721.

Richardson, Sarah S. 2013. *Sex Itself: The Search for Male and Female in the Human Genome*. University of Chicago Press.

Riggs, E. R., et al. 2014. "Chromosomal Microarray Impacts Clinical Management." *Clinical Genetics* 85(2):147–53.

Rimland, Bernard. 1964. *Infantile Autism: The Syndrome and Its Implications for a Neural Theory of Behavior*. Taylor & Francis.

Rineer, Suzanne, Brenda Finucane, and Elliott W. Simon. 1998. "Autistic Symptoms among Children and Young Adults with Isodicentric Chromosome 15." *American Journal of Medical Genetics* 81(5):428–33.

Ritvo, Edward R., and B. J. Freeman. 1977. "National Society for Autistic Children Definition of the Syndrome of Autism." *Journal of Pediatric Psychology* 2(4):146–48.

Roberts, Jane E., et al. 2009. "Mood and Anxiety Disorders in Females with the *FMR1* Premutation." *American Journal of Medical Genetics, Part B* 150B(1):130–39.

Roberts, Nicholas J., et al. 2012. "The Predictive Capacity of Personal Genome Sequencing." *Science Translational Medicine* 4(133/133ra58).

Robin, Nathaniel H. 2006. "It Does Matter: The Importance of Making the Diagnosis of a Genetic Syndrome." *Current Opinion in Pediatrics* 18(6):595–97.

Robin, Nathaniel H., et al. 1995. "Opitz-Syndrome Is Genetically Heterogeneous, with One Locus on Xp22, and a 2nd Locus on 22q11.2." *Nature Genetics* 11(4):459–61.

Rodriguez-Revenga, Laia, et al. 2009. "Penetrance of *FMR1* Premutation Associated Pathologies in Fragile X Syndrome Families." *European Journal of Human Genetics* 17(10):1359–62.

Roeltgen, D. P., and J. L. Ross. 2010. "XYY Syndrome: A Possible Model for Autism Spectrum Disorder (ASD)." *Neurology* 74(9):A243–44.

Roettger, Michael E., Jason D. Boardman, Kathleen Mullan Harris, and Guang Guo. 2016. "The Association between the *MAOA* 2R Genotype and Delinquency Over Time among Men: The Interactive Role of Parental Closeness and Parental Incarceration." *Criminal Justice and Behavior* 43(8):1076–94.

Ropers, H. Hilger, and Ben C. J. Hamel. 2005. "X-Linked Mental Retardation." *Nature Reviews Genetics* 6(1):46–57.

Rose, Hilary. 2007. "Eugenics and Genetics: The Conjoint Twins?" *New Formations* (60):13–27.

Rose, Nikolas. 1998a. *Inventing Our Selves: Psychology, Power, and Personhood.* Cambridge University Press.

———. 1998b. "Medicine, History and the Present." In *Reassessing Foucault: Power, Medicine and the Body,* edited by C. Jones and R. Porter, 48–72. Routledge.

———. 2007a. "Molecular Biopolitics, Somatic Ethics and the Spirit of Biocapital." *Social Theory & Health* 5(1):3–29.

———. 2007b. *The Politics of Life Itself.* Princeton University Press.

Rose, Nikolas, and Carlos Novas. 2007. "Biological Citizenship." In *Global Assemblages,* edited by A. Ong and S. J. Collier, 439–63. Blackwell.

Rosenberg, Charles E. 1966. "Cholera in Nineteenth-Century Europe: A Tool for Social and Economic Analysis." *Comparative Studies in Society and History* 8(4):452–63.

———. 2009. *The Cholera Years: The United States in 1832, 1849, and 1866.* University of Chicago Press.

Rosenberg, Charles E., and Janet Lynne Golden. 1992. *Framing Disease: Studies in Cultural History.* Rutgers University Press.

Ross, Judith L., et al. 2012. "Behavioral and Social Phenotypes in Boys with 47,XYY Syndrome or 47,XXY Klinefelter Syndrome." *Pediatrics* 129(4):769–78.

Rossen, Michael L., and Harvey B. Sarnat. 1998. "Why Should Neurologists Be Interested in Williams Syndrome?" *Neurology* 51(1):8–9.

Roubertoux, Pierre L., and Bernard Kerdelhué. 2006. "Trisomy 21: From Chromosomes to Mental Retardation." *Behavior Genetics* 36(3):346–54.

Rousseau, F., et al. 1991. "Direct Diagnosis by DNA Analysis of the Fragile X Syndrome of Mental Retardation." *New England Journal of Medicine* 325(24): 1673–81.

Rowan, Rob, and Dennis A. Powers. 1991. "A Molecular Genetic Classification of Zooxanthellae and the Evolution of Animal-Algal Symbioses." *Science* 251(4999):1348–51.

Royce, Kenneth. 1973. *The XYY Man.* HarperCollins.

———. 1977. *The XYY Man: The Concrete Boot.* Mayflower.

Ruangdaraganon, N., C. Tocharoentanaphol, P. Khowsathit, T. Sombuntham, and B. Pongpanich. 1999. "Chromosome 22q11 Deletion Syndrome: The First Three Cases Reported in Thailand." *Journal of the Medical Association of Thailand (Chotmaihet Thangphaet)* 82 (supp. 1):S179–85.

Rutter, Michael. 1978. "Diagnosis and Definition of Childhood Autism." *Journal of Autism and Developmental Disorders* 8(2):139–61.

———. 2000. "Genetic Studies of Autism: From the 1970s into the Millennium." *Journal of Abnormal Child Psychology* 28(1):3–14.

Rutter, Michael, Anthony Bailey, Patrick Bolton, and Ann Le Couteur. 1994. "Autism and Known Medical Conditions: Myth and Substance." *Journal of Child Psychology and Psychiatry* 35(2):311–22.

Sabol, S. Z., Stella Hu, and D. Hamer. 1998. "A Functional Polymorphism in the Monoamine Oxidase A Gene Promoter." *Human Genetics* 103(3):273–79.

Sacks, Oliver. 2007. *Musicophilia: Tales of Music and the Brain.* Knopf.

Sahin, Mustafa, and Mriganka Sur. 2015. "Genes, Circuits, and Precision Therapies for Autism and Related Neurodevelopmental Disorders." *Science* 350(6263):926.

Salk Institute. 2011. "NIH Awards Salk Institute $5.5 Million Grant to Study Williams Syndrome." *Salk News*, May 20. http://www.salk.edu/news/press release_details.php?press_id=488.

Sandberg, Avery, Takaaki Ishihara, Lois H. Crosswhite, and George F. Koepf. 1963. "XYY Genotype—Report of a Case in a Male." *New England Journal of Medicine* 268(11):585–89.

Sandberg, Avery, G. F. Koepf, T. Ishihara, and T. S. Hauschka. 1961. "An XYY Human Male." *Lancet* 2(7200):488–89.

Santiago-Sim, Teresa, et al. 2017. "Biallelic Variants in *OTUD6B* Cause an Intellectual Disability Syndrome Associated with Seizures and Dysmorphic Features." *American Journal of Human Genetics* 100(4):676–88.

Sarasua, Sara M., et al. 2011. "Association between Deletion Size and Important Phenotypes Expands the Genomic Region of Interest in Phelan–McDermid Syndrome (22q13 Deletion Syndrome)." *Journal of Medical Genetics* 48(11):761–66.

Saul, Robert A., and John B. Moeschler. 2009. "How Best to Use CGH Arrays in the Clinical Setting." *Genetics in Medicine* 11(5):371.

Scambler, Peter, et al. 1991. "Microdeletions within 22q11 Associated with Sporadic and Familial DiGeorge Syndrome." *Genomics* 10(1):201–6.

———. 1992. "Velo-Cardio-Facial Syndrome Associated with Chromosome 22 Deletions Encompassing the DiGeorge Locus." *Lancet* 339(8802):1138–39.

Schachar, Russell. 2014. "Genetics of Attention Deficit Hyperactivity Disorder (ADHD): Recent Updates and Future Prospects." *Current Developmental Disorders Reports* 1(1):41–49.

Schneider, A., et al. 2016. "Broad Autism Spectrum and Obsessive–Compulsive Symptoms in Adults with the Fragile X Premutation." *Clinical Neuropsychologist* 30(6):929–43.

Schneider, Maude, et al. 2014. "Psychiatric Disorders from Childhood to Adulthood in 22q11.2 Deletion Syndrome: Results from the International Consortium on Brain and Behavior in 22q11.2 Deletion Syndrome." *American Journal of Psychiatry* 171(6):627–39.

Schopler, Eric, Robert Reichler, Robert DeVellis, and Kenneth Daly. 1980. "Toward Objective Classification of Childhood Autism: Childhood Autism Rating Scale (CARS)." *Journal of Autism and Developmental Disorders* 10(1):91–103.

Schwartz, C. E., et al. 1994. "Obstetrical and Gynecological Complications in Fragile X Carriers: A Multicenter Study." *American Journal of Medical Genetics* 51(4):400–402.

Sebat, Jonathan, et al. 2004. "Large-Scale Copy Number Polymorphism in the Human Genome." *Science* 305(5683):525–28.

Seltzer, Marsha Mailick, et al. 2012. "Prevalence of CGG Expansions of the *FMR1* Gene in a US Population-Based Sample." *American Journal of Medical Genetics* 159(5):589–97.

Sequenom. 2013a. "Sequenom CMM's MaterniT21 PLUS LDT Now Reporting on Gender-Specific Chromosomal Abnormalities." PR Newswire, February 4. https://www.prnewswire.com/news-releases/sequenom-cmms-maternit21-plus-ldt-now-reporting-on-gender-specific-chromosomal-abnormalities-189627021.html.

———. 2013b. "Sequenom Laboratories Launches the Enhanced Sequencing Series for the MaterniT21™ PLUS Test." PR Newswire, October 22. https://www.prnewswire.com/news-releases/sequenom-laboratories-launches-the-enhanced-sequencing-series-for-the-maternit21-plus-test-228746901.html.

———. 2014. "Sequenom, Inc. Reports Financial Results for the Fourth Quarter and Full Year of 2013." PR Newswire, February 27. https://www

.prnewswire.com/news-releases/sequenom-inc-reports-financial-results-for-the-fourth-quarter-and-full-year-of-2013-247622741.html.

Sergovich, F., G. H. Valentine, A. T. L. Chen, R. A. H. Kinch, and M. S. Smout. 1969. "Chromosome Aberrations in 2159 Consecutive Newborn Babies." *New England Journal of Medicine* 280(16):851–55.

Service, Robert F. 2006. "The Race for the $1000 Genome." *Science* 311(5767):1544–46.

Sewell, William H., Jr. 1992. "A Theory of Structure: Duality, Agency, and Transformation." *American Journal of Sociology* 98(1):1.

———. 1996. "Three Temporalities: Toward an Eventful Sociology." In *The Historic Turn in the Human Sciences*, edited by T. J. McDonald, 245–80. University of Michigan Press.

Shaffer, Brian L., Aaron B. Caughey, and Mary E. Norton. 2006. "Variation in the Decision to Terminate Pregnancy in the Setting of Fetal Aneuploidy." *Prenatal Diagnosis* 26(8):667–71.

Shaffer, Lisa G. 2009. *ISCN 2009: An International System for Human Cytogenetic Nomenclature (2009): Recommendations of the International Standing Committee on Human Cytogenetic Nomenclature*. Edited by L. G. Shaffer, M. L. Slovak, and L. J. Campbell. Karger Publishing.

Shaffer, Lisa G., et al. 2007. "The Discovery of Microdeletion Syndromes in the Post-genomic Era: Review of the Methodology and Characterization of a New 1q41q42 Microdeletion Syndrome." *Genetics in Medicine* 9(9):607–16.

Shah, Saleem Alam. 1970. *Report on the XYY Chromosomal Abnormality*. National Institute of Mental Health, Center for Studies of Crime and Delinquency.

Shakespeare, Tom. 1998. "Choices and Rights: Eugenics, Genetics and Disability Equality." *Disability & Society* 13(5):665–81.

Shapira, S. K., et al. 1997. "Chromosome 1p36 Deletions: The Clinical Phenotype and Molecular Characterization of a Common Newly Delineated Syndrome." *American Journal of Human Genetics* 61(3):642–50.

Shattles, Ashley. 2016. "Florida Dad Inspires Legislation That Benefits PMS Families." Phelan-McDermid Syndrome Foundation. https://web.archive.org/web/20160801041558/http://22q13.org/j15/.

Shaw, Alison, Joanna Latimer, Paul Atkinson, and Katie Featherston. 2003. "Surveying 'Slides': Clinical Perception and Clinical Judgment in the Construction of a Genetic Diagnosis." *New Genetics and Society* 22(1):3.

Sherman, Stephanie L. 2000. "Premature Ovarian Failure in the Fragile X Syndrome." *American Journal of Medical Genetics* 97(3):189–94.

Shim, Janet K. 2010. "Cultural Health Capital: A Theoretical Approach to Understanding Health Care Interactions and the Dynamics of Unequal Treatment." *Journal of Health and Social Behavior* 51(1):1–15.

Shostak, Sara, Peter Conrad, and Allan V. Horwitz. 2008. "Sequencing and Its Consequences: Path Dependence and the Relationships between Genetics and Medicalization." *American Journal of Sociology* 114(S1):S287–316.

Shprintzen, Robert J. 1998. "The Name Game." *Perspectives on Speech Science and Orofacial Disorders* 8(1):7–11.

Shprintzen, Robert J., et al. 1978. "A New Syndrome Involving Cleft Palate, Cardiac Anomalies, Typical Facies, and Learning Disabilities: Velo-Cardio-Facial Syndrome." *Cleft Palate Journal* 15(1):56–62.

Silverman, Chloe. 2011. *Understanding Autism: Parents, Doctors, and the History of a Disorder*. Princeton University Press.

Simon, Tony J. 1997. "Reconceptualizing the Origins of Number Knowledge: A 'Non-numerical' Account." *Cognitive Development* 12(3):349–72.

Singer, Emily. 2002. "Study Links Antisocial Behavior to Abuse, Variant Gene." *Los Angeles Times*, August 2.

Singh, Jennifer. 2010. "Autism Spectrum Disorders: Parents, Scientists and Interpretations of Genetic Knowledge." PhD diss., UC San Francisco.

———. 2015. *Multiple Autisms: Spectrums of Advocacy and Genomic Science*. University of Minnesota Press.

Singh, Jennifer, Judy Illes, Laura Lazzeroni, and Joachim Hallmayer. 2009. "Trends in US Autism Research Funding." *Journal of Autism and Developmental Disorders* 39(5):788–95.

Skotko, Brian G. 2009. "With New Prenatal Testing, Will Babies with Down Syndrome Slowly Disappear?" *Archives of Disease in Childhood* 94(11): 823–26.

Slaughter, Louise. 2008. Genetic Information Nondiscrimination Act. Available at https://www.congress.gov/bill/110th-congress/house-bill/493.

Smith, A. C., et al. 1986. "Interstitial Deletion of (17)(P11.2p11.2) in Nine Patients." *American Journal of Medical Genetics* 24(3):393–414.

Smith, David W., Klaus Patau, Eeva Therman, and Stanley L. Inhorn. 1960. "A New Autosomal Trisomy Syndrome: Multiple Congenital Anomalies Caused by an Extra Chromosome." *Journal of Pediatrics* 57(3):338–45.

Smith, Laurie D., et al. 2013. "Exome Sequencing Reveals De Novo Germline Mutation of the Mammalian Target of Rapamycin (MTOR) in a Patient with Megalencephaly and Intractable Seizures." *Journal of Genomes and Exomes* 2013(2):63–72.

Soden, Sarah E., et al. 2014. "Effectiveness of Exome and Genome Sequencing Guided by Acuity of Illness for Diagnosis of Neurodevelopmental Disorders." *Science Translational Medicine* 6(265/265ra168).

South, Sarah T., et al. 2013. "ACMG Standards and Guidelines for Constitutional Cytogenomic Microarray Analysis, Including Postnatal and Prenatal Applications: Revision 2013." *Genetics in Medicine* 15(11):901–9.

Star, Susan Leigh. 2010. "This Is Not a Boundary Object: Reflections on the Origin of a Concept." *Science, Technology & Human Values* 35(5):601–17.

Star, Susan Leigh, and James R. Griesemer. 1989. "Institutional Ecology, 'Translations' and Boundary Objects: Amateurs and Professionals in Berkeley's Museum of Vertebrate Zoology, 1907–39." *Social Studies of Science* 19(3):387–420.

Steele, M. W., and W. R. Breg Jr. 1966. "Chromosome Analysis of Human Amniotic-Fluid Cells." *Lancet* 1(7434):383–85.

Steinbock, Bonnie. 2008. "Designer Babies: Choosing Our Children's Genes." *Lancet* 372(9646):1294–95.

Stern, Alexandra Minna. 2005. *Eugenic Nation: Faults and Frontiers of Better Breeding in Modern America*. University of California Press.

St. George, Marie. 1998. "What Studying Genetically-Based Disorders Can Tell Us about Ourselves." *Trends in Cognitive Sciences* 2(6):203–4.

Stock, Robert W. 1968. "The XYY and the Criminal." *New York Times*, October 20.

Stokes, Jon. 2006. "Maori 'Warrior Gene' Claims Appalling, Says Geneticist." *New Zealand Herald*, August 10.

Stromme, P., P. G. Bjornstad, and K. Ramstad. 2002. "Prevalence Estimation of Williams Syndrome." *Journal of Child Neurology* 17(4):269–71.

Sunder Rajan, Kaushik. 2006. *Biocapital: The Constitution of Postgenomic Life*. Duke University Press.

Sutherland, G. R., and E. Baker. 1992. "Characterisation of a New Rare Fragile Site Easily Confused with the Fragile X." *Human Molecular Genetics* 1(2):111–13.

Swidler, Ann. 1986. "Culture in Action: Symbols and Strategies." *American Sociological Review* 51(2):273–86.

———. 2001. *Talk of Love: How Culture Matters*. University of Chicago Press.

Tabor, Holly K., and Martine D. Lappé. 2011. "The Autism Genetic Resource Exchange: Changing Pace, Priorities, and Roles in Discover Science." In *Achieving Justice in Genomic Translation*, edited by W. Burke and K. Edwards, 56–71. Oxford University Press.

Tager-Flusberg, H., and K. Sullivan. 2000. "A Componential View of Theory of Mind: Evidence from Williams Syndrome." *Cognition* 76(1):59–89.

Tao, Victoria Q., et al. 2014. "The Clinical Impact of Chromosomal Microarray on Paediatric Care in Hong Kong." *PLOS One* 9(10):e109629.

Tarquinio, Daniel C., Marilyn C. Jones, Kenneth Lyons Jones, and Lynne M. Bird. 2012. "Growth Charts for 22q11 Deletion Syndrome." *American Journal of Medical Genetics, Part A* 158A(11):2672–81.

Tartaglia, Nicole R., Susan Howell, Ashley Sutherland, Rebecca Wilson, and Lennie Wilson. 2010. "A Review of Trisomy X (47,XXX)." *Orphanet Journal of Rare Diseases* 5(1):8.

Tartaglia, Nicole R., et al. 2006. "Attention Deficit Hyperactivity Disorder and Autism Spectrum Disorders in Males with XXY, XYY and XXYY Syndromes." *Journal of Intellectual Disability Research* 50(11):787.

———. 2007. "Autism Spectrum Disorders in XXY, XYY, and XXYY Syndromes: Abstract 28." *Journal of Developmental and Behavioral Pediatrics* 28(4):S8.

———. 2008. "A New Look at XXYY Syndrome: Medical and Psychological Features." *American Journal of Medical Genetics, Part A* 146A(12):1509–22.

Ta-Shma, Asaf, et al. 2017. "Mutations in TMEM260 Cause a Pediatric Neuro-developmental, Cardiac, and Renal Syndrome." *American Journal of Human Genetics* 100(4):666–75.

Tassone, Flora, Paul J. Hagerman, and Randi J. Hagerman. 2014. "Fragile X Pre-mutation." *Journal of Neurodevelopmental Disorders* 6(1, art. 22).

Taussig, Karen-Sue, Rayna Rapp, and Deborah Heath. 2003. "Flexible Eugenics: Technologies of the Self in the Age of Genetics." In *Genetic Nature/Culture: Anthropology and Science beyond the Two-Culture Divide*, edited by A. H. Good-man, D. Heath, and M. S. Lindee, 58–76. University of California Press.

Telfer, Mary A., David Baker, Gerald R. Clark, and Claude E. Richardson. 1968. "Incidence of Gross Chromosomal Errors among Tall Criminal American Males." *Science* 159(3820):1249–50.

Terry, Sharon F., Patrick F. Terry, Katherine A. Rauen, Jouni Uitto, and Lionel G. Bercovitch. 2007. "Advocacy Groups as Research Organizations: The PXE International Example." *Nature Reviews Genetics* 8(2):157–64.

Tilly, Charles. 1993. "Contentious Repertoires in Great Britain, 1758-1834." *Social Science History* 17(2):253–80.

———. 2003. *The Politics of Collective Violence.* Cambridge University Press.

———. 2004. *Social Movements, 1768–2004.* Paradigm.

Timmermans, Stefan. 2015. "Trust in Standards: Transitioning Clinical Exome Sequencing from Bench to Bedside." *Social Studies of Science* 45(1): 77–99.

———. 2017. "Matching Genotype and Phenotype: A Pragmatist Semiotic Ana-lysis of Clinical Exome Sequencing." *American Journal of Sociology* 123(1): 136–77.

Timmermans, Stefan, and Marc Berg. 1997. "Standardization in Action: Achiev-ing Local Universality through Medical Protocols." *Social Studies of Science* 27(2):273–305.

Timmermans, Stefan, and Mara Buchbinder. 2010. "Patients-in-Waiting: Living between Sickness and Health in the Genomics Era." *Journal of Health and Social Behavior* 51(4):408–23.

———. 2011. "Improving Expanded Newborn Screening." *Journal of Health and Social Behavior* 52(2):279–81.

———. 2012. "Expanded Newborn Screening: Articulating the Ontology of Diseases with Bridging Work in the Clinic." *Sociology of Health & Illness* 34(2):208–20.

———. 2013. *Saving Babies? The Consequences of Newborn Genetic Screening.* Uni-versity of Chicago Press.

Timmermans, Stefan, and Steven Epstein. 2010. "A World of Standards but Not a Standard World: Toward a Sociology of Standards and Standardization." *Annual Review of Sociology* 36(1):69–89.

Timmermans, Stefan, and Steven Haas. 2008. "Towards a Sociology of Dis-ease." *Sociology of Health & Illness* 30(5):659–76.

Tingley, Kim. 2015. "'Food Is a Death Sentence to These Kids.'" *New York Times,* January 21.

Tirrell, Meg. 2014. "Illumina DNA Test Has More Accurate Down Syndrome Diagnosis (2)." *BusinessWeek*, February 27.

Tjio, Joe Hin, and Albert Levan. 1956. "The Chromosome Number of Man." *Hereditas* 42(1–2):1–6.

Tonelli, Adriano R., Kalyan Kosuri, Sainan Wei, and Davoren Chick. 2007. "Seizures as the First Manifestation of Chromosome 22q11.2 Deletion Syndrome in a 40-Year Old Man: A Case Report." *Journal of Medical Case Reports* 1:167. https://doi.org/10.1186/1752-1947-1-167.

Torre-Ubieta, Luis de la, Hyejung Won, Jason L. Stein, and Daniel H. Geschwind. 2016. "Advancing the Understanding of Autism Disease Mechanisms through Genetics." *Nature Medicine* 22(4):345–61.

The Trans-NIH Fragile X Research Coordinating Group and Scientific Working Groups. 2008. *National Institutes of Health Research Plan on Fragile X Syndrome and Associated Disorders*. US Department of Health and Human Services, National Institutes of Health.

Trent, James W. 1995. *Inventing the Feeble Mind: A History of Mental Retardation in the United States*. University of California Press.

Trivedi, Bijal P. 2017. "Is Health Care Ready for Routine DNA Screening? A Massive New Trial Will Find Out." *Science*, October 26.

Turkheimer, Eric, Andreana Haley, Mary Waldron, Brian D'Onofrio, and Irving I. Gottesman. 2003. "Socioeconomic Status Modifies Heritability of IQ in Young Children." *Psychological Science* 14(6):623–28.

Turleau, Catherine. 2008. "Monosomy 18p." *Orphanet Journal of Rare Diseases* 3:4. https://doi.org/10.1186/1750-1172-3-4.

Turner, G., et al. 1996. "Prevalence of Fragile X Syndrome." *American Journal of Medical Genetics* 64(1):196–97.

Turpin, Raymond, and Jérôme Lejeune. 1969. *Human Afflictions and Chromosomal Aberrations*. Pergamon.

UC Davis Health. 2016. "Fragile X drug trial gets $11.5 million in NIH funding." UC Davis Health press release, December 15. https://health.ucdavis.edu/publish/news/newsroom/11686.

Unique. [2008]. "XYY Study Day Report." http://www.rarechromo.org/files/XYYStudyDayReport.pdf.

US Food and Drug Administration. 2017. "Statement from FDA Commissioner Scott Gottlieb, M.D., on Implementation of Agency's Streamlined Development and Review Pathway for Consumer Tests That Evaluate Genetic Health Risks." FDA Statement, November 6. https://www.fda.gov/NewsEvents/Newsroom/PressAnnouncements/ucm583885.htm.

Vailly, Joëlle. 2008. "The Expansion of Abnormality and the Biomedical Norm: Neonatal Screening, Prenatal Diagnosis and Cystic Fibrosis in France." *Social Science & Medicine* 66(12):2532–43.

Varga, Elizabeth A., Matthew Pastore, Thomas Prior, Gail E. Herman, and Kim L. McBride. 2009. "The Prevalence of PTEN Mutations in a Clinical Pediatric Cohort with Autism Spectrum Disorders, Developmental Delay, and Macrocephaly." *Genetics in Medicine* 11(2):111–17.

Venkitaraman, A. R. 2002. "Cancer Susceptibility and the Functions of BRCA1 and BRCA2." *Cell* 108(2):171–82.

Verinata Health. 2012a. "Verinata Health Announces New Findings at the American Society of Human Genetics." PR Newswire, November 9. https://www.prnewswire.com/news-releases/verinata-health-announces -new-findings-at-the-american-society-of-human-genetics-178078611 .html.

———. 2012b. "Verinata Health's Non-Invasive verifi® Prenatal Test Now Includes Unique Ability to Detect Additional Fetal Chromosomal Abnormalities." PR Newswire, December 3. https://www.prnewswire.com/news -releases/verinata-healths-non-invasive-verifi-prenatal-test-now-includes -unique-ability-to-detect-additional-fetal-chromosomal-abnormalities -181820331.

———. 2012c. "Verinata Health's verifi® Prenatal Test Expanded to Include the Most Common Sex Chromosome Abnormalities." PR Newswire, November 6. https://www.prnewswire.com/news-releases/verinata-healths-verifi -prenatal-test-expanded-to-include-the-most-common-sex-chromosome -abnormalities-177457771.

Verkerk, Annemieke J. M. H., et al. 1991. "Identification of a Gene (*FMR-1*) Containing a CGG Repeat Coincident with a Breakpoint Cluster Region Exhibiting Length Variation in Fragile X Syndrome." *Cell* 65(5): 905–14.

Verp, Marion S., et al. 1988. "Parental Decision Following Prenatal Diagnosis of Fetal Chromosome Abnormality." *American Journal of Medical Genetics* 29(3):613–22.

Vorstman, Jacob A. S., et al. 2017. "Autism Genetics: Opportunities and Challenges for Clinical Translation." *Nature Reviews Genetics* 18(6):362–76.

Wade, Nicholas. 2009. "Genes Show Limited Value in Predicting Diseases." *New York Times*, April 16.

Wailoo, Keith. 2001. *Dying in the City of the Blues: Sickle Cell Anemia and the Politics of Race and Health*. University of North Carolina Press.

Walzer, S., and P. S. Gerald. 1975. "Social Class and Frequency of XYY and XXY." *Science* 190(4220):1228–29.

Walzer, S., P. S. Gerald, and S. A. Shah. 1978. "The XYY Genotype." *Annual Review of Medicine* 29(1):563–70.

Wang, John M., et al. 2012. "Male Carriers of the *FMR1* Premutation Show Altered Hippocampal-Prefrontal Function during Memory Encoding." *Frontiers in Human Neuroscience* 6:297. https://doi.org/10.3389/fnhum.2012 .00297.

Wapner, Ronald J., et al. 2012. "Chromosomal Microarray versus Karyotyping for Prenatal Diagnosis." *New England Journal of Medicine* 367(23): 2175–84.

Warburg, Mette. 1960. "Anophthalmos Complicated by Mental Retardation and Cleft Palate." *Acta Ophthalmologica* 38(4):394–404.

Warburg, Mette, and M. Mikkelsen. 1963. "13-15 Trisomy with Severe Ocular Malformations." *Archives of Ophthalmology* 69(3):420.

Warkany, Josef. 1960. "Etiology of Mongolism." *Journal of Pediatrics* 56(3):412–19.

Waterhouse, Lynn. 2013. *Rethinking Autism: Variation and Complexity*. Academic Press.

Waterhouse, Lynn, Lorna Wing, Robert Spitzer, and Bryna Siegel. 1992. "Pervasive Developmental Disorders: From *DSM-III* to *DSM-III-R*." *Journal of Autism and Developmental Disorders* 22(4):525–49.

Watson, M. S., et al. 1984. "Fragile X in a Survey of 75 Autistic Males." *New England Journal of Medicine* 310(22):1462.

Webb, T. P., S. Bundey, A. Thake, and J. Todd. 1986. "The Frequency of the Fragile X Chromosome among Schoolchildren in Coventry." *Journal of Medical Genetics* 23(5):396–99.

Weber, Max. 2011. *Methodology of Social Sciences: Max Weber*. Edited by E. Shils and H. Finch. Transaction Publishers.

Weiss, Lauren A., et al. 2008. "Association between Microdeletion and Microduplication at 16p11.2 and Autism." *New England Journal of Medicine* 358(7):667–75.

Weiss, Philip. 1975. "Ending the Test for Extra Chromosomes." *Harvard Crimson*, September 15.

Wenger, Tara L., Charlly Kao, et al. 2016. "The Role of MGluR Copy Number Variation in Genetic and Environmental Forms of Syndromic Autism Spectrum Disorder." *Scientific Reports* 6:19372.

Wenger, Tara L., Judith S. Miller, et al. 2016. "22q11.2 Duplication Syndrome: Elevated Rate of Autism Spectrum Disorder and Need for Medical Screening." *Molecular Autism* 7:27.

Wentzel, C., M. Fernström, Y. Öhrner, G. Annerén, and A. C. Thuresson. 2008. "Clinical Variability of the 22q11.2 Duplication Syndrome." *European Journal of Medical Genetics* 51(6):501–10.

"What Is to Be Done with the XYY Fetus?" 1979. Editorial. *British Medical Journal* 1(6177):1519–20.

Wheeler, Anne C., et al. 2014. "Associated Features in Females with an *FMR1* Premutation." *Journal of Neurodevelopmental Disorders* 6(1):30.

Whooley, Owen, and Allan V. Horwitz. 2013. "The Paradox of Professional Success: Grand Ambition, Furious Resistance, and the Derailment of the DSM-5 Revision Process." In *Making the DSM-5*, edited by J. Paris and J. Phillips, 75–92. Springer New York.

Williams, J. C. P., B. G. Barratt-Boyes, and J. B. Lowe. 1961. "Supravalvular Aortic Stenosis." *Circulation* 24(6):1311–18.

Wilson, Jacque. 2014. "Kids Who Don't Cry: New Genetic Disorder Discovered." CNN.com, March 20. http://www.cnn.com/2014/03/20/health/ngly1-genetic-disorder/index.html.

Wing, Lorna. 1973. "Concepts of Autism: A Review." *Journal of Paediatrics and Child Health* 9(4):246–47.

———. 1980. "Childhood Autism and Social Class: A Question of Selection?" *British Journal of Psychiatry* 137(5):410–17.

Wing, Lorna, and Judith Gould. 1979. "Severe Impairments of Social Interaction and Associated Abnormalities in Children: Epidemiology and Classification." *Journal of Autism and Developmental Disorders* 9(1):11–29.

Wolfson, Elijah. 2014. "My Genes Did It!" *Newsweek*, March 5.

Wong, A. C., et al. 1997. "Molecular Characterization of a 130-Kb Terminal Microdeletion at 22q in a Child with Mild Mental Retardation." *American Journal of Human Genetics* 60(1):113–20.

Woodin, Michael, et al. 2001. "Neuropsychological Profile of Children and Adolescents with the 22q11.2 Microdeletion." *Genetics in Medicine* 3(1):34–39.

Wright, Jessica. 2016. "DNA Doubling on Chromosome 22 Shows Strong Ties to Autism." *Spectrum*, May 30. https://spectrumnews.org/news/dna-doubling-on-chromosome-22-shows-strong-ties-to-autism/.

Wulfsberg, E. A., J. Leana-Cox, and G. Neri. 1996. "What's in a Name? Chromosome 22q Abnormalities and the DiGeorge, Velocardiofacial, and Conotruncal Anomalies Face Syndromes." *American Journal of Medical Genetics* 65(4):317–19.

———. 1997. "What's in a Name? The 22q11.2 Deletion—Reply." *American Journal of Medical Genetics* 72(2):248–49.

"The XYY Chromosome Defense." 1968. *Georgetown Law Journal* 57:892–922.

XYY Man. 1976. Television series. Produced by Granada Television. See https://en.wikipedia.org/wiki/The_XYY_Man#The_XYY_Man_%E2%80%94_The_TV_Series.

Yong, Ed. 2010. "Dangerous DNA." *New Scientist* 205(2755):34–37.

———. 2013. "'We Gained Hope': The Story of Lilly Grossman's Genome." *National Geographic*, March 11. https://www.nationalgeographic.com/science/phenomena/2013/03/11/we-gained-hope-the-story-of-lilly-grossmans-genome/?user.testname=none.

———. 2015. "How Genome Sequencing Creates Communities around Rare Disorders." *Atlantic*, September 21. https://www.theatlantic.com/science/archive/2015/09/how-genome-sequencing-gave-lilly-grossman-an-answer-a-future-and-a-community/406345/.

Young, Susan E., et al. 2006. "Interaction between *MAO-A* Genotype and Maltreatment in the Risk for Conduct Disorder: Failure to Confirm in Adolescent Patients." *American Journal of Psychiatry* 163(6):1019–25.

Yu, S., et al. 2008. "Familial 22q11.2 Duplication: A Three-Generation Family with a 3-Mb Duplication and a Familial 1.5-Mb Duplication." *Clinical Genetics* 73(2):160–64.

Yunis, Jorge J. 1977. *New Chromosomal Syndromes.* Academic Press.

Yunis, Jorge J., and O. Sanchez. 1974. "A New Syndrome Resulting from Partial Trisomy for the Distal Third of the Long Arm of Chromosome 10." *Journal of Pediatrics* 84(4):567–70.

"The YY Syndrome." 1966. *Lancet* 287(7437):583–84.

Zeaiter, Zaher, Zhongxing Liang, and Didier Raoult. 2002. "Genetic Classification and Differentiation of Bartonella Species Based on Comparison of Partial *FtsZ* Gene Sequences." *Journal of Clinical Microbiology* 40(10): 3641–47.

Index

The letter *t* following a page number denotes a table, and the letter *f* denotes a figure.